"In an era when traditional psychiatry risks reducing the human being to diagnoses and protocols, this book offers a breath of fresh air. The author, with solid scientific training and profound spiritual sensitivity, invites us to reconsider psychiatric disorder as part of an inner process of transformation—at times painful, yet intrinsically creative: the awakening of consciousness.

With clear language and rich references to masters such as Dante and Jung, the text weaves together ancient wisdom and modern knowledge, showing how the 'dark night of the soul' can become a passage toward rebirth. Far from aiming to return the patient to a fragile previous equilibrium, the author opens the way to accompanying them toward a new identity—more aware, more free.

It is a courageous invitation to the psychiatry of the future—a 'conscious psychiatry', alchemical in nature, capable of transforming lead into gold. A precious manual for professionals and researchers, but also for anyone who, in the midst of pain, senses that within it lies the key to their own liberation."

Giulia Jordan, *transpersonal psychologist, explorer of consciousness and guide, writer*

Psychiatry and Spiritual Awakening

Psychiatry and Spiritual Awakening reimagines the landscape of mental healthcare by integrating traditional psychiatric approaches with Transpersonal Psychology and spiritual insight.

Written from the perspective of a seasoned psychiatrist and transpersonal therapist, the book offers an innovative synthesis that bridges biological, psychological, and spiritual understandings of mental suffering. It highlights the limitations of the biomedical paradigm and the chronic, stigmatizing identity it often imposes on patients, instead reframing psychiatric suffering as a potential catalyst for personal and spiritual growth. Through a historical and conceptual overview, the author traces the evolution of psychiatry and psychology, examining how modern practice has become dominated by symptom-focused, pharmacological interventions. The book then introduces the principles of Transpersonal Psychology, drawing on the work of figures such as Jung, Assagioli, Wilber, and Grof, and integrating Eastern contemplative traditions and spiritual frameworks with Western clinical practice and contemporary neuroscience. Through detailed case studies, the book demonstrates how Transpersonal Therapy differs from conventional approaches and comprehensively illustrates the clinical application of the transpersonal point of view. The author explores different psychiatric syndromes and their models of diagnosis, treatment, and recovery according to different approaches, bridging the gap between biological psychiatry and holistic, meaning-centered approaches. Techniques such as deep guided relaxation through chakra-focused energy work in the sessions are described in detail and the therapist's own state of presence and energetic awareness is emphasized as a key factor in facilitating healing. The book calls for a paradigm shift: to move beyond symptom management and toward an integrative model that honors the complexity—and possible purpose—of altered states.

Both authoritative and accessible, this practical, compassionate guide charts a path toward a more holistic, humane, and hopeful vision of mental healthcare for any clinician or researcher, providing technical details on Transpersonal Psychotherapy.

Claudio Maddaloni is an Italian psychiatrist and Jungian analytical psychologist, with over 40 years of professional experience. He is a strong proponent and active disseminator of Transpersonal Psychiatry, a field that uniquely integrates spiritual and transcendent aspects into the healing process, viewing psychiatric disorders as part of consciousness evolution.

Psychiatry and Spiritual Awakening

Psychopathology Through the Lens of Transpersonal Development and Energy Transformation

Claudio Maddaloni

Routledge
Taylor & Francis Group
NEW YORK AND LONDON

Designed cover image: *Gallerie Nazionali di Arte Antica, Roma (MiC) – Bibliotheca Hertziana, Istituto Max Planck per la storia dell'arte/Enrico Fontolan*

First published 2026
by Routledge
605 Third Avenue, New York, NY 10158

and by Routledge
4 Park Square, Milton Park, Abingdon, Oxon, OX14 4RN

Routledge is an imprint of the Taylor & Francis Group, an informa business

ISBN: 978-1-041-14855-5 (hbk)
ISBN: 978-1-041-14853-1 (pbk)
ISBN: 978-1-003-67646-1 (ebk)

DOI: 10.4324/9781003676461

Typeset in Sabon
by Newgen Publishing UK

To Gianpaolo, who jumped down from the sky,
and to Elio, who hung himself to the sky,
and to many others
who never knew why...
And to the sky,
which watches all of this

Contents

Foreword

Reading Claudio Maddaloni's book, one soon gets the impression of an "eagle of Psychiatry" soaring above the field, discerning its details while keeping a global perspective—grounded with detailed references. The author observes the whole field of psychiatry from a general perspective that encompasses Past and Present—and, later, in the text, Future. His vision is integrative, open to the new sciences but also to the ancient wisdom traditions.

Being a deep knower and lover of Dante's Divine Comedy, he masterfully uses it at as a metaphor for an ensouled Psychiatry—one that acknowledges and uses the spiritual dimension of man and its mystery.

There is very sound scholarship in this book. References, notes, and a careful articulation, together with a broad scope. Maddaloni acknowledges the merits and denounces the limits of modern psychiatry, largely stemming from its medicalized origins, and its attempts to objectify a science which is, in reality, the most subjective of all. This is why he presents to us divergent or convergent other rivers of this delta, humanistic psychology, Jungian perspectives—and transpersonal psychiatry as a new way of integrating transpersonal psychology (that is too far from the central point of psychiatry: psychoses)—and classical psychiatry, that has been separated from its healing purpose from its very methodology.

To the author, some models for cosmogenesis and the macrocosm, to be found in spiritual traditions such as Hinduism, may also apply to the microcosm of human individuals as they relate to an infinitely larger ecosystem. Maddaloni dedicates a chapter to redefine consciousness, psychic energy, and the maps of the psyche that tradition has handed down to us: the central and peripheral nervous system physically replicate the eastern tantric maps of energy channels. He also mentions the western symbolic maps or representations of these "*other worldly*" things, like the three realms of Divine Comedy or the astrological map, where planets represent consciousness symbols of qualified energy flowing in the inner sky, according to the long-accepted truth that the microcosm replicates the macrocosm. We share with him a fundamental idea: that consciousness, in the microcosm, becomes what we call individual self-awareness as it *identifies with a specific mind-body system*—a person. In this process, consciousness becomes sort of dormant in what concerns its higher possibilities, being *separated* from them, until awakening (that is, the fruit of our inner evolutive drive), restores us into union with the larger Cosmos.

He then discusses scientific references about the assumption that consciousness is but a product of brain activity.

Maddaloni warns us about the need for inner experience with modified states of consciousness before we can understand what such big maps of the human mind and experience might mean.

For example, the eastern concept of *Kundalini* is after all not so far away from the libido concept we find in the west, in mystics referring to the sacred fire; in the Divine Comedy, this ascending fire that brings you back to the inner sky is Beatrice, elevating consciousness through the planets-*Chakras* to the candid Rose of the Empyrean. He emphasizes that not only theoretical but also practical knowledge about the *Chakras*, *Kundalini* and their psychic functions is fundamental to understanding a Transpersonal Psychiatry perspective; their blockages, their overstimulation and unbalances or their harmony might find intense correspondences in symptoms but also in healing processes.

Thus, psychopathology is understood through the lens of spiritual awakening and energy activation: the movements and blockages that arise from the ego's resistance to this death–rebirth process. A powerful analogy is drawn between the birth process and psychiatric crisis, illustrating how both situations can benefit from a non-pathological interpretation and wise accompaniment. Such crises, when viewed as outcomes of *Kundalini* awakening and *Chakra* stimulation, frequently present as identity crises. If navigated skillfully, these can yield new, more integrated forms of self—though not without the turmoil that results from the ego's fears and attachments. Paradoxically, the birth of a new, less separated (or even non-separated), livelier, more awakened, identity, might bring with it intense fear of death and resistance to identity change: this, in turn, may bring with it a powerful constellation of symptoms, making for a great part of psychiatry.

Maddaloni proceeds to classify the different types of psychiatric crises according to whether identity, energetic, or reactive components predominate. He introduces a novel framework for psychopathological understanding anchored to the axes of identity, energy, and egoic response. This framework is elaborated in chapters dedicated to "energetic disturbance prevalence syndromes" and "identity disturbance prevalence syndromes," where he offers transpersonal interpretations of classical conditions—such as anxiety disorders, bipolar disorder, depression, personality disorders, obsessive–compulsive disorder, and psychosis.

The author also underlines here something not to be missed: that, to traditional psychiatry, the objective is to restore the patient back from turmoil and dissociation, disorientation, anguish, confusion, and the like, to the old coherent, adapted self—whereas, to a transpersonal psychiatry perspective, this would imply totally missing an evolutionary opportunity.

The *Kundalini* syndrome is discussed in depth as one variety of energetic syndromes, often mistaken for panic attacks or other pathological conditions (such as depersonalization syndrome). Differential diagnosis is also addressed as the author provides considerable detail about this syndrome and its possible evolution over time, noting that its psychiatric correlates may be cyclical and encompass motor, somatosensory, psychological, and even psychic–paranormal manifestations. He also brings to our attention that inner trauma not infrequently can have roots on unprocessed, highly scary, manifestations of *Kundalini* awakening: knowledge about the process of *Kundalini* awakening can amount to "a critical bridge between spirituality and psychopathology".

Mainstream psychiatry reduces the profound spiritual experiences of mystics such as the Buddha, Christ, St. John of the Cross, St. Teresa of Ávila, or Muhammad to mere psychosis and biochemical alterations in the brain. Such an outdated approach amounts to "psychiatry without hope, without future, without soul". That is why a whole chapter is devoted to understanding the experiences of well-known mystics or Masters as they achieved "successful awakenings," working with the *Kundalini* fire and attaining profound transformation and states of enlightenment—sometimes after considerable inner turmoil.

As for therapy—which occupies the last, but also most interesting, part of the book from the standpoint of Transpersonal Psychiatry's practical contributions—the author advocates a gentle use of medication to help patients manage subtle energy processes occurring during psychiatric crises, rather than suppressing them. Psychotic patients, he notes, "are people who fly but are not quite ready, and they often fall or fragment." Psychiatry, in this view, is essentially a catalogue of those who should already be able to fly but are blocked (as in neuroses), or of those who fly poorly and get hurt (as in psychoses).

In the therapy chapter, the author goes on to characterize Transpersonal Psychiatry on what he calls a rather "radical condition," namely "the centrality attributed to the transpersonal psychiatrist's state of consciousness within the therapeutic relationship"—a state of consciousness not identified with the ego. The therapist must remain in a centered and present state, attuned to the energetic perception in their own *Chakras*, thereby helping the patient to do the same. "The essence of the method," Maddaloni emphasizes, "is deep listening." This includes "listening to the energy" and the energy phenomena going on with them, the patients and the energy field including both.

We truly appreciate how radical is the view presented here, where "The *real actor and driver of the process, however, is the therapy itself*, the *therapeutic field (...)*, a *unified 'field'* in which emotions and psychological dynamics are transmitted and transformed, a '*morphogenetic field*', endowed with 'memory', information."

In this same chapter, we may find a very specific methodology for helping the patients work through their *Chakras* and energy system and deal with their crisis in a very constructive and deep way—eventually reaching states of deep and healing peace. A detailed case study is then presented and discussed. We find here a lot of guidance about how to proceed, and we end up, one would say, witnessing the way Maddaloni dances with his patients and the energy and consciousness flow. We notice how daring but also how respectful he may be while doing this, trusting himself within the process, trusting the field—and probably, above all, just flowing from some non-egoic stance. For the Author, the ultimate therapeutic goal is going beyond suffering—and, to attain such a goal, healing the disconnection of the patient from his pure being and, with this, "achieving ultimate health". In that sense, cure is yoga, reconnection, and "baptism into the inner river, which restores life".

In sum, this book is commendable for its depth, its aim, the way it has been built, its clear structure and discussion, the grounded and careful references, and, of course, its novel and bold presentation of Transpersonal Psychiatry as a field to be developed and as a hope towards shaping a future towards a better Humanity.

Beauty is to be found in the shape of the text, the poetic quality of its language, and the breadth of its vision. I am grateful for the opportunity to engage with this work and to reflect on its valuable contribution to contemporary psychiatry.

Dr Vitor Jose F. Rodrigues, Psychologist, Psychotherapist, and writer, taught Educational Psychology at the Faculty of Psychology and Educational Sciences, University of Lisbon, for 14 years and then lectured at the Nursing school in Evora and at the Faculty of Humanities and Social Sciences at the University of Algarve (Developmental Psychology). He was President of the European Transpersonal Association (EUROTAS) from 2005 to 2009 and of the Luso-Brazilian Transpersonal Association between 2003 and 2009. He was the Coordinator of the European Committee for Certification and Accreditation of EUROTAS, 2000–2013. He has written 16 books, see https://vitorrodriguespsicologo.weebly.com/index.html

Preface

Over years of clinical practice and research, I have increasingly felt the urgent need for a psychiatry capable of embracing the totality of human experience—a discipline that recognizes the depth and multiplicity of states of consciousness, without reducing them to mere anomalies of brain functioning. This book arises precisely from this need: to understand what happens during psychiatric crises, and to propose a model that includes the dimension of consciousness—the "subtle heart" of psychic life—as a key to interpreting crisis and transformation in the modern individual. This book has been written to help people overcome suffering.

My perspective is grounded in the daily observation that many psychiatric situations, regarded as purely pathological within psychiatry, in fact contain a spiritual and evolutionary potential hidden behind the suffering and misunderstandings of patients and clinicians who interpret them exclusively through a materialistic lens.

In many cases, Non-ordinary States of Consciousness (here abbreviated as NOSC)—which include identity crises, dissociative states, sudden awakening experiences—can represent critical passages, at times painful but potentially transformative, in which consciousness awakens to itself (the famous "*I found myself...*" from the Divine Comedy), The mental and psychological upheaval observed in these situations is a consequence of this a true identity crisis occurs, powerful energetic currents are activated inwardly, and defensive reactions arise in an effort to preserve fragments of the old world that is collapsing.

What is at stake, as can be seen, is a different interpretive framework.

In this book, I deliberately employ the paradigm of Dante's Divine Comedy: just as the poet traverses Inferno and Purgatory before ascending to a unifying vision, so too the psychiatric journey, in this view, should be able to accompany the patient from chaos and crisis to a possible conscious rebirth. The psychiatrist or therapist thus becomes a guide who, "*with skill and with art*", supports this courageous crossing. The aim is not to "normalize" at all costs, nor to repress, but to recognize that the journey through the mind's dark regions can become a path of transformation and meaning.

In the chapters dedicated to disorders of control, such as OCD—a symbol of a society that fears the void and seeks to control the uncontrollable—I consider how these conditions can also be read as collective signals of an epochal transition. My view is that some prevalent disorders today are not just deficits or deviations, but indicators of an impasse and transition of consciousness, and of the new possibilities and obstacles our civilization is called to face.

The chapters therefore explore the phenomenology and clinical management of NOSC, offer practical criteria to distinguish them from organic psychiatric crises, and propose a transpersonal therapeutic approach to therapy that values symbolic, energetic, and relational dimensions. The underlying conviction is that only by integrating the scientific rigor of psychiatry with the wisdom of spiritual traditions and a genuinely open attitude toward the mystery of consciousness will it be possible to help patients to transform crisis into an opportunity for growth.

This volume is intended for to all those who, working in clinical practice, research, or theoretical reflection—or who, as patients find themselves involved in or swept up by these processes—wish to explore new horizons and the future challenges of psychiatry.

It is an invitation to regard every crisis not only as a risk but as a symbolic initiation to a new potential for humanity.

AI acknowledgment statement

I acknowledge the use of artificial intelligence tools (Perplexity) to assist with reference verification, language improvement, definition clarification, and translation support during the preparation of this manuscript. All AI-generated content was thoroughly reviewed and edited by me. The ideas, analysis, and conclusions presented remain entirely my own work.

Chapter 1

Psychiatry yesterday, today, and tomorrow

"*I am in crisis,*" says the patient who sits before me. Examining his story, one soon sees that the crisis is disproportionate to the reported facts, which play more of a triggering, or concausal role, and do not seem to constitute the real reason for the *psychiatric crisis.*

It is clear, however, that this is not a *psychological crisis,* due to external factors; as regards both quality and intensity, in the first case the subject's inner and outer reactions are normal, whereas in the second they are altered, exaggerated, abnormal.

For a psychiatric crisis (henceforth *PC*) *to occur*, there has to be something extra-ordinary that has happened '*within*': precisely, a state of consciousness out of the ordinary.

The patient recognizes that something has changed, something fundamental; something big has emerged, something alien to oneself, something irreversible.

The person in crisis is disorientated, agitated, sleepless, anxious; he does not control his mind, he has new sensations which are worrying and intense, unexplainable. He usually has an intense fear, of dying, of *going mad*, which is a bit like *dying* since he fears losing himself completely: the fear of entering a crisis and never coming out, of going insane[1] and never returning to normal. The psychiatric crisis is like a *shipwreck*, like that of Ulysses.

PC is usually characterized by a sudden change, involving the *appearance of signs (objectively observable) and symptoms (subjectively perceived), i.e. a syndrome.*

In medicine, a pathognomonic grouping of signs and symptoms, i.e. a syndrome, identifies a clinical picture, a *disease;* in the case of a PC, psychiatry speaks of *mental illness.*

In this text, we consider the PC to be the basic unit, the fundamental brick, the building block of every psychiatric syndrome in its various forms. Psychiatry as a whole is thus made up of so-called syndromes, i.e.

DOI: 10.4324/9781003676461-1

psychological conditions or manifest behaviours considered critical, often dysfunctional, often worrying (because unknown), constituting a *pathology*.[2]

> *Symptoms may be positive*, i.e. previously absent, such as the onset of intense distress, of a quality and intensity quite different from any previous inner difficulties the person may have experienced.
>
> *Symptoms may also be negative*, with discomfort or reduction or loss of a previous function or capacity, such as sociability, concentration, etc, i.e. a *pathology*.

The study and treatment of mental illness fall within the field of study of psychology and psychiatry.

The *criterion* by which to assess whether certain types of behavior are symptoms of mental illness has *changed over time*, as the boundaries of mental illness are conditioned by the evolution of society, its tolerance of deviance.[3]

In these definitions of mental distress, however, there is never any mention of an alteration of ordinary consciousness. For mainstream psychiatry, and for ordinary people, the problem is a "mental" problem: what needs to be investigated and treated is the "mind", i.e. the set of psychic phenomena (thoughts emotions dreams, memories, etc.), that are altered.

However, on closer inspection, *it is not the phenomena* (which are perceived *objects*, internal or external), *but the individual state of consciousness*, (i.e. the percipient *subject*), *that has changed,* that has passed from one state to another: there has been a shift *from an ordinary state of consciousness to a non-ordinary state of consciousness* (henceforth *NOSC)*.

To use an analogy the individual consciousness is poetically described as *a sleeping beauty in the woods*, *awakened* by the Solar, celestial principle, to the state of *clear consciousness*.[4]

So in this book we will deal with altered, non-ordinary states of consciousness, how they manifest, how they generate alterations in mood, in identity, as a crisis, a rupture.

In fact, it is a matter of *death and rebirth*, of a transformation, of a *shift from the* "me" *to the* "Self"*:* the subject shifts from the *small I* the *me-person* (the *perceived* one), to the *big I* the Self, the *percipient consciousness.*

This shift is usually not painless, and that is why we speak of symptoms, of a crisis (PC).

PC possesses in itself a duplicity: *opportunity and danger*, and can lead to an opening towards a higher consciousness, as well as being the beginning of a sinking towards a state of suffering and personal disintegration.

- Thus, *eulogies of madness* have been woven.

  For example, Plato argues that mania brings one closer to divinity.

  Erasmus of Rotterdam weaves a eulogy of madness by personifying it, speaking to it as if it were a friend, a wealth.

  A proverb says: *Only madmen can know the truth.*

  Crisis *survivors* sometimes say they feel changed for the better, to the point of being grateful, of never wishing to go back to the way they were.
- However *going mad is no picnic*: those who went through it often had to suffer greatly, something not to be wished on the worst enemy!

  The madman has often *lost everything*, the world, and *even himself.*

  In this sense he may be a liberated one, but he has also passed through death.

  He is liberated from himself.
- An ancient saying goes that "in the world there are three kinds of men: the living, the dead, and those who go by sea."[5]

  The *dead* are the majority of humanity, those who have yet to set out on the inner journey: the *sleepers* (Plotinus).

  The *living* are those who have crossed over, and they are few in number.

  The madmen we know in psychiatry are *those who go by sea*, often *drifting* away. They have left the shore, willingly or unwillingly, summoned by awakening.

  And going by sea one meets all kinds of people in distress: some of them are still near the shore, and some are almost at the other shore; some are sailing in precarious little boats, and others do not know how to sail at all, and many go in the wrong direction.

  Therapists also go by sea, and in attempting to bring help one has to assess well who are they facing, and what situation they are in.

1.1 A few words of history

The study of the mind has always fascinated mankind; philosophy, psychology, spirituality investigate the human experience, feelings, desires and passions, the deceptions and potentialities of the soul. *The history of psychiatry is complex and intertwined with the development of medicine, philosophy, and the social sciences.* Over the centuries, it has moved from primitive and often cruel approaches to more humane methods, approaching medicine and psychology after the 19th century. The modern medical orientation focuses on the biological basis of psychic distress, looking for the cause of disorders in biochemistry, anatomy, neurons, and molecules.

Let us briefly recount how we arrived at the current situation.

The study of mental illnesses dates back to ancient times, when they were attributed to *supernatural or spiritual causes* to the action of gods and demons.

In ancient Greece, Plato, in Phaedrus, distinguished two types of madness (mania): *pathological,* caused by human illnesses, and "divine," arising from a change brought about by the gods. Divine madness was seen as a privileged condition, capable of bringing humanity the greatest gifts: wisdom, creativity, love, and self-knowledge.

It was cathegorised in four main forms, each linked to a deity: *Prophetic* (*Apollo*): oracular inspiration and divination; *Initiatory* (*Dionysus*): mystical ecstasy and purification rites; *Poetic* (*Muses*): artistic and poetic creativity; *Erotic* (*Aphrodite/Eros*): love that elevates the soul toward the divine.

Hippocrates proposed a theory that linked human behavior to *imbalances in the humors of the body* (bile, phlegm, blood, and black bile). Depression, for example, was called *melancholia*, i.e., a disturbance due to Black bile.

During the Middle Ages, mental illness was often viewed through the lens of *religion*. Many patients were accused of witchcraft or possession and underwent exorcisms or other religious practices; many women who practised natural cures were considered witches and burnt at the stake for this.[6]

With the Renaissance, there was a slow revival of interest in scientific medicine.

The Swiss physician *Paracelsus* (1493–1541) was one of the first to argue that mental illnesses had *natural causes* and should be treated like any other illness.

In the Modern Era (*17th and 18th century*), psychiatry began to take shape as an autonomous discipline. Initially, the mentally ill were *segregated together with the poor and delinquents*, in rather inhuman conditions. Over time, psychiatry became more and more a medical speciality, and the *asylums* where these patients were housed and segregated (the forerunners of our mental hospitals) became more and more *dedicated* to mental disorders, and these sufferering ones were more and more considered as sick people. Attempts were made to humanize these asylums: in the 18th century, *Philippe Pinel* in France and *William Tuke* in England pioneered the "moral treatment," an approach that promoted the humane and compassionate care of mental patients.

We thus come to the 19th century: *the 1800s* saw the birth of psychiatry as a distinct *medical* field, developing with neurology. *Esquirol*, a pupil of Pinel, contributed greatly to the classification of mental illnesses. In Germany, *Emil Kraepelin* developed a classification of mental illnesses that profoundly influenced modern psychiatry, distinguishing between manic-depressive psychosis (today known as bipolar disorder) and schizophrenia[7]. *Eugene Bleuler* coined the terms "schizophrenia" and "autism."

1.2 Modern psychiatry and psychology

In the 20th century, psychiatry took a decisive step forward, when the medical approach became prevalent, and psychiatry became a much *more considered* science; it was at this stage that a tendency towards the meticulous classification of all kinds of deviance from the norm began.[8]

1.2.1 Psychotropic drugs

Before 1950, there were no psychotropic drugs; natural substances (opium, cannabis, herbs, alcohol) or drugs (such as morphine, barbiturates, and reserpine) were used for sedative or anxiolytic purposes, often with serious side effects and risks of addiction.

Modern psychopharmacology emerged in the late 1940s and early 1950s.[9]

A true "psychopharmacological revolution" took place between 1950 and 1960, with the discovery and marketing of the main classes of psychotropic drugs: *antipsychotics*, *antidepressants*, *anxiolytics*, *mood stabilizers*, and *sedatives*.

The introduction of psychotropic drugs radically changed the therapeutic landscape, allowing many patients to live outside psychiatric hospitals.

In the 1970s and 1980s, attempts were made to *improve the safety and efficacy profile* of psychotropic drugs. Antidepressants with fewer side effects (SSRIs such as Prozac, launched in the 1980s), new (atypical) antipsychotics and additional mood stabilizers were developed; these *second-generation* drugs (i.e. more evolved and effective, with fewer side effects), gave the illusion of having found the key for the cure of psychiatric disorders, believed in the bio-medical view to be due exclusively to biological factors. These drugs saw a vertiginous development in the second half of the century[10]; in the following decades, however, the search for new drugs yielded less striking results than the initial ones.

Today, bio-medically oriented psychiatry continues to evolve *with the progress of neuroscience and genetics*. Functional magnetic resonance *imaging* (fMRI) and other brain imaging technologies make it possible to study the brain in vivo, providing new insights into the pathophysiology of mental illness.

Modern psychiatry adopts an integrated approach, i.e. it considers biological, psychological and social factors as competing in the genesis and treatment of mental disorders, while always giving preeminent importance to the biological factor.

1.2.2 Phenomenological psychiatry

The phenomenological psychiatry developed at the end of the 19th and beginning of the 20th century, intertwining with philosophy[11] in an attempt to overcome the organicist ("biomedical") paradigm in psychiatry. For the phenomenological current, *intuition* is a fundamental cognitive modality, a bridge between subjectivity and objectivity, between science and life, between individual and collectivity.

From Husserl's phenomenology to Bergson's philosophy, from Jung's depth psychology and Hillman's to the phenomenological and transpersonal clinic, intuition emerges as an indispensable tool for an authentic understanding of the other and of oneself.

In the clinical context, intuition allows access to levels of reality not reducible to rational analysis, to grasp atmospheres, energy states, and deep meanings that manifest themselves in the therapeutic encounter.[12]

The great pioneers of phenomenological psychiatry were *Karl Jaspers*[13], *Eugene Minkowski*, and *Ludwig Binswanger.* They proposed the idea that understanding the psyche should start from the patient's subjective experience rather than from rigid, objective categories.

For example, *Rümke* recognized the validity of the "early feeling" (Praecox-Gefühl) in the diagnosis of schizophrenia: a kind of immediate perception of the patient's radical otherness, not reducible to objective criteria, but based on a pre-verbal and global feeling.[14]

The phenomenological method, applied to psychiatry, opens up interesting perspectives, and has anticipated many of the central practices of transpersonal psychotherapy by decades and prepared the ground for its emergence.

The *methodological foundations* laid by psychiatric phenomenology are:

- The *state of non-judgmental awareness* (called *epoché): there is* "suspension of judgement" in therapy, which puts pre-conceived knowledge and theoretical and diagnostic prejudices aside.
- *The openness to experience* moment by moment: there is an acceptance of experience as it presents itself, moment by moment, an empathic understanding that transcends the I–other separation.[15]
- The *overcoming of dualism*[16]: phenomenology has revolutionized the understanding of *intersubjectivity* in psychiatry, showing how the therapeutic encounter can become a space of *existential sharing* that transcends individual boundaries.
- The *therapist* is called upon not only on a theoretical level to *go beyond* the concepts of normality and pathology, to *go beyond* any rigid and formal technical articulation, but also practically to an *authenticity of being and total commitment of the person.* The therapist must be "open to the ineffable, to the mystery of existence, in a state of consciousness receptive to the unexplainable and the non-rational."

Despite the innovations, the phenomenological approach in psychiatry has certain *limitations* compared to the transpersonal: it lacks *specific techniques* for the induction of non-ordinary states of consciousness, it does not include the spiritual dimensions of experience; a descriptive aspect predominates in this approach, as opposed to an active intervention to help transformation of consciousness.

1.2.3 Psychotherapies

While biologically oriented psychiatry proceeded at a fast pace in its discoveries, great *advances in the psychological understanding of mental illnesses* were emerging towards the end of the 19th century and especially in the 20th century, so that psychology also became a science in its own right, intersecting with and diverging from the emerging psychiatry.

Many schools of thought thus emerged. Each psychological school of thought offers a unique perspective on the causes of mental disorders and a specific intervention method, reflecting its fundamental theories and principles.

1. *The psychoanalytic movement* was *the forerunner* of a new psychological approach in Europe (later moving to the United States), with regard to the origin and treatment of mental disorders. Psychoanalysis was considered the *first force* in psychology, taking the first major step towards an evolution beyond biological psychiatry. In psychoanalysis, the emphasis was no longer on the organic disorder, but on intrapsychic dynamics. There were a few main strands: Freud, Jung, Adler, Reich, and others.

- *Freudian psychoanalysis*: *Sigmund Freud (1865–1939)*, (and, later, the neo-freudians), proposed an approach that sought to understand mental disorders through the analysis of the subconscious mind and childhood experiences, especially sexual ones (a psychogenetic aproach). Here the role of trauma (unresolved traumatic experiences during childhood can lead to mental disorders), defense mechanisms (excessive or inappropriate use of defense mechanisms such as repression or projection can cause psychopathological symptoms), the foundations of therapeutic relationship (transference and counter-transference), dream analysis, and much more were studied.
- Freud regarded sexual drive (libido) and its frustration or deviations as central to the genesis of mental disorders. In this view, mental disorders arise from unconscious conflicts between the different components of the psyche (id, ego, superego).[17]
- *Jung (1875–1961), Adler, Reich, and many others* laid the foundations for a different interpretation of clinical practice by founding schools of psychoanalysis that diverged from Freud's approach. They emphasized alternative mechanisms behind the formation of psychiatric conditions, and different strategies for treatment.

- For *Adler*, mental disorders can result from feelings of inferiority and overcompensation for these feelings (inferiority complex).
- In this approach, the basis of mental disorders can be found in the patient's maladaptive lifestyle (i.e. maladaptive way of coping with life and its problems), the setting of unrealistic or fictitious goals, which are not in tune with the person's abilities and possibilities.[18]
- For W. *Reich*, at the basis of mental disorders we can find blockages in the life energy (which he called *orgone*), e.g. repression of sexuality and natural emotional expression; this generates defenses, such as chronic muscle tension and *character armour* (rigid ways of behaving), which contribute to mental disorders.[19]
- *Jung* in particular extends the Freudian view by arguing that libido is not only sexual, but vital energy, even spiritual. He argues that in addition to the personal unconscious, content from the collective unconscious, archetypes (collective structuring forms for symbols and deep dynamics) and complexes (i.e., feelings, thoughts, and memories associated in active nuclei that can become autonomous and interfere with behavior and well-being), can cause mental disorders. Obstacles in the individuation process (the process of becoming one's true self) can cause psychological problems.[20]

2. *Behaviorism* represents one of the most influential currents in 20th century psychology, arising as a reaction to introspection and psychoanalysis, shifting the emphasis to environment and learning. This psychological movement was called the *second force in psychology*, due to its methodological break with the psychodynamic approach and its application impact.[21]

This school of thought redefined psychology as a science of observable behavior, rejecting the analysis of consciousness.[22] The studies on conditioning evolved through time:

- *Classical conditioning*, studied in the early 1900s by *Pavlov* (Russian physiologist, Nobel prize winner for medicine in 1904 for this discovery), is a process by which a *neutral stimulus* is associated with an *unconditioned stimulus* that already provokes an automatic response. He discovered that if one associates a sound stimulus such as a bell with a natural stimulus such as food, which naturally causes the dog to salivate, the reflex phenomenon occurs after repeated associations, whereby the neutral stimulus alone is able to provoke the same response (the bell sound makes the dog salivate even without food).[23] These are *involuntary and reflexive responses*. [24]
- Later studies have evolved conditioning; *E. Thorndike* (1905, with the Law of Effect) showed how voluntary behavior can be reinforced or

weakened according to its consequences (reward or punishment). *F. Skinner (1930s–1950s)* developed the concept and term "*operant conditioning*," which is based on *voluntary, actively chosen behavior* by the organism (e.g. a mouse pressing a lever to obtain food).[25] *Edward Tolman* integrated cognitive elements (e.g., mind maps), while maintaining the focus on behavior.[26]

- *Operant conditioning reinforces classical*: *classical conditioning* creates associations between stimuli, "preparing" an emotional/automatic response. *Operant conditioning* uses consequences (reinforcements or punishments) to reinforce or weaken behavior that can be influenced by those same associations. Operant conditioning acts on voluntary behavior, reinforcing or weakening actions that can be made more likely by prior classical associations; the combination of the two mechanisms explains many forms of learning and the persistence of behavior in both animals and humans.

Studies on conditioning have been *applied in the clinic*; for example, it has been seen that certain dysfunctional behaviors and attitudes can be learnt by observing models (e.g. parents behaviour), and are maintained by operating conditioning through negative reinforcement, or lack of positive reinforcement; this is the case of anxieties and phobias. When a feared stimulus is avoided, relief is experienced; consequently, avoidance behavior is reinforced. *Obsessive disorders* are based on such a dynamic.

However, studies on conditioning have become increasingly sophisticated because, *applied on a social level*, they make it possible to condition, to control, people and their social and mental behavior: one can intervene on a large scale on education, on how people think and act, react, condition them on what to fear, what to buy (this is the basis of marketing).

3. *Humanistic psychology, which was called the* "Third Force" (as opposed to behaviorism and psychoanalysis); it focuses on the study of the human being as a whole, emphasizing self-fulfilment, creativity, and subjective experience, in a more positive view of the human being. The *focus here is on subjective experience and self-realization*, the valorization of human dignity and the development of latent potential; much emphasis was placed on group therapy and shared experiences.

Humanistic psychology sees the ego as an autonomous centre of consciousness, capable of free and responsible choices, and believes that the search for the meaning of existence is fundamental to the individual's well-being. The causes of mental disorders, in this approach, are often linked to factors that prevent or hinder personal fulfilment, authenticity, and realization of one's potential.

One of the most representative figures of this movement was *Abraham Maslow* (1908–1970) (who coined the term in 1954). He founded the *Association of Humanistic Psychology* in the United States in 1962; he was interested in studying the positive and not just the pathological potential of the human being.[27]

Maslow argued that a person's basic needs are hierarchically ordered in a *pyramid* culminating in self-fulfilment. If basic needs (physiological, security, love and belonging, esteem) are not met, the individual may develop mental disorders. Repression of authentic emotions and desires, experiences of trauma or abuse, lack of unconditional acceptance from significant figures such as parents or partners, and social isolation can all contribute to feelings of inadequacy and low self-esteem and to the development of mental disorders.

For *Carl Rogers* (1902–1987), founder of "client-centered" *non-directive therapy*, the *incongruence between the real self and the ideal self* plays a pathogenetic role in mental disorders. This condition arises when there is a significant discrepancy between how a person perceives him/herself and how he/she would like to be, as happens for example when external expectations and pressures lead people to behave in ways that are not authentic. Living authentically, in accordance with one's values and needs, is therefore considered crucial for mental health.

In the 1960s and 1970s, there was a spread of numerous *humanistic therapies* such as *Gestalt, Bioenergetics* and *existential psychology. Gestalt* or "form psychology," was founded by *Fritz Perls,* and studies perception and experience as global and organized processes. The cardinal principle is that "the whole is more than the sum of the parts": the mind tends to organize stimuli into meaningful and structured forms, not as simple aggregates of elements. In this view, mental disorders are caused by a lack of awareness of the present and of one's own emotions and needs. Avoiding parts of oneself or uncomfortable situations, rather than facing them directly, and failing to take responsibility for one's actions and choices (interrupted or incomplete experiences ("incomplete gestalten") can lead to inner conflict and psychological dysfunction.

- *Viktor Frankl* is an important exponent of existential psychology, which is closely related to humanistic psychology, who emphasizes the importance of individual freedom and responsibility. He argued that a lack of purpose or meaning in life can lead to a "noogenic neurosis" or existential crisis characterized by anxiety and depression.
- *Bioenergetics* is a psycho-body discipline developed in the 1950s by *Alexander Lowen*, which integrates work on the body and mind. It is

based on the idea that psychological disorders also manifest as energy blocks and tensions in the body.[28]

4. *From humanistic psychology emerged* (shortly afterwards), *the Fourth Force, transpersonal psychology*, which we will discuss at length in this book.

Born in the 1960s by *Maslow* (the same man who had founded humanistic psychology), *S. Grof* (whom we will discuss at greater length in a moment), *Sutich*, and *Vich*; these and others advocated the integration of among those who have integrated the spiritual and transcendent aspects of human experience with modern scientific psychology. Transpersonal psychology *focuses on personal growth, self-realization, and the exploration of non-ordinary states of consciousness*, going beyond the individual personality to include universal and spiritual dimensions of existence. Other important authors who contributed to this direction were *K. Wilber* and *R. Assagioli*.

The Association of Transpersonal Psychology was founded in 1969, and shortly afterwards The *Journal of Transpersonal Psychology* was published.

The founding texts of Transpersonal Psychology explore personal growth, non-ordinary states of consciousness and self-realization.[29]

5. *Anti-psychiatry*

Within the field of psychiatry, besides phenomenological psychiatry, a number of *other strands diverging from mainstream psychiatry* have developed, which, for example, insist more on the *importance of the social in the determinism of mental disorders.*

Experiments in *therapeutic communities* and those of *anti-psychiatry*, in England and the United States, insist on the importance of not merely medicalizing psychiatric crises, and insist on the importance of welcoming and supporting the patient.[30]

Some orientations even go so far as to deny the very existence of mental illness, shifting the cause of distress exclusively to society (*Szasz*).[31]

In Italy, law 180, also known as the Basaglia law, has greatly changed the landscape of public psychiatry with the closure of mental hospitals since 1978.[32]

1.3 The scientific method and its limits

As we have seen, 19th-century positivist psychiatry (organicist psychiatry) developed as an autonomous discipline from the late eighteenth century onward, and saw madness as a somatic illness (to be treated by the physician in an appropriate place, such as the asylum). The first studies on mental illnesses came from neurologists who sought biological evidence of correlation with mental disorders.

In establishing itself as a scientific discipline, psychiatry *modelled its method on the example of the natural sciences.*

With the evolution of technology and studies in this direction, there has been a shift from the old anatomo-pathological studies to the study of *alterations in neurotransmitters, communication pathways between neurons, and brain structures.* The many biological factors that have been studied include *genetic*[33], *neurochemical*[34], *structural*[35], *endocrine*, *prenatal*, *immune*, and *neuroplasticity*-related factors.[36]

The field is complex and the factors are clearly interconnected, and in the modern psychiatric view they interact with psychological and environmental elements, which contribute to the manifestation and severity of mental disorders (see studies on *epigenetics*).[37] *The application of the scientific method and procedures of medicine to the field of psyche, soul, and consciousness requires caution and suffers from limitations.*

Although the scientific method has brought important advances in modern science, its trasposition in the field of psychiatric disorders remains open to substantial criticism:

a. *The naturalistic scientific method has a major limitation: it cannot conceive of the psychic*, since that method never allows us to understand the experience of the individual patient.
b. *The method of observation that we apply in the natural sciences is in fact characterized by the separation of subject and object,* where a subject, the experimenter, observes an object, which would have nothing to do with the observer. When, on the other hand, the observing subject observes itself as an object (its own mind, for example), we find ourselves in a short circuit: we use the observed instrument for the observation itself.

   In psychiatry, *a main methodolgical issue* is that the very object of "knowledge" coincides with the "knowing" subject itself, a situation that in no way exists in the scientific method.[38]

   Consciousness, the soul, eludes the objective study of the natural sciences, and imposes a different cognitive approach that includes but transcends the scientific method of the natural sciences.
c. *The scientific method is not as scientific as we believe*; *it is based on reliability, and reproducibility.*[39] However, this procedure is not applicable to the living matter of the psyche, which is by nature changeable, inexplicable, creative, and mysterious.

   Moreover, the scientific method does not propose certain and reproducible results even in the materialistic field.[40]

d. *In the scientific method, it is taken for granted that the experimenter is neutral* with respect to the experiment, that he neither falsifies nor modifies the observation.

In reality, subject and object are not distinct, and this supposed neutrality does not exist; moreover, the very fact of observing modifies what is being observed.

e. *The organicist psychiatrist*, in defining a mental disorder, in order to be able to guarantee the objectivity of his observation, *refers to a clinical*, "nosographic" *method*, as a way of classifying mental disorders.

Our psychiatric classifications describe groupings of symptoms, syndromes: they are catalogues of syndromes, i.e. constellations, symptomatological groupings, in continuous evolution. In other words, they *are not diseases*, characterized by evidence comparable to those studied by medicine using the objectivizing scientific method.

Thus, psychiatric nosography *appears to be based on firm foundations* as if it described "entities" with pathological substance, *when in fact* it arbitrarily brings together, changeably (many new syndromes arise and many disappear in subsequent classifications), symptoms and psychic signs whose origin remains unknown.

f. *Cataloguing syndromes by attributing to them the label of disease suggests a biological cause of mental disorders, which has yet to be proven.* Convincing evidence of a "sick" organ has not been found, neither at the macroscopic nor at the biochemical level; although in some cases biological alterations (i.e. cerebral, neurocirculatory, biochemical conditions specific to different psychopathological pictures) which were concomitant to psychic disorders have been traced, this does not directly prove a *cause and effect* relation. The coexistence of biological findings and psychic syndromes leaves the field of study open to the synchronic appearance on different planes of an unknown process.[41]

Tracing a coexistence of stabilized psychiatric syndromes and existing organic alterations in the brain does not indicate a cause and effect relationship, but rather a circularity of conditions. Coincidences and correlations are often interpreted as causal relationships.

An *example* is the observation of alterations in brain areas with elevated specific neurotransmitter activity as the cause of mental disorders detected in the symptomatic picture; the causal relationship is added to demonstrate the thesis, rather than scientifically proven.[42] When doing research, we should think differently, openly; it is a matter of including (but not concluding!), the findings of neuroscience, maintaining an open model.

g. *The clinical syndromes studied and catalogued most often belong to patients treated with psychotropic drugs*, sometimes for a long time. Consequently, the biological terrain is certainly altered. Also, patient's history and relationships with family and environment will also have been influenced by psychotropic drugs and psychiatric interventions (e.g. due to the stigma of being mentally ill, with which the patient has identified).
h. *The intervention we use in psychiatry is pharmacological and symptomatic, not curative.*

   Well, we know that in medicine symptomatic treatment is permissible, and only temporarily, when the cause of the disorder is unknown. This implicitly admits thus that the causes of these psychiatric conditions are not known.
i. *In medicine, intervention aims at a cure in the sense of a* "restitutio ad integrum", at the *status* "quo ante", that is "as before".

For these various reasons, starting in the early 1900s, the need was felt for a *different method in psychiatry.*

1.4 The biological psychiatry of the future

1.4.1 Meanwhile, the future is already here

The world is changing at a speed of which we are generally unaware of.

It is a *change in the way power is managed in the world*, in the economic and financial, military and religious spheres, which is changing social policy and the quality of life of humanity. *Power* is also changing face and strategy: it requires an updated, more advanced control of the body and mind of individuals (and therefore of the masses), a *more subtle control.*

The new rule is the *conditioning of human consciousness in a more profound and systematic manner than in the past*, while the violent control of social behavior (prevalent until recent times, and to some extent still active in many places or at certain moments in history) will recede more and more into the background, as it is less efficient, more costly, and in the long run less effective; this is already happening.

The change we observe in *medicine and psychiatry* is closely linked to this general change, to the new order in the world. Science in general, and medicine and psychiatry very much so, are increasingly becoming a point of reference, playing their part in a modern and post-modern era. They have *married the modern* "scientific" *view*, which studies nature and man as an inert, external, inanimate object, not as a conscious subject.

1.4.2 Science

In the modern world, the collective consciousness has developed a materialistic conception of man. No longer a religious vision, of man as a child of God, endowed with spirit; he is now seen as matter, and psyche and consciousness as emerging as a product of brain functioning: a biological machine that must be studied by refining the technical instruments of investigation. The idea is that by knowing every part of man thoroughly, human suffering will eventually disappear, and we will conquer death.

It is a project of domination over nature, of absolute power; science is the *new religion.*

This is a major fundamental change that has an enormous impact on freedom, individuality, and the critical and social consciousness of man.

1.4.3 Transhumanism

Together with society, the vision of man is changing: of man, as we have known him for millennia, only a few traces may soon remain.

Transhumanism proposes the use of scientific and technological discoveries to increase physical and cognitive capabilities, and improve those aspects of the human condition that are considered undesirable, such as illness and ageing, also with a view to a possible post-human transformation. These new technologies will change the world to such an extent that our descendants will not be "human" in many respects: we will have a *post-Darwinian humanity.*[43]

Transhumanistic ideology emerged from the scientific, moral, and philosophical tradition of the 19th century, influenced by the Enlightenment and positivism. A new transhumanist movement has developed.[44]

The modern world and modern medicine seem to be moving towards a new man, transformed in body, and racing towards a future that has already begun. Will we sacrifice everything on this new altar? Sacrifice has always been demanded of the many, for the benefit of the few.

These ideas are, however, controversial: some dissonant voices are being raised, even cautious or sceptical authoritative voices, which argue that human beings following this path will probably end up extinct through the transformations advocated by transhumanism.[45]

1.4.4 The singularity

Kurzweil's contribution on the singularity is interesting in this regard. This term refers to a *point in the development of a civilization where technological progress accelerates beyond the capacity of human beings to understand and predict.*[46]

Kurzweil argues that the speed of change increases exponentially and non-linearly, and that we would collectively be in the hyperbolic steepening phase of the curve at this point. This would correspond to a fundamental change in human history, to a *singularity* already almost achieved.

To take one example, the development of artificial intelligence in the last few years and months has made such progress that Artificial General Intelligence (AGI) is now very close.[47] *The singularity is near!*[48]

1.4.5 Medicine

Much has changed in recent years in the world of medicine. This vision translates into an ever-increasing power to separate, replace, and condition any parts of the body as a separate and at least partly technically replaceable and manipulable biological object.

Thus, the new paradigm will be *epigenetics and genetic manipulation, immuno-modulation, nutrition, transplants of stem-generated organs, the invasion of nanotechnology.*

There have been discoveries in the field of *biology* (stem cells, biochemistry, nutrition), the implementation of *information technology* in the organization of medical services and data, in drug research, in diagnosis, in communication.

Health services, hospitals, have profoundly changed, starting from organization (increasingly based on political and economic *corporate* profit logics), as well as health givers: the doctor–patient and doctor–institution relationship has profoundly changed; the old figure of the accessible and human family doctor, and humanly accessible nurses, has largely disappeared. *University education* has become increasingly sectoral, technological, and not global; super-specialists are being trained who are less and less able to see and treat man as a whole.

In this political and social economic development, we are also witnessing a *decline in the founding principles of health*, since the business rationale is profit, not the needs of citizens.

1.4.6 Mainstream psychiatry

Official, academic, mainstream (MS) psychiatry, which adheres to the dominant mono-paradigmatic biomedical model, *is changing along with medicine*, to which it is increasingly wedded.

As we have seen, this view holds that mental disorders are diseases of the brain: we can eliminate them as we have already done with many physical diseases.

MS psychiatry tends to disregard mental *distress as a transformation of consciousness*, and to *deny the importance of the human soul* in favor of an enhancement of knowledge of the human body, and a medicalization of psychiatric diagnosis and treatment.

This MS psychiatry is driven by a great need to intervene with more advanced means, since mental disorders, such as depression, are on the rise today, constituting the main cause of disability and expenditure in the world.[49] As distress and mental illnesses are increasing, psychiatry is moving more and more towards a technocratic world, favouring specialization and techniques over the integration of knowledge typical of the humanistic approach of the past.[50]

1.4.7 Technology

Moving in this direction, *great changes are already coming, and they are under way from the technology sector, which will have a major transformative impact on how treatment for mental disorders can be administered.*[51]

Let us take a look[52] at some features of this accelerated development, as proposed and dreamt up by neuroscience:

- Psychiatry is undergoing an unprecedented technological evolution, with *telemedicine* expanding: *online visits, computerized data management, and remote monitoring of patients in psychiatric facilities.*
- Drugs with smart sensors to *monitor* therapeutic *compliance* are being studied, and wearable devices to track emotional and cognitive parameters.
- Technology is increasingly present in psychiatric treatment, leading to *precision psychiatry*, which *analyzes biological, genetic, and environmental variables* to personalize treatment.
- *Virtual reality* is being used to treat phobias, PTSD, and addictions. *Therapeutic avatars* are already being used to replace specialists in underserved areas; these are able to look at us, analyze our language, our body movements, make even emotional contact with us, and respond to us in a very human-like manner.
- Parallel, *asynchronous telepsychiatry*[53] *and artificial intelligence* are transforming the role of the physician, *automating clinical decisions and rationalizing resources* according to business logic.[54]
- *Psychiatric apps* are on the rise: they can monitor symptoms, language, and behavior, alerting doctors in case of deterioration.[55]
- *New molecules* for psychiatric disorders are being studied and the *roles of the glutamatergic system, neurohormones, and brain inflammation*

are being investigated, identifying *biomarkers of suicide* with great precision.
- *Microbiota, nutrition, and lifestyle are* receiving increased attention, *while electromagnetic therapies (EMT)* are being tested.[56]
- Modern *psychotherapies* are being revised from a biomedical perspective, and some equate them with pharmacological treatments.

In conclusion, the *transhumanist vision* permeates the entire field, with extreme perspectives such as human–machine interfaces, brain pacemakers, and even the possibility of interconnecting human brains.

Instead of opposing the dehumanization of care, this type of psychiatry of the future seems to embrace a transhumanist vision of man.

Certainly there is some benefit in how technology can help health care. However, technological research seems to mask psychiatry's inability to deal with human suffering in an authentic way. Despite progress, the suicide rate has not changed in the last 40 years. This type of psychiatry risks distancing the patient from his or her inner experience, favoring laboratory solutions over a humanistic and relational approach.

Moreover, the evolution of society in this techno-bureaucratic direction will most likely lead to a *major reorganization of man's work and social life* and to major *social problems*. Perhaps, who knows, by favoring this direction *the very existence of the psychiatric specialist will come to be nullified.*

Notes

1 The terms *madness* and *insane* are not entirely equivalent. Madness now denotes a more or less permanent mental disorder. The term *insane* is now an informal term denoting mental instability; in the medical profession the term is now avoided, and in disuse, in favor of more specific diagnoses of mental illness. The term *insanity* is more about how much we are or are not within the norm, and insists more on the side of altered behavior than the mental functions that determines it.

2 *Pàthos*, from the verb πάσχω 'to suffer' is *a* 'tormenting condition caused by the assiduousness of pain.'

3 The evolution of the DSM, from edition to edition, is proof of this. For example, homosexuality was considered a mental disorder until 1973, when the evolution of research and clinical reflection led the international scientific community to leave this old interpretation.

4 In the Divine Comedy, it is described as the "medium" in which life flows; it is here that the Awakening, the "I found myself again" occurs: awakening, finding one's true self, thus pertains to the true self, and involves the individual identity undergoing a great disaggregation.

5 This saying probably derives from an ancient proverb, perhaps of Greek origin; it is generically linked to the philosophical environment of Plato or classical Greece, but without a precise textual confirmation in his known writings.

6 *Witch hunts* in Europe came to an end between the end of the 18th and the beginning of the 19th century, with the case of the burning of Anna Göldi (1782) in Switzerland, symbolically marking the end of this tragic page in European history. The "witches" were often women who practiced natural medicine, sometimes with the help of *enteogenous* plants.

7 See his treatise "Compendium der Psychiatrie: Zum Gebrauche für Studirende und Aerzte" ("Compendium of Psychiatry: for the Use of Students and Physicians"), first published in 1883; this text was later expanded and updated in numerous subsequent editions, until it became a monumental multi-volume work entitled "Ein Lehrbuch der Psychiatrie," the latest edition being published in 1927.

8 "The threatening ambiguity of mental disorder (Who is insane? Who is sane?) leads us to take our system of perception of mental illness for granted, when it is precisely that system that should be the object of study, since it defines our experience of mental illness" (J.D. Blum).

9 In 1949, lithium was introduced for the treatment of mania, in 1952 chlorpromazine inaugurated the category of antipsychotics, and in 1957 imipramine launched the era of tricyclic antidepressants.

10 The production and sale of psychotropic drugs have grown exponentially from the mid-20th century to the present. From 2008 to 2019 it grew by 4% per year.

11 In particular that of Edmund Husserl and that of Martin Heidegger.

12 For *Husserl*, a philosopher considered to be the founder of phenomenology, eidetic intuition (the ability to directly grasp the essences of phenomena) is a form of immediate, pre-conceptual knowledge of the essence of things, overcoming the dichotomy between inside and outside. This approach founds the possibility of a science of subjectivity, in which truth is not given by correspondence with an objective world, but by experienced and intersubjectively shared evidence. For *Bergson*, also a philosopher, intuition is the only way to come into contact with the absolute, with life in its fullness, a privileged means of access to the profound meaning of existence and subjectivity. *Jung* considers intuition as the "*perception through the unconscious*", one of the four fundamental functions of the psyche (thought, feeling, sensation, intuition). Intuition, an "irrational" function, allows us to grasp possibilities, connections, and meanings that escape rational analysis. For *Hillman*, intuition is the way one perceives one's calling, one's destiny; in this perspective, it is the bridge between the unconscious and consciousness, between personal myth and reality.

13 Karl Jaspers, *Allgemeine Psycopathologie* (1913).

14 He argued that the doctor grasps, in a pre-rational and intuitive way, a "diversity" in the schizophrenic patient's way of being, moving, and being in space, which manifests itself even in the simplest gestures, such as crossing the room from the moment he enters.

15 *Binswanger* rigorously applies epoché in his *Daseinsanalyse*, recommending the "suspension of one's own knowledge in order to apprehend each phenomenon," to "be-with" (*Mitsein*), to "live-with." Psychotic experience in this view is considered a distorted mode of "being-in-the-world." For Biswanger, phenomenological psychiatry "intends to gain direct access to psychopathological phenomena: to consider them in their semantic immediacy and in their radical giving of meaning."

16 Barison: "In hermeneutic dialogue there is not a subject and an object, but there is the meeting of two horizons, which merges into a new horizon, constituted by a change of both at the moment of interpretation." This description is strikingly similar to what we find in transpersonal practices, where therapist and patient share a *unified field of consciousness* that transcends the apparent individual separation. From www.psychiatryonline.it/psicoterapie/la-fenomenologia-nella-sua-teoria-e-nella-sua-prassi-in-psichiatria/

17 Sigmund Freud (1899, translated by Bollati Boringhieri), *The Interpretation of Dreams*, *Three Essays on Sexual Theory* (1905, Bollati Boringhieri) and *The Ego and the Id* (1923, Bollati Boringhieri).

18 Carl Gustav Jung: *Man and his Symbols* (1964, Longanesi), *Psychological Types* (1921, Bollati Boringhieri).

19 For Alfred Adler see *Il senso della vita* (1933, Astrolabio Ubaldini), *Il medico come educatore* (1904, Rivista di Psicologia Individuale).

20 Wilhelm Reich: *The Function of the Orgasm* (1927, SugarCo Editions), *Character Analysis* (1933, SugarCo Editions).

21 This address introduced revolutionary techniques in therapy (behavior modification), education (structured learning), and research (rigorous experimental methods).

22 *Psychology as seen by a behaviourist* by John B. Watson, 1913 article.

23 Pavlov, I. (1927): *Conditioned reflexes* (studies on classical conditioning).

24 Pavlov, I. (1927): *Conditioned reflexes* (studies on classical conditioning).

25 Skinner, B. F. (1938): *The behavior of organisms.*

26 Tolman, E. (1932): *Purposeful behaviour in animals and man* (intentional behaviorism).

27 A. Maslow, *Toward a Psychology of Being* (1962), and *Motivation and Personality* (1954); C. Rogers: *On becoming a person* (1961), and *Client-centred therapy* (1951).

28 See Alexander Lowen: *The Language of the Body* and *Bioenergetics.*
Rollo May and J. Bugental who integrated elements of existential psychology.

29 A. Maslow: *Toward a Psychology of Being* (1962), *The Farther Reaches of Human Nature* (1971); S. Grof: *The Adventure of Self-Discovery, The Holotropic Mind, Transpersonal Psychology* (with Christina Grof). Ken Wilber: *The Transformations of Consciousness* (with Jack Engler and Daniel P. Brown), *A Theory of Everything, The Spectrum of Consciousness.* R. Assagioli: *Psychosynthesis, The Act of Will.*

30 The British *anti-psychiatry movement* emerged in the 1960s and 1970s, criticizing traditional psychiatry in both theory and practice. Its leading exponents were R.D. Laing and David Cooper. These psychiatrists argued that mental illness, particularly schizophrenia, was a reasonable reaction to an "unhealthy" family context and not a simple biological disorder. They founded alternative therapeutic communities like *Kingsley hall* in London, where patients lived freely, without forced pharmacological interventions, and experimented with new forms of personal confrontation and group therapy (see Laing's books, *The Divided Self*, or Ken Loach's film, *Family Life*, which chronicles the Kingsley Hall residential experience). In the US, the anti-psychiatry movement consolidated from the 1950s and 1960s, as a reaction to the abuses of psychiatric hospitals and invasive therapies such as lobotomy and electroshock. (See *One Flew Over the Cuckoo's Nest*, a 1975 novel/film.) Let us remember the experiences of Perry, who founded the therapeutic community of *Diabasis* in

1971 (he recounts his experiences in *The Far Side of Madness* (1974)), and *Soteria House* in San Jose, California (1971), by L. Mosher; and see also in this panorama the positions of T. Leary, and the survivors' movement (Mental Patients Liberation Front), and others.

31 T. Szasz, with the publication of *The Myth of Mental Illness* (1961), denied the very existence of "mental illness" and attacked psychiatry as an instrument of social control; he promoted the right to refuse treatment and abolish forced hospitalization.

32 Franco Basaglia was inspired by English and American developments; he criticized asylum as a repressive institution and contributed to the "Law 180" (1978) which led to the closure of mental asylums in Italy.

33 *Genetic factors*: Many mental disorders, such as schizophrenia, bipolar disorder, and major depression, appear to have a significant genetic component, as people with a family history of these disorders have a higher risk of developing them. However, it does not appear that a single gene is responsible, but rather a combination of genetic variants that increase susceptibility.

34 *Neurochemical factors*: Imbalances in neurotransmitters, such as serotonin, dopamine, noradrenaline, and GABA, have been associated with various mental disorders. For depression, low levels of serotonin and noradrenaline have been found, for schizophrenia an excess of dopaminergic or imbalances of serotonin and GABA in anxiety disorders.

35 *Structural Factors and Brain Function*: Changes in the structure and function of specific brain areas associated with mental disorders have been found, such as a reduction in the volume of the hippocampus in depression, alterations in the prefrontal cortex and in the cerebral ventricles in schizophrenia. In bipolar disorder, abnormalities in emotion regulation were found, with involvement of the amygdala and prefrontal cortex.

36 *Endocrine factors*: Abnormal cortisol levels are often associated with disorders such as depression and anxiety. It is believed that dysfunction of the HPA (hypothalamus pituitary) axis may contribute to an altered stress response, influencing the development of mental disorders. Recent studies have also suggested a link between *chronic inflammation* and mental disorders such as depression and schizophrenia; in fact, an abnormal *immune response* may affect brain function and contribute to the development of mental disorders. It is also believed that the brain's ability to adapt and reorganize itself (*neuroplasticity*) may be impaired in various mental disorders. Alterations in synaptic connectivity and synaptic plasticity have been observed in autism and schizophrenia. It is believed that the risk of mental disorders in children may also depend on exposure to *infections, stress, or toxic substances during pregnancy, or even on possible complications at birth*, such as oxygen deficiency during delivery.

37 *Epigenetics* is a branch of biology that studies heritable changes in the expression of genes that do not involve alterations in the DNA sequence; in other words, while genetics deals with the information encoded in the DNA (*genotype*), epigenetics focuses on how this information is "read" and used by cells, thus determining the *phenotype*, i.e. the observable characteristics of an organism. *Epigenetics is the bridge between the genetic heritage and the environment.*

Epigenetic mechanisms act as chemical "tags" that are added to DNA or the proteins that envelop it (histones), influencing the activation or silencing of genes without changing the genetic sequence itself. A key feature of epigenetics is the possibility of *certain modifications being passed on to daughter cells* during cell division and, in some cases, even to subsequent generations (*intergenerational* transmission) modulating their expression.

38 Let us recall that the verb *scio*, in Latin, from which the term "scientific," refers to knowing about the deep nature of man, to *know thyself* of the Delphic oracle, to that *I found myself* of the Divine Comedy. "Knowing" therefore does not only mean knowing how certain mechanisms of the conditioned mind work, but rather "*knowing the knower.*"

39 *Reliability* is the consistency and precision of the results obtained: an experiment is reliable if *it produces the same results when replicated under the same conditions.*

Reproducibility is the ability to obtain similar or identical results when a study is replicated by independent researchers using comparable methods, data, and starting conditions.

40 Recently *Nature*, one of the most prestigious scientific journals in the world, published an article in which it was shown that *more than 70% of the scientific research examined had failed reproducibility tests*; despite this, that research involved was published, disseminated, and cited by other researchers as the basis of their own experiments. The study also showed that scientists often have an interest in publishing for the sake of their careers: almost 14% of the scientists surveyed said they knew colleagues who had totally fabricated data, and 34% said they had purposely selected data to bring out results they were interested in. (www.nature.com/articles/533452a). An article, published on "Science", 2015, with the title "Estimating the reproducibility of psychological science," coordinated by the "Reproducibility Project" in psychology, attempted to replicate 100 studies published in leading journals, finding that only about 40% of these results were replicable.

41 We can study "how" things happen, not "why."

42 For example, the efficacy of antipsychotics is tested in the laboratory on cells and animals, but the complexity of the human mind and the verification of the actual effects on neurotransmitters in vivo remain largely indirect. In vitro tests allow the study of individual receptors or pathways, but not the complex interactions in the living brain. Changes in neurotransmitters cannot be directly studied "live" in the human brain during antipsychotic use. Functional magnetic resonance imaging and PET techniques offer important data (for example, they can assess changes in blood flow/metabolic activity, or receptor "occupancy" using radioactive ligands), but they do not precisely show what happens to synaptic neurotransmitters in the living human brain. These techniques do not directly measure synaptic neurotransmitter levels and provide only indirect data. Dold, M., Leucht, S. (2014). "Pharmacotherapy of schizophrenia: Recent advances and future prospects".

43 In particular because of AI, but also of biotechnological innovations and nanotechnological, artificial prostheses, cryonics, the use of artificial wombs, cloning, and interfaces between the mind and machines.

44 Already G. Orwell (with *1984*, written in 1949) warned against the developments of a technological society guided not by love and wisdom but by the principle of power, a dystopia of human civilization already foreshadowed 40 years before him by Aldous Huxley.

45 See Bill Joy, co-founder of Sun Microsystems, who states this in his article "Why the Future Doesn't Need Us", and the wide discussions on internet on the rapid development of AI and the dangers of misuse of it.

46 Raymond Kurzweil (New York, February 12 1948) is an inventor, computer scientist and essayist from US. He is the author of *The Singularity Is Near*, Viking Press, 2005, and numerous other books on health, artificial intelligence, transhumanism, and the technological singularity. Founder *of Singularity University*.

47 Artificial General Intelligence (AGI) is an AI system capable of performing any human cognitive task with performance equal to or better than that of a person, demonstrating learning, reasoning, and adaptation capabilities in new and unforeseen contexts during training.

48 The presence of singular situations is all the more likely the more complex the system, such as a society, a civilization: the study of the collapse of ancient civilizations has indicated that the difficulty of finding solutions in a complex system was a determining cause of their downfall.

49 As a cause of disability, psychiatric and neurological disorders are in fact in first place (18%), followed by cardiovascular disorders, cancers, and on to traffic accidents (3%).

50 Although it now seems clear that we may not be able to keep up with a future that has begun to run, (madly, we might say), there are those who advocate speeding up in that direction anyway, rather than stopping for a moment to consider which is the best direction to take.

51 Insel, 2015, writes: "Technology can fulfil the task of diagnosing many processes.... moreover, many mental health treatments are psychosocial interventions, and these can be carried out through a smartphone."

52 I take for this paragraph and the previous one the clear exposition of the salient points of this development as set out in a video by Dr. Valerio Rosso, (www.youtube.com/watch?v=ZN_w-8ew9yA) and in the videos of Dr. Arshya Vahabzadeh, www.youtube.com/watch?v=2ZxW8N68CBw .

In this view of the future, it is implied and accepted that this development is inevitable, and is also accepted as favorable, although it often is not.

53 For instance, a psychiatrist could in fact review many interviews, many sessions at the end of a day, recorded and processed by the computer, which has become capable of learning and analyzing emotions through the recognition of facial expressions, and the analysis of sensor data, which allow emotions to be assessed and monitored.

54 The AI will increasingly manage machines and relationships to the point of at least partially replacing it; it will make choices instead of the doctor, for example, it will choose which data to consider important, and which to neglect, it will dictate the timing and manner of interventions, allying itself with corporate profit and political policies.

55 Applications for mobile phones or PCs are already in use that help patients identify symptoms, follow strategies, keep a diary of symptoms, and alert the caregiver if things worsen beyond a certain degree. In the future, for example, we will be able to monitor language, behavior, digital parameters, changes in sleep, appetite using mobile phone apps, i.e. smartphone technology and other sensors.

56 Transcranial Magnetic Stimulation (TMS) and other forms of non-invasive neuro-modulation are becoming increasingly central to the psychiatry of the future. These techniques use low-intensity magnetic or electric fields to modulate the activity of neurons in specific brain areas. TMS is already approved for drug-resistant major depression and is also showing interesting results for anxiety disorders, obsessive-compulsive disorder, addictions and chronic pain.

However, especially for high-intensity fields, there is no certainty that they are not harmful; for example, acute exposure to very high-intensity electromagnetic fields (EMFs), such as those used in the military or in experimental applications, has been shown to induce significant effects on neurons and the central nervous system, as they can induce electric currents in networks in neurons. Extreme pulsed fields (e.g. *EMPs*, *Electromagnetic Pulses)* can cause disorientation or temporary loss of cognitive functions, and can interfere with brain rhythms (alpha, beta waves); whereas low intensity PEMFs (e.g. While low-intensity PEMFs (e.g. 1–10 mT) show therapeutic effects (reduction of inflammation, neuronal repair), high-intensity PEMFs (> 50 mT) may have opposite outcomes, such as excitotoxicity and damage to the blood-brain barrier, facilitating the entry of neurotoxins into the brain parenchyma.

Chapter 2

Transpersonal psychology, the psychology of the future

2.1 The transpersonal field

2.1.1 Psychiatry and consciousness

A different conception of psychiatry, one that includes the soul, the spirit, energy, alchemy, requires a different conception of man, of psyche, of spirit.

In a Transpersonal (henceforth TP) view, man is *an indivisible and complex being, a mystery that manifests* itself in multiple dimensions: spiritual, psychic, and also material, in a *continuum*.

We would thus like to revisit psychiatry and psychology from a point of view which is more aware of this complex and mysterious, spiritual, cosmic nature of man.

We advocate a "psychiatry with a soul", a *more* "conscious psychiatry", and not just a more "technological psychiatry."

To do this, we shall now examine the contribution of the TP field, of that psychology which is more open to the spiritual world. We shall soon recognize a different method, and also a different language: in order to listen to and understand the nature of the soul and its transformations, we shall consider images and symbols in our investigation.

We shall go to sea, without the compass of the scientific method, but with the compass of the soul. This will be the way to reach the other shore, to arrive in the "new world," to understand these other-worldly things, these crazy things of our patients.

But how did we arrive at this soulless science?

The most significant answer, though not the only one, is that we are at this point because Western culture has removed spiritual experience, that is, mysticism, confining it to a field of exceptionality: since then, there has remained only an alleged knowledge of the soul, entrusted to psychology ...

DOI: 10.4324/9781003676461-2

In our societies, the hierarchy of anthropological knowledge has its summit in psychology ... but psychology and psychiatry know nothing about the spirit: psychology has only some knowledge of the faculties of the soul (better to say of the psyche, given the religious-spiritual meaning of soul), but not of its spiritual 'foundation', which is only experienced in absolute detachment – in the 'night' of nothingness, in the 'death of the soul' ... the experience of the spirit is as unknown to psychology as it is to religion in its prevailing sociological aspect...[1]

Modern medicine and psychiatry seem to have *lost the way of true knowledge long ago*: these sciences have embraced the materialist view of man and consciousness.

Thus, *some fundamental questions are no longer asked*, such as: *What is man? Where does he come from, and where does he go? What is the nature of mind, symbols, and consciousness? And what is the origin of the world*? These sciences no longer ask these questions, because they consider them to be connected to religion or philosophy: old, outdated and superfluous stuff.

However, especially *for psychiatry, these are fundamental questions* for the cure of souls, for happiness.

As we said, this is why a number of scholars in psychology and psychiatry have turned to *other fields*, especially to *alternative ways of knowing, to a different kind of knowledge.*

I am referring to *humanistic, historical, philosophical, anthropological, and religious* fields that are useful for better understanding the nature of the human being the mind, its purpose, and its potential.

The models and wisdom of traditional spiritual systems—such as *hinduism, buddhism, tantra and kashmiri yoga, alchemy,* or works like the *Divine Comedy*—offer substantial and profound contributions to understanding the mind, its functioning, mental disorders, and ego-consciousness.

This kind of knowledge mantains an openness to other possibilities, an interest in the psyche as "*reality*," and—above all—a focus on the *subject*: consciousness.

2.1.2 Non-ordinary states of consciousness (NOSC)

As we have seen, the *seeds* of a new psychology and psychiatry can already be traced in psychoanalysis (especially with Jung), psychosynthesis (Assagioli), and humanistic psychology.

Furthermore, over the past 60 years, a *TP psychology movement* has developed in the USA from humanistic psychology. The term *T-P* stands for those areas of psychic reality that extend beyond identification with the individual personality.

By Transpersonal Psychology (henceforth TPP) we mean a *psychological approach that addresses the study and culture of spirituality and spiritual experiences within a psychological context.*[2] This definition is widely accepted in TPP, but it has its limitations, as we shall see.

TPP could also be called "spiritual psychology", as it is interested in the "realization of the Self" for the awakening of each individual's spiritual nature.[3]

In the above-mentioned sense, TPP emphasizes *changes in consciousness, and* "anomalous" *psychic experiences*, including those of a *spiritual and mystical* nature. Inner experiences of a mystical and ecstatic order, in fact, as well as the ego's yearning for transcendence, constitute a significant aspect of human experience, and are therefore worthy of study by psychology.

In a deeper sense of the term, however, TP indicates *states of consciousness beyond the personal* identification, and, even, beyond the me and the Self: that is, states of non-dual consciousness. This approach is close to the teachings of non-duality in the spiritual field.

From this perspective, the "ordinary me" (that is, the identity we experience in everyday life) is a contracted and conditioned form of identification of a broader, deeper, *Self,* which is what we truly are: consciousness; it is infinite in finite form, not different in nature.

As we shall see later, these distinctions are of great importance in the diagnostic and therapeutic approach to mental disorders.

Consciousness, in this view, although based on the biological support of man, is ultimately independent of it, transcending the division of spiritual and material; for biological psychiatry, as we have seen, consciousness is instead a product of the brain.

Research in TPP is still tied to integrating spirituality into the developing ego, focusing on the idea of a "spiritual ego." In this view, only the awakening of the individual ego is sought, not that of the Self.

A different conception of TPP, on the other hand, proposes a non-dualistic view of reality, operating a true reversal of the point of view. It is not enough to recognize that the "me" must be open to the "Self," but it is also necessary to recognize that it is the "Self" that recognizes itself in the me.[4]

These *experiences of transcendence* have, over the centuries, been given many names in the various traditions: *mystical ecstasy*, *cosmic experience*, *cosmic consciousness*, *oceanic experience*, *peak experience*, *nirvana*, *satori*, *samadhi*, *kingdom of heaven*, *dream body*, *nagual*, and so on.[5]

These states of superconsciousness have also been referred to as *non-ordinary states of consciousness*, (henceforth *NOSC*). S. Grof in the 1970s also referred to them as *Holotropic States of Mind*[6], i.e. evolutionary stages towards a more unified, non-dual, more evolved consciousness: conditions for the emergence of a new state of consciousness, a new being.

2.1.3 Role of the TPP

TPP *has played an important role in the renewal of psychology*, with the recognition of the nature and value of transpersonal experiences, of subjective realities, previously regarded as belonging exclusively to the mystical, religious, metaphysical area.

Transpersonal Psychology shares with humanistic psychology the view that psychic and psychiatric crises contain an evolutionary potential in human consciousness. However, it *takes it a step further* by asserting that the personal ego (or self) is only a reflection of a transcendent self, of a transpersonal center of consciousness that is the unity underlying the apparent multiplicity. In doing so, it makes a significant contribution to the development of man and psychology.

In psychiatry in particular, which has always dealt mainly with madness, (that is, with major disorders, such as psychosis and manic depressive forms), a new vision was opportune, necessary, urgent, so as to reinterpret and intervene differently on these processes.

TPP also recognizes how crises are not only potentially evolutionary conditions for the individual, but at the same time *an expression and stimulus for social, collective change*, necessary to face life in the third millennium. It therefore contributes to reviewing the role of social psychology.

TPP also gave voice to and *integrated into itself the crisis and then the development of new horizons of thought*.[7]

The TPP has also made its part in *influencing culture and academic circles*, so that there is now an increasing acceptance of a radically new world view, of what is scientific, and a revaluation and new understanding of ourselves, nature, and the universe.

Furthermore, there is an *increasing demand* for therapies and therapists open to new developments from patients, who are now more aware and informed.

However, it must be noted that *TPP is still not very well known and accepted by the medical and psychiatric world*, and that (in Italy in particular) the biological orientation of psychiatry is increasingly asserting itself, tending to stifle these promising new developments.[8]

2.1.4 Psychosis or transcendence?

Mainstream psychology and psychiatry define transcendental experiences as fantasies or pathologies.

Depending on the personal approaches one considers, transpersonal psychology would represent "an attempt to satisfy the desire to be cared for by a 'good mother,' or the sign of a fragile ego unable to distinguish between internal images and external reality."

In the "scientific" community, spirituality is seen as a result of ignorance, superstition, or primitive and childish magical thinking. Here, consciousness, mystical images, and experiences are believed to *derive from biochemical changes in the brain* and may even be considered *manifestations of severe mental illness.*[9]

The psychiatric literature contains numerous articles and books discussing *what might be the appropriate clinical diagnosis for many of the great figures of spiritual history.*

For example, as Harner reports[10], "*St. Anthony* has been called *a schizophrenic*, *St. John of the Cross* has been labeled a "hereditary degenerate"; *St. Teresa of Ávila* has been dismissed as a "severe hysterical psychotic," and *Muhammad*'s mystical experiences have been attributed to *epilepsy*. Many other religious and spiritual figures, such as the *Buddha*, *Jesus*, *Ramakrishna*, and *Sri Ramana Maharshi* have been seen as suffering from *psychosis* due to their visionary experiences and beliefs, and even Buddhist meditation is described in psychopathological terms and referred to as "artificial catatonia."[11] Similarly, some anthropologists believe that *shamans* are *schizophrenics*, *walking psychotics*, *epileptics*, or *hysterics*.

Western psychology and psychiatry describe the rituals and spiritual life of ancient and native cultures in pathological terms: and yet, *the madness of our world*, (which risks self-extinction) is considered normal to the point of not being recognized as pathological by doctors and researchers.[12]

2.2 The authors

R. Assagioli and *C. G. Jung*, although part of the psychodynamic and personal psychoanalysis movement, were the first psychiatrists to propose a transpersonal approach in Western psychiatry far before the development of humanistic psychology or the transpersonal movement overseas. *Phenomenological psychiatry*, distinguishing itself from biological psychiatry, had previously laid some foundations for these future developments.

In more recent times, we will focus especially on the contribution of two important figures in the development of psychology and TP psychiatry, namely *K. Wilber* and *S. Grof*. But let us start further back.

2.2.1 Dante Alighieri, saving one's soul

Dante Alighieri was an illustrious Italian poet and sage, who lived at the turn of the 14th century; in his work the *Divine Comedy* (but even earlier in the *Vita Nova*), he describes in detail *the awakening of the Self at the level of the individual consciousness.*[13]

The work describes a symbolic *journey into* the afterlife, that is, beyond-life, (i.e. beyond the ordinary state of consciousness), into a symbolic space, where after going astray, one finds the *direct path*; a journey where one goes from suffering to peace, from darkness to light, where one is reborn.

The symbolism, present in the *Christian resurrection myth*, starts from the bewilderment and pain experienced emerging from the "the dark forest," and which matures by visiting the three realms of this spiritual world.[14]

The journey begins by visiting *Hell* (the condition of the obscured consciousness), accompanied by a spiritual guide (Virgil); it proceeds in a descending left-handed spiral, where circles (i "cerchi" , corresponding to the Chakras in an anagogic, i.e. alchemical-spiritual, vision) are progressively and successively visited; in each circle one makes contact, experiences, and abandons that specific downward bound energy, thus practically reversing its action.

The descending journey ends by inverting the direction of the two pilgrims (Dante and Virgil) on the very source of that attractive force, i.e. a 180-degree inversion of Lucifer's own body, placed at the center of the Earth (Earth in the sense of planet and humanity as a whole, but also in the sense of inner Earth, one's own ego), at the Earth's center of gravity.

One initially visits regions with boiling waters (the blood river of Phlegethon) to arrive at the bottom of the pit at regions with icy waters (Cocytus); these hellish rivers are a transparent metaphor for the energy that cools and imprisons souls in inanimation and suffering.15

This descending force is then also activated and accompanied in the second cantica by ascending the Purgatory, the Sacred Mountain, this time proceeding along a rightward ascending spiral; here the operation will be to rectify from frame to frame the vices by applying the corresponding corrective virtues, so as to finally reach the earthly Paradise, the apex of the cone now straightened.

Immediately after passing through the gate of Purgatory, and past the guardian angel, the energy that supports and drives the process manifests itself in the form of an undulating ascending path, which opens up in the mountain-consciousness, and which fully manifests itself near its apex as a wall of fire that juts out from the mountain.

Here Virgil is succeeded by the guidance of Beatrice, who is the true driving force behind the entire process of salvation from pain, and who will bring about the definitive purifying process; the exit from suffering and evil is thus concluded. [16]

Beatrice represents the driving force in the Divine Comedy[17] that will lead him through the planetary *heavens* with a direct and ecstatic path to the highest heaven, in the Empyrean, where the reunion with the cosmic consciousness itself will finally take place.

The author himself declares that the work is *polysemous*, i.e. it possesses several levels of meaning, and advises the use of progressively deeper keys of interpretation: *literal, allegorical, moral and anagogical or spiritual.*

An anagogic, or alchemical, reading reveals the *here-and-now operation* of the alchemical transmutation of consciousness, and demonstrates the therapeutic value of this path.

We will thus see how the symbolic journey, described in the text, recounts the awakening of consciousness in the present, the "rediscovering" of clear, transcendental consciousness, the pure Self *finding* itself again.

This journey is a call from Heaven (in other words, it is activated by a call from the Higher Self) and, as the text describes in detail, requires special preparation and guidance.

It is in fact not an easy path, but the birth of a new being, a new consciousness: a death, rebirth, a transformation. Although awakening in fact occurs before and outside the mind, a gradual integration (of this progressive dis-identification from the "me," from the body-mind) is subsequently necessary, a process that is then described in detail in stages, transformative steps, of death and rebirth. This will allow the individual consciousness to gradually *shift* from the narrow consciousness of identification with the body-mind, the "me," into a wider consciousness, the "Self."

The suffering experienced on the path to self-realisation (or enlightenment) is due to the *resistance* to this process of death on behalf of the old identity, creating conflict, lamenting depression and refusal of the felt sense of death, preventing rebirth. In Inferno this opposition, in agreement with the primary opponent, Lucifer, maintains chronic suffering, as in chronic illnesses (*fire that torments*); in welcoming the process, understanding that it is part of a higher purpose, in Purgatory, the suffering is diluted, as in Psychotherapy (*fire that refines*) until it is extinguished, and finally in Paradise this fire radiates as pure love (*fire that illuminates*).[18]

These NOSC are also the states of consciousness that we encounter in psychiatry, where most often they are ego-dystonic, i.e. rejected, unwelcome, tragic, because consciousness does not understand and accept them.

Precisely because of the difficulty and confusion one goes through on this contrasted path of awakening, in psychiatry, it will be appropriate and necessary to make use of an "expert guide" (of a Virgil), a role delegated to the *therapist*, sent "from heaven" to help.[19]

The therapist-guide is thus invested with a sacred role, that is, to help the process of the reunion of the separated ego (the patient) with itself (*I found myself*).

The therapeutic process in psychiatry, seen from the TP perspective, is thus not only the relief of (mental) suffering of a person, who frees himself from it by becoming more spiritual.

It is rather about the awakening of self-consciousness in that character: a rediscovery of consciousness (*I found myself*); and this is the reason why the character goes into deep and irreversible crisis.[20]

We thus see in the Divine Comedy a detailed exposition of the stages and methods of consciousness transformation, described and recounted in poetic, symbolic, sublime, and unsurpassed language. We have here a non-dualistic vision of consciousness, and of its evolution and difficulties, which heals from suffering by rediscovering itself.[21]

2.2.2 Roberto Assagioli and psychosynthesis

We have seen how TPP was officially born in the 1960s in America. However, at least 60 years earlier, transpersonal models of psychology and psychotherapy existed in Europe, such as *Assagioli's Psychosynthesis*, *Frankl's Logotherapy*, and *Jung's Analytical Psychology*.

R. Assagioli's contribution thus precedes in time the American development of TPP and anticipates and accompanies an evolution towards spirituality in the psychologies of the time, helping psychoanalysis to open itself differently to spiritual evolution and awakening. There are documents testifying that Assagioli was already speaking about Transpersonal Psychology around 1914, and then founded the Psychosynthesis Institute in Rome in 1926.

Psychosynthesis (henceforth *PS*) is a psychological theory and praxis that developed from psychoanalysis, to evolve on one side and in parallel with Humanistic Psychology (Assagioli and Maslow had exchanges and clinical interests in common), and opening up on the other side into existential and transpersonal psychology (which focuses on spiritual development and higher states of consciousness). This is how Assagioli defined it:

> a method of self-training and psycho-spiritual realization for all those who do not want to accept remaining slaves to their inner phantoms and external influences, to passively undergo the play of psychological forces taking place within them, but want to become masters of their own inner realm.
>
> Assagioli, 1973

Assagioli maintained that PS was not a school that had to maintain an orthodoxy, and that different psychosynthetic currents could coexist within it:

> there is no orthodoxy in psychosynthesis and no one, starting with myself, can proclaim himself its true or authentic representative. Therefore, in a broader sense, "psychosynthesis" can be defined as any

> attitude oriented towards increasingly broader integrations and syntheses, any attitude that takes man to heart in his entirety and uniqueness, up to the realization of his spiritual dimension.
>
> Adapted from Assagioli, 1973 (personal translation)

Human suffering results from man being out of tune with his own evolutionary project, due to the sleep of consciousness, or the active resistance of the ego, his opposition, sometimes due to previous wounds of the soul.[22]

PS is a method that uses *specific tools and techniques* to help this evolutionary process, such as meditation, guided imaginations, and other techniques. This therapeutic orientation is concerned with helping self-realization, aimed at the full development of its four dimensions: *physical*, *emotional*, *mental*, and *spiritual*.

According to Assagioli, the individual is inseparably composed of body, psyche, and spirit, is endowed with *consciousness and will*, and is capable of developing a conscious and volitional orientation, after having known and mastered his or her unconscious world.[23]

For this pioneer, it is essential in the process of spiritual development to *come into contact with the transpersonal Self*. Assagioli clearly distinguishes the *study of the superconscious* (the true territory of Transpersonal Psychology) from what he calls the *experience of the transpersonal Self* (also called "peak experience").[24] About the experience of the Transpersonal Self he writes:

> ...it is a state of consciousness that can be, and is, experienced, at certain moments of elevation, of stepping outside the limits of ordinary awareness. One experiences in this experience a sense of enlargement, of limitless expansion, pervaded by intense joy and bliss. It is essentially ineffable, not expressible in words.
>
> Here one comes into contact with the Mystery, with the supreme Reality. Of this I cannot speak; it is beyond the boundaries of science, of psychology.
>
> But Psychosynthesis can help to get closer, to reach that threshold, and that is already a lot.[25]
>
> Assagioli, 1973 (personal translation)

A founding point of this direction is that in the "cure of the soul", the *analytical phase* must be followed by a *synthetic phase*, that is, a more active phase oriented towards the discovery of the personal will. In other words, there is a path of *personal psychosynthesis*, which concerns the integration and harmonization of the various psychic functions, and a path of *transpersonal psychosynthesis*, which allows man to access higher dimensions of the psyche.

In the psychotherapeutic sense, it is therefore possible to speak of a phase psychotherapy at the level of the ego, and one at the level of the self.

As we can see, this is an orientation that really has a potential to go beyond personalization, to be considered a trans-personal psychotherapy. PS does not break with the ancient tradition of teachings on the mind, but provides it with a new language, and makes other original contributions. It does not place psychology in another sphere than spirituality, but rather maintains the profound significance of human life in relation to the cosmos.

Of Assagioli's conception, many may be familiar with the *diagram of the egg*, where one can see the inner way indicated: the contact between the personal self and the higher Self is nothing other than the opening of an inner healing way.[26]

2.2.3 C. G. Jung

Although this author initially joined the Freudian psychoanalytic movement, he departed from it very early on to found an orientation called *analytical psychology*.

His conception of the libido as not only sexual, the theory of symbols and archetypes, differed substantially from the Freudian view of the unconscious and of therapy.

In his writings, he claimed to be interested in studying and describing the reflection of the spirit that is present and active in the human psyche, rather than the absolute reality, which in itself is indescribable.[27] His interest was to understand and accompany the transcendental experiences, which he and psychiatric patients experience in an often incommunicable manner.

In his *Red Book*, Jung recounts the process of awakening and the psychic turmoil he himself had undergone on an individual level in the period from 1913 to 1930 to which the text refers.[28] The text is autobiographical, and uses both the written word and numerous beautiful illustrations by his own hand, which evoke significant unconscious images. It constitutes an example of what Jung himself would later refer to as "active imagination," and testifies to his effort in consciously going through this experience.

By his own admission, all of his later work is based on this period of individual transmutation, investing his studies in alchemy and spirituality as much as his earlier therapeutic practice. The Red Book in fact marks *the turning point in Jung*, as perhaps for each of us, towards a true *transpersonal direction*, stemming from the experience of losing oneself and finding oneself as a different consciousness, which he recounts in those pages.

At that juncture he is reduced to impotence, and his knowledge is no longer valid: and the Soul, beyond any category of judgement, kills him and regenerates him as a new man.

Luigi Aurigemma, in a fine article in 2004,[29] explores this transformation, arguing that perhaps at that time Jung's process was not fully and definitively completed, and notes how a partial identification with the body-mind and knowledge still remained. Indeed, Jung argues (as does Kant) that "the spirit can neither establish nor prove anything that exists outside its boundaries ...," and that "our psychology is a science of pure phenomena devoid of any metaphysical implications," an almost "prison-like" psyche.[30]

On the one hand, therefore, Jung is fascinated by the Indian *Upanishads*, where the basis of everything, the *ontology*, is the consciousness of being: it is all about inner experience.

Jung seems to share these views: "To know whether it is so or not, look into your own spirit."[31]

On the other hand, there is the inescapable reality of the body as support: *We cannot know anything that is not separate from us.* "Even when I say, 'I know myself,'" says Jung, "there remains an infinitesimal 'I', the 'I who knows', always separate from 'myself."[32]

Carl Gustav Jung, through his writings, played a pioneering role in interpreting the Indian concept of *Kundalini* from a Western psychological perspective. He wrote extensively on numerous spiritual traditions, Western and Eastern; we are particularly interested though in his series of *lectures on Kundalini Yoga* from 1932 in Eranos, Switzerland.

Together with an Orientalist, Dr. H. Zimmer, he held a number of seminars later collected in the book *Kundalini Yoga* (see Bibliography).

Jung considered the *Kundalini* not only a spiritual concept, but a powerful psychological metaphor that helps to understand the deep levels of the human unconscious.

Jung argued that the *Kundalini* is a force within each of us, that connects the individual mind to the collective unconscious and, more broadly, to the universe.

In those seminars, Jung spoke of the *Chakras* as symbols of stages of psychological development, as places of transition to greater self-awareness, in parallel with personal growth and inner transformation.

For Jung, the *ascent of the Kundalini symbolizes the path of* "individuation," a progressive journey that leads the individual to confront and integrate unconscious contents, passing through various psychological levels (*Chakras*), until the attainment of a unified and realized personality.

Jung emphasizes that the images and symbols of the *Kundalini* are not exclusive to the Indian tradition, but *universal archetypes* that every culture can recognize, emerging spontaneously in the dreams and symbols of people all over the world.

Aware of the West's difficulties in integrating the *Kundalini* without risk of psychic imbalance, Jung repeatedly emphasizes the need for a precautionary and psychological approach rather than a dogmatic or purely practical one, since the forced awakening of the *Kundalini* can lead to imbalances such as ego inflation or even psychotic states. The integration of the contents of the unconscious must therefore be conducted gradually and consciously.

Jung's texts on the Indian East all tend to take us into the depths of the "self," to recognize the unique conscious being, that is, to recognize the most universal roots of our feeling and knowing, the archetypes.[33] In his theory of the archetypes they are *psychic processes of the* "objective psyche," *linked to the collective unconscious, the primary activity of the objective, transpersonal psyche.*

2.2.4 Ken Wilber[34]

Ken Wilber is a central figure in the development of transpersonal psychology. His work has allowed TPP to gain fame and acceptance and influence, thanks to a great breadth of vision, a capacity for rigorous and systematic analysis, combined with excellent synthesis and intellectual rigor. He succeeds in clearly communicating and disseminating complex ideas.

2.2.4.1 The "spiral dynamics" model

This model describes *the evolution of human value systems and consciousness* through a series of *developmental stages*, each characterized by specific psychological patterns, values, cognitive structures, and worldviews.[35] Each stage represents a way of adapting to reality according to historical, social, or personal context. The stages are not "better" in an absolute sense, but more complex and adaptive.

The *higher stages transcend and include the previous ones (they do not negate them)*. This is not a rigid progression: people and societies can regress at times of crisis.

Psychopathology in this context is considered a developmental disorder, at different stages of its developmental arc.

Let us look at these levels in some detail, because they will serve us to assess the mode of expression of awakening in psychiatric patients (see Table 2.1).

As can be seen, the visions of psychology change according to the level of consciousness, individual and collective developmental stages.[36]

Table 2.1 Evolutionary Stages

Stage Name & Color	*Psychology*	*Values*	*Cognitive Structure*	*Worldview*	*Examples*
Archaic-Instinctual (Survival), Beige	Instinctive, focused on pure survival (food, water, shelter)	Preservation of life, physical safety	Pre-logical, linked to instincts and biological needs	No conscious reflection on oneself; one lives in the here and now	Infants, primordial tribes, people in extreme survival conditions
Magical-Animistic (Tribal Security), Purple	Magical, animistic thinking, tribal dependence	Protection of ancestors and spirits, respect for traditions, superstitions	Pre-rational, dominated by myths and rituals	The universe is governed by spirits and supernatural forces	Shamanism, tribal cults, mythological worldview
Egocentric-Power (Strength), Red	Impulsive, aggressive, seeks control over others	Honor, respect based on strength, unbridled individualism	Egocentric, oriented towards personal power	"I win, you lose"; the strongest dominates	Warrior leaders, criminal gangs, feudalism, conquering empires
Traditional (Authority), Blue	Dogmatic, devoted to a greater cause	Discipline, morality, order, duty, obedience to rules	Linear logic, but rigid and absolutist	The world has a divine order and one must follow the rules	Traditional religions, monarchies, theocratic states, nationalism
Modern, Rational-Scientific (Success), Orange	Competitive, oriented towards material success	Merit, individualism, innovation, market freedom	Logical-rational, empirical, data-oriented	The world is a resource to be exploited for progress	Capitalism, Enlightenment, science, industrialization

(Continued)

Table 2.1 (*Continue*)

Stage Name & Color	*Psychology*	*Values*	*Cognitive Structure*	*Worldview*	*Examples*
Post-Modern, Pluralist (Community), Green	Empathetic, post-materialist, seeks harmony and equality	Diversity, social justice, inclusion, respect for the environment	Relativist, systemic, oriented towards collective well-being	All points of view are valid and worthy of respect	Ecological movements, human rights activism, post-modern society
Integral, Systemic (Adaptive), Yellow	Holistic, able to integrate different perspectives	Autonomy, adaptability, systemic intelligence, continuous learning	Complex thinking, metacognitive, self-organizing	All systems have value, but must be integrated effectively	Wilber's integral approach, systemic management, complexity science
Holistic-Transpersonal (Unity), Turquoise	Transpersonal, feels the interconnectedness of everything	Spirituality without dogma, intuitive wisdom, global consciousness	Non-dual, transcends and includes all previous stages	Reality is a great field of unified consciousness	Advanced Mysticism, enlightened leaders, Unified Field Theory

Table 2.2 The Four Quadrants

Quadrant	*Main Question(s)*	*Refers to*	*Clinical/Intervention Approach*
Individual Interior (Subjective Self)	"How do I feel?" "What is my intention?" "How do I feel inside?"	Emotions, thoughts, personal values, intimate motivations, insight, states of consciousness, symptom experience	Psychotherapy, introspection techniques
Individual Exterior (Objective Ego)	"What can be seen from the outside?" "What are the objective signs?" "What does the body show?"	Physical symptoms, observable behavior, neurological data, test results, brain activity, physiological parameters	Objective examination, medical diagnosis, neuroimaging, pharmacotherapy, behavioral observation
Collective Interior (Subjective Us)	"What are the beliefs of my group?" "What values do we share?" "What meaning does it have for our community?"	Social norms, language, myths, symbols, religion, customs, shared worldview, stigma	Analysis of cultural context, group therapy, focus on social meaning of the symptom, work with family or community
Collective Exterior (Objective We)	"What institutions are involved?" "How does the system work?" "What are the objective group dynamics?"	Family, school, hospital, laws, economy, environment, infrastructure, health policies	Systemic analysis, policy intervention, institutional collaboration

The complete trajectory of human development can thus be seen as the progressive decline of egocentrism.[37]

Wilber integrates the scientific conceptions of psychology with the *perennial philosophy*,[38] i.e. with the Western and Eastern non-dualist meditative tradition.

2.2.4.2

In time, Wilber addressed the limitations of transpersonal psychology by developing a *broader and more articulated vision*. His main critique was that *it focused almost exclusively on the spiritual dimension, neglecting other fundamental aspects of psyche and reality*. In the 1980s and 1990s, he thus proposed the *Integral Model* (or *Integral Psychology*)—an attempt to unify psychology, philosophy, religion, and science in a single paradigm.

Thus was born the AQAL (All Quadrants, All Levels) model, which seeks to integrate all dimensions of human experience. *The four quadrants* make it possible to place each phenomenon, each experience according to more individual or collective, inner or outer perspectives, and to differentiate clinical approaches according to them.

Let us briefly look at the characteristics of the four quadrants, which phenomena they refer to, and which clinical approach is most appropriate in each area.

In Ken Wilber's integral model, human development is seen as the *transition from pre-egoic to egoic to transegoic; from pre-conventional morality, to conventional morality, to post-conventional morality; from egocentric, to socio-centric, to cosmo-centric behavior; from subconsciousness, to self-consciousness, to superconsciousness.*[39]

The four quadrants answer different questions, as described in Table 2.2.[40]

Wilber is also a keen observer and scholar of the modern world seen in its negative and positive aspects.[41]

Wilber's Integral Model is also important because *it has influenced several areas*, including:

- *Integral Psychotherapy* (combination of cognitive, psychodynamic, body, and spiritual therapy)
- *Education* (learning systems based on different levels of development)
- *Integrative Medicine* (holistic approaches that consider mind, body, emotions, and culture)
- *Leadership and Organizational Development* (models for personal and social growth based on the development of consciousness)

He is one of the founders of the *Integral Institute in 1998*.

Ken Wilber's work has attracted not only plaudits but also serious criticism from various sources.[42]

2.2.5 Stanislav Grof

Stanislav Grof, together with Ken Wilber, is today among the most representative figures of the transpersonal movement. Of Czech origin (Prague, 1931), he began his training as a Freudian psychoanalyst. Here he began his first experiments with LSD, which was legal at the time, on *psychotic patients and other clinical subjects*, as part of official psychiatric research, in the then Czechoslovakia, mainly in the 1950s and 1960s, at the Prague

Psychiatric Institute. He obtained encouraging results especially with neurotic patients undergoing psychotherapeutic treatment, in the treatment of terminally ill patients, and as a contribution to the training of therapists.[43]

He then moved to the United States (Johns Hopkins University in Baltimore, then Director of Psychiatric Research at the Maryland Psychiatric Research Center) and experimented with LSD as a means of *alleviating the suffering of terminally ill cancer patients*.[44]

In 1973, Grof was invited to the *Esalen Institute* in Big Sur, California, where he lived until 1987 as a resident teacher, meeting all kinds of prominent people and giving numerous seminars. There, dissatisfied with the current state of psychology which, in his opinion, did not duly take into account the spiritual sphere of the psyche, *he founded transpersonal psychology together with Maslow, Anthony Sutich, and other researchers.*

After the prohibition of using hallucinogenic substances in research, he experimented (with his wife Cristina) with a *breathing method, called holotropic* (i.e. aimed at the integration of being), capable of inducing non-ordinary states of consciousness without the administration of drugs.

Grof was one of the first to elaborate a *transpersonal psychodynamic model*, as well as *a map of inner experience and a psychotherapeutic methodology with a transpersonal approach*. Through the observation of non-ordinary states of consciousness, *Grof amplified the cartography* of the unconscious beyond the known limits of official science by adding two trans-biographical levels to the biographical level: the *perinatal level*, related to the birth experience, and the *transpersonal level*, which implies crossing the space-time boundary.[45]

Grof's thought contributed to a new and *broader interpretation of mental illness*. He argues that at least some of the crises diagnosed by medicine as psychotic are actually psychic states endowed with great evolutionary potential, defined as "spiritual emergence" (emergence in the sense of emergence). These are in reality often dramatic episodes in which, however, an enormous evolutionary potential and inner renewal is hidden (and emerges, precisely).

By diagnosing these states as pathologies and treating them with drugs, in order to suppress the psychiatric crisis rather than accompany it, official psychiatry does not differentiate between the various psychotic states and risks hindering the natural process of healing and psychological development of those cases in which the crisis is evolutionary.[46] On the other hand, it has been argued, "not all 'expansive' experiences are signs of awakening or spiritual realization."[47]

Stanislav Grof therefore considers psychological issues from an evolutionary perspective and believes that the current global crisis, which threatens the depletion of the planet's vital resources and our very survival, is the collective result of individuals' current level of consciousness. He recognizes the transition to a higher state of consciousness as essential, both individually and collectively.

In conclusion, although still evolving, *TP psychology* is the school that today perhaps comes closest to the *psychology of the future.*

However, while approaching NOSC in a different way from other schools of psychology and psychotherapy, TPP today shows interpretative and applicative limits, and needs a renewal, a refounding, to return to be more in tune with its original principles, and to cross the clinical bridge that still separates TPP from psychiatry.

Notes

1 "But it is not just ignorance: it is also hostility. The hostility of one who senses that the thing is profoundly, intimately distant – indeed contrary – to what one claims, ... something capable of unmasking all the lies one feeds on and of leaving one, so to speak, naked, bereft of all power and self-assertion ..."
From https://marcovannini.it/volumi-collettanei/sulla-follia-divina
2 From Lattuada, https://pierluigilattuada.com/psicologia-transpersonale/
3 See e.g., *Tart.* Spiritual does not mean belonging to some religious denomination. However, in a deeper sense of the term TP indicates states of consciousness beyond the personal plane, states of nondual consciousness.
4 This is the deepest meaning of Dante's "I found myself": it is not Dante who recognizes himself, it is the true Self that recognizes itself in the individual consciousness, which awakens, while Dante gets lost, loses the old way in order to find the straight path he has lost.
5 Reported by Lattuada, in www.psicologia-psicoterapia.it/articoli-psicoterapia/lattuada-che-cos-e-la-psicologia-transpersonale.html. Moreover, "Recent studies show that the majority of Americans report having had some form of mystical experience (Greeley 1987), while in another research (Davis, Lockwood, and Wright, 1991) 79% of a large sample report having had peak experiences and define them as the most profound and important experiences of their live."
6 From the Greek *holos* ("totality") and *trepein* ("moving towards"), indicating a condition in which consciousness is oriented towards the integration of biographical, perinatal and transpersonal aspects: "tending towards the One."
7 In the field of science and philosophy, for example, in the late 20th century (i.e. in the early years of TPP's life) there were important *developments in the philosophy* of traditional Western science, which challenged the Newtonian-Cartesian paradigm that had been in force until then.
8 Partially taken up again and modified from the cited article of Lattuada.
9 For example, during a psychotic delusional crisis the person might believe he is the new messiah, God himself, due to a biochemical alteration.
10 V. Harner: "The way of the shaman" (Harner 1980). *Michael Harner* was an American anthropologist with good academic credentials, who experienced, in his fieldwork in the Amazon, a powerful shamanic initiation. I paraphrase the text.

11 v. Franz Alexander, 1931, psychoanalyst physician (Budapest 1891–USA 1964), considered one of the founding fathers of psychosomatics and psychoanalytic criminology.
12 Harner, summarizing the imperfections of academic psychology, suggests that the understanding of the psyche in industrial civilization is severely biased, i.e. *ethnocentric and cognicentric*, in the sense that they consider only rationality as valid, ignoring the other dimensions of human experience.
13 This is the alchemical transformation of the ordinary state of consciousness (that of the *sleepers*), due to the awakening of self-consciousness, to finally realize the "clear consciousness" of enlightenment. For many italians, Dante is "Father Dante."
14 Translating "la selva oscura," as "the dark forest" is incorrect; it is difficult for non-Italian readers, but it refers to the symbolic and anagogic meaning, i.e., the obscuration of individual consciousness, a sort of a sleeping condition of consciousness. Also, the direct path is frequently translated as the right path, bur it refers to the central channel of the subtle body, *Sushumna.*
15 The hot and cold hell domains of Buddhists' *wheel of life.*
16 In the earthly paradise there is no more suffering, because there is no more opposition in the ego, there is no more blemish, and one comes to be pure (the word comes from the Greek "piur," meaning fire, and is the root of the verb *to purify*), through immersion in the two rivers flowing from one source. And at this point one is also disposed, oriented, to the ascent of energy towards paradise.
17 Beatrice is the rectified *Kundalini* energy, as we shall see later on, which at first coiled as a descending spiral and then rectified as an ascending spiral carries Dante along the rediscovered direct path, the central channel, up to the seventh heaven and beyond.
18 The purification from these contrary egoic tendencies takes place in the first two canticles, with the renunciation of the egocentric view, and the development of a transpersonal consciousness. Through this purification of the "medium," of the subtle body of consciousness, one will be able to know and experience the higher states of consciousness, that is, pure consciousness.
19 One patient told me: "Doctor, you are not a layman!"
20 This is the essence of PC, as we shall see more clearly in the dedicated chapter, and which we shall only hint at here.
21 Assagioli insists on the psychosynthetic process that the Divine Comedy indicates, in *Principles and Methods of Therapeutic Psychosynthesis* (Astrolabium, 1973, pp. 174–176) and in other texts to Psychosynthesis. The pilgrimage to the Underworld, the ascent along the mountain of Purgatory, the final illumination in the presence of the divinity, indicate *the stages of the exploration of the unconscious until the* "gradual awakening" *of consciousness.* It is therefore a profoundly Christian, and anti-Catholic, non-dualistic vision. As we shall see, Assagioli's approach is in harmony with the message of the Divine Comedy.
22 Roberto Assagioli (Venice, 1888–1974) was the first Italian psychiatrist to take an active interest in psychoanalysis: his graduation thesis, prepared in 1907 in the Burgholzi psychiatric hospital in Zurich (where C.G. Jung operated, with whom he developed a personal friendship) was entitled "Psychoanalysis." Subsequently, he introduced psychoanalysis to Italy; in 1912 he founded, together with others, the journal "Psiche," of which he was the editor-in-chief and animator; the second issue was dedicated entirely to psychoanalysis. As

early as 1914, however, Assagioli began to *move away from Freudian thought*, which he considered too reductive and rigid with respect to the breadth and complexity of the human psyche. Assagioli was an active member of and contributed to a number of transpersonal or spiritual groups, including *Theosophy*. He gave impetus to the *School of Esoteric Studies; he was a freemason*, initiated into the famous "Lucifero" Lodge in Florence (From https://it.wikipedia.org/wiki/Psicosintesi).

23 Assagioli gives much importance to the individual will (*good, strong, skillful*) in favoring, for example, the integration of the *sub-personalities* of which each of us would be composed (i.e., the complex configurations that express inner positions and identifications, ancient or recent) around a unifying center. See Assagioli's book "L'atto di volontà," Astrolabio Ubaldini, 1978. in his view, will is at the center of human personality, as the psychological function most closely adherent to the ego; it is closely linked to the experience of the self and thus regarded as the fundamental element upon which the method of self-realization is hinged. The will derives ultimately from the transpersonal and superconscious experience, which is fundamental to the self-realizing process of psychosynthesis.

24 By Andrea de Marsanich, from www.psicosintesiamo.it/category/psicologia-transpersonale/

25 This shows that Assagioli had an "opening," an awakening to the higher self, where he experienced non-duality, that is, a state in which he, as a distinct person, was no longer there.

26 The model of the structure of the human psyche proposed by Assagioli can be represented, very briefly, with an *ovoid* figure: inside is the personal unconscious in its different components (lower, middle, and upper unconscious), outside the egg is the collective unconscious. Inside the egg is a central core corresponding to the field of consciousness with at its center the ego, which is nothing other than a reflection of the Self.

The Self is depicted on top of the egg, transcending the individual psyche, it is transpersonal. The superconscious is for Assagioli a latent aspect of the human dimension, a potentiality that normally remains unconscious, and thus corresponds to a "higher unconscious." This includes man's higher values and possibilities, but also everything that elevates man above reason (such as *love*, *beauty*, *justice*, *piety*, *creative impulses*, *artistic intuition*, *scientific intuition*, and beyond) to the *divine* within us.

As we shall see later, we can recognize in this opening of the inner path a parallelism with the opening of the path of the central channel of the *Chakras;* here is a somewhat disguised, indirect way of conveying the ancient knowledge of the path.

27 These are in fact inexpressible experiences, which go beyond language and understanding, transcending precisely into the divine, the sacred, the absolute. We are dealing here with experiences of transmutation of consciousness, of *Transhumanation*, Dante would say.

28 *The Red Book* of C. G. Jung Libro Rosso, also known as *Liber Novus* ("New Book" in Latin), is a work of over 400 pages written and illustrated by Carl Gustav Jung approximately between 1913 and 1930, but published posthumously at his explicit request, 50 years after his death, in 2009. The text includes an introduction, references, and notes edited by the historian of psychology Sonu Shamdasani (published in Italy by Bollati Boringhieri in 2010).

29 From www.arpajung.it/wp-content/uploads/2015/07/L.-Aurigemma-Jung-fra-critica-kantiana-and-ontologism-vedantic-relation-held-at-the-conference-Jung-and-theOrient-organised-by-ARPA-and-by-the-Publisher-Bollati-Boringhieri-on-29-May-2004.pdf

30 The Kantian critique intended to demonstrate the *radical illegitimacy of any claim to break through the heavens beyond the limits of the human psychic faculty of knowing, in whose structures and laws the said claim is inexorably constrained.* The "Thing in itself" is and *cannot but remain a* "mystery". And the "Thing in itself", which is the ultimate substance, *is* "pure divine Reality."

31 Sentence taken from the Tibetan book of the great liberation.

32 Jung, leaning on Kant's thesis, will argue, that *psychology assumes that* "spirit can neither establish nor prove anything that exists outside its boundaries..." That is, "'our psychology is a science of pure phenomena devoid of any metaphysical implications'"; our psyche thus "is almost a prison". (in *Psychological Commentary on the Tibetan Book of the Great Liberation*, 1939), "... Beyond the psychic instrument one cannot go, and therefore one must not even try to go: there is no more metaphysics, there is only psychology: and all analytical psychology, with its typology and its doctrine of dreams, and so on, is founded on this Kantian basis."

33 However, in doing so, the boundaries between the psychic and the metaphysical on which Jung wanted to insist no longer have any real reason to exist, in essence, and thus effectively disappear. Again from Aurigemma: Psychological Commentary on the *Bardo Thoedol*, "To the Western spirit ... the psyche appears as something very small, of inferior quality, personal, subjective, and so on ... [But in reality] it is the psyche that pronounces metaphysical assertions by virtue of its innate divine creative force ... It is not only the condition of metaphysical reality, but this reality itself." Jung thus eventually finds himself exposed, often lost, inwardly doubtful .... forced at times to confess, he a famous psychologist, that he no longer knows for certain what the psyche is. "... we neither know nor claim to know what the psyche is."

34 Kenneth Earl Wilber Jr. (Oklahoma City, 31 January 1949) is an essayist and American philosopher. Reprinted in part by V. Salles, on her website page dedicated to K. Wilber.

35 The model was first developed by Clare Graves (Maslow's friend and colleague), and then extended by Don Beck and Christopher Cowan, while Ken Wilber later integrated it into his theory of the development of consciousness within the Integral Approach.

36 In the spiral, the lower stages can also be related to the first *Chakras*, as the higher ones to the upper *Chakras*; they are different maps of stages of consciousness, but in the case of the *Chakras* they refer to the degree of solarization of the *Chakras* as well as their ascending position.

37 Wilber criticises some transpersonal authors for *confusing pre-rational experiences with transrational experiences (pre/trans fallacy)*, emphasizing the need for an orderly progression of consciousness development. Otherwise one risks *spiritual by-pass*, i.e. believing one has reached a higher level when in fact one has not passed through the lower one, and *ego inflation*, due to residual identification with the *ego* during the expansion of consciousness.

38 A term originally introduced by Leibniz and later popularized by Aldous Huxley, this worldview *considers only the One, the unmanifest Spirit, the Absolute, transcendent, which becomes Manifest, immanent, which is indivisible and indestructible, to be real.* The illuminative experience of this

fundamental reality is witnessed by the great sages of all time. "The fulcrum of perennial philosophy consists in the conception that reality consists (is composed) of various levels of existence, levels of being and knowing (the great chain of being) that unfold from matter to body, from body to mind, from mind to soul, from soul to spirit. Each larger dimension transcends and includes the smaller dimensions. So it is a conception of totality within totality, within totality, infinitely. In other words, the great chain of Being of the Perennial Philosophy is actually a 'Great Nest' (a spiral, tangle) of Being. The Great Nest is essentially a 'morphogenetic field' (Sheldrake) or space of general development." See also V. Salles' website page dedicated to Ken Wilber.

39 "For an integral psychology the deepest thrust is to actualise the entire evolutionary field of personality, so that one can become, in full realization, a vehicle of the radiantly shining Spirit in the world" (Ken Wilber).

40 The four quadrants intersect and complement each other. This framework allows for integrating not only developmental levels (evolutionary stages of consciousness) but also lines of development (cognitive, moral, emotional, spiritual), temporary states (ordinary, meditative, mystical), and typologies (personality differences, cognitive styles, and so on).

41 For its dark sides (environmental disasters and the loss of values in ethics and science, the death of God (or the Goddess), the loss of the meaning of life and values, existential terror, the levelling of qualitative distinctions and the substitution of quality for quantity, capitalism, industrialization, and unbridled and vulgar materialism, scientific imperialism, the various forms of world domination, the "disenchantment of the world"). For its positive sides, such as the development of liberal democracies, the ideals of equality, freedom, and justice; the advancement and positive contribution of modern medicine, physics, biology, and chemistry; the end of slavery (at least of a certain kind), feminism, human rights)

42 For example, Grof himself, while acknowledging Wilber's value ("... he is to be regarded as undoubtedly the most prolific living transpersonal theorist"), nonetheless criticized "the absence of the pre- and perinatal stages from the spectrum of consciousness" treated by Wilber, and of having "ignored the psychological importance of biological birth and death." Wilber's writings have "often an aggressive polemical style that also contains vicious ad personam attacks and does not contribute to debate/dialogue. Wilber has no clinical experience and the main sources of his data come from his extensive readings and experiences from his personal spiritual practice."

43 His work was part of an official project to evaluate the effectiveness of LSD in the treatment of various mental disorders. In that context, Grof proposed LSD to *psychotic patients (mainly schizophrenics and severely depressed), other psychiatric patients with severe neuroses, mental health workers (psychiatrists, psychologists, nurses), and healthy volunteers, including students, to increase empathic understanding of altered states.*

The results of those experiments were that there was "promise" as a psychotherapeutic catalyst *in neurotic patients* (it facilitated the recall of childhood traumas, perinatal experiences, and unconscious contents, often more quickly and effectively than classical psychoanalysis). According to Grof, the experiences that emerge during this activation of the unconscious possess therapeutic qualities in that, through the "removal of psychological blocks," they could bring out unconscious contents with a strong emotional charge. This method, later modified, was used in the experimental treatment of *bipolar and psychosomatic forms*. Some patients reported lasting relief from symptoms, with profound restructuring of the personality.

The use on health professionals was considered extremely useful for empathic training, helping therapists to better understand patients' psychotic experiences.

However, *in chronic psychotic patients*, the results were less encouraging: experiences tended to be chaotic, fragmented, and difficult to integrate, and LSD could accentuate dissociation and loss of ego boundaries, already fragile in these subjects; in some cases, acute crises occurred that required containment.

44 *Stanislav Grof's experiments with LSD on the terminally ill in the USA* were conducted mainly at the Maryland Psychiatric Research Center (formerly Spring Grove Clinic) between 1966 and the early 1970s.

The results (published in 1972) were very interesting: Patients who experienced "psychospiritual death/rebirth experiences and cosmic unity" showed a profound reduction in fear of death; many patients reported significant pain relief, "even pain that did not respond to narcotics." The result was that the treatment enabled patients to live the rest of their lives "one day at a time," with greater serenity. See bibliography for studies on LSD in the clinic.

45 For example, Grof reports on a clinical case in which a young patient with depression and anxiety resistant to conventional therapy underwent a session with LSD (100 mcg). "During the experience an intense experience of constriction and suffocation emerges, symbolically associated with the birth process (perinatal matrix II). The experience culminates in a symbolic rebirth with marked and lasting improvement of symptoms. This confirms therapeutic access to deep levels of the unconscious not accessible by verbal techniques" (Clinical case from *LSD: Doorway to the Numinous,* 1975). See also S. Grof's book: *Psychology of the Future. Developments in Modern Consciousness Research*, Inner Space, 2015.

46 Many researchers in the field of transpersonal psychology believe that the growing interest in spirituality and the increased incidence of spontaneous mystical experiences represent an *evolutionary trend toward a new level of human consciousness*. This perspective is only apparently utopian, because in reality nature seems to have provided the necessary means and conducted pilot experiments in this direction. Recognizing the difficulty and fear of being considered crazy when an awakening occurs, Grof and his wife Cristina created an international support network for those experiencing a spiritual awakening crisis in 1980: the "Spiritual Emergence Network" (SEN). From V. Salles.

47 Capriles emphasizes that many Western transpersonal theories (Wilber, Washburn, Grof) *fail to adequately distinguish between truly liberating states of consciousness* (nirvanic) *and seemingly* "superior" *states* (samsaric or neutral). According to him, experiences that appear spiritual or transpersonal may actually be merely altered states that do not lead to true liberation from suffering. In his view, true realization does not follow a fixed structure or hierarchy of stages, but consists of the direct recognition of the nature of the mind, without intermediate stages, as in Dzog Chen Buddhism. (See "Beyond Mind III: Further Steps to a Metatranspersonal Philosophy and Psychology" by Elías Capriles).

Chapter 3

Consciousness and energy

In order to understand psychiatric crises from a different perspective, we need to start from a new foundation—one that allows for a different understanding of the human mind and psychic suffering.

To this end, we shall now look at various sources concerning the *nature of mind and psychic energy*—a great wealth of knowledge passed down through spiritual and philosophical wisdom traditions, especially, though not exclusively, those of the East.

We shall now introduce concepts and models that have been excluded from the predominant scientist model and that belong to ancient wisdom.

This material is generally *well known* at various levels in *philosophical or spiritual* circles, but on the contrary is often *little known by those who deal with mental disorders* (psychiatrists and psychologists), who believe (wrongly in my opinion) that this knowledge is of little relevance to the study of the treatment of psychiatric disorders.

Many of these teachings seem incomprehensible or useless, in reality, simply *because we do not understand them and do not know what to do with them*. But *why do* these messages not speak to us, *why do we not understand them?*

In general, one reason can be found in the *symbolic or metaphorical language* with which this knowledge has often been expressed. A *literal interpretation* of them makes them absurd or outdated; a profound understanding of this knowledge requires that we go beyond the literal, superficial understanding, and requires us to read more deeply, to understand the symbolic aspects, and behind them the concrete operations to which they allude, i.e. the alchemical, or *anagogical* meaning. We must use a different, deeper key of interpretation.

However, to access these teachings at a deeper level, one should *already possess a deeper*, or higher, broader *level of consciousness* to be able to use and understand this different level of interpretation. As in matryoshkas,

DOI: 10.4324/9781003676461-3

the deeper meanings lie hidden inside and beyond the most superficial understanding: to read them, one must go beyond, that is, *beyond our ordinary level of consciousness*, enter into non-ordinary states of consciousness (SNOC). Only then will these texts (such as the Bible, the Indian scriptures, but also texts like the Divine Comedy, or even proverbs) reveal their secrets to us.

This indication is also valid for understanding psychiatric disorders, and NOSC in general. The material remains incomprehensible until we use a symbolic and anagogic key.

To give an example, the understanding of *medieval Western alchemy texts* were incomprehensible and unusable when read in a literal sense, as operational indications of physical substances to be manipulated with physical fire. It was only after *Jung*'s work on this subject in the first half of the last century, understanding the symbolic and operative level in consciousness (allegorical and anagogic or spiritual meaning), that a way was opened for their applicative understanding and possible use in psychotherapy, understood as an alchemy of consciousness.

The same applies to understanding the map of awakening and labor described in the Divine Comedy[1]; to be able to understand the treasure hidden in it, one needs to read it with another level of consciousness, a NOSC, possessed only by those who have experienced it and thus possess the necessary qualification to lead others on the path. Only those who have passed through certain conditions of consciousness recognize and understand them. Thus, these teachings are open to all, yet also secret; and what might be understood on one level might be contradicted by what is affirmed on another level.

But what are the *universal symbols, the archetypes*, that show and explain to us how the world and man are made? His inner world (our mental world, made up of images, feelings, memories), or his outer world outside the body, which appears objective, external, separate, solid, and material? *What are the symbols* recounting us, representing the perceptual *consciousness*, which generates the phenomenal world, *and of the energy* that constitutes and transforms the world?

In Hinduism, the founding symbols of the world, of cosmogenesis, are the male and female principles, Shiva and Shakti. We could equate them with the concepts of consciousness and energy.[2]

Understanding these symbols in depth is fundamental to understanding psychiatry, disorders of consciousness, and all the phenomena that we observe.

For this reason, we will now set out some general concepts that will later serve us to understand the clinical practice.

We will start with how traditions tell us about the birth of the world, the big world (macrocosm) and the small world, man (microcosm), and their rcognized correlation (or perhaps identity).

We will then describe the maps of energy flow in the microcosm, which describe how energy divides and transforms in the psyche, in the inner world of man (microcosm).

3.1 Shiva Shakti. How the world comes into being. The macrocosm[3]

In Hinduism, the two constitutive principles of the manifest world are *Shiva and Shakti*:

- On the one hand *Shiva* the male principle, represents in the world the still, creative consciousness, *the Being*, the *One* in the world.[4]
- On the other hand *Shakti*, the female principle, represents the *Becoming*, i.e. the *Energy*; she represents the *activity* of Shiva, the *manifestation* of all forms of consciousness, i.e. the world, the *duality* of every manifestation of the One, the sacred feminine.[5]

In Tantric traditions, there is no hierarchical distinction or separation between the unmanifest consciousness (Shiva) and the manifested energy (Shakti). *Shakti is the power of Shiva.*

In this tradition, the *great Shakti*, i.e., *MahaShakti*, *the great Goddess*, *the great Mother*, is the energy that creates the world, by taking every manifested form, the macrocosm, and the microcosm, energy that maintains and destroys it.[6]

Shakti, in this context, is the energy that manifests the universe and all its forms, which are the play or dance of *Shakti; Shiva* remains the unchanging, silent background.

Shiva and Shakti are represented in *constant sexual union*, indicating the intimacy, the non-separability of the two principles.[7] Both are essential and always present in every aspect of existence.

Through Shakti, the consciousness, *Shiva* would perform five basic actions in creation:

create, maintain, dissolve, forget, remember.

3.2 Reflections on cosmic and individual consciousness (Shiva)

The problem of consciousness is a complex conundrum of contemporary science and philosophy. Let us first better define the terms.

3.2.1 Pure consciousness

Mystical traditions (e.g., *Advaita Vedanta, Mahayana Buddhism)* and *transpersonal psychology* speak to us of a pure, impersonal consciousness (*pure awareness*), or rather *non-dual* "awareness": it corresponds to "pure perception" without subject-object separation (non-dual).[8]

In these traditions, pure awareness corresponds to the *true Self* (Atman/Brahman), to the unlimited and undifferentiated nature of the individual, the ultimate goal of spiritual awakening. It is that which cannot be defined and pre-exists behind everything. It is a *luminous, conscious, detached, unconditioned, universal and eternal presence*, completely free from the influence of conditions and memories associated with personal identity.[9] Eckhart Tolle calls it "Presence," a state of pure awareness beyond the ego.

Consciousness in the microcosm becomes *individual consciousness by identifying with the body-mind, with the person.* It emerges during childhood development through interaction with the environment and the internalization of cultural patterns, an identification that gives rise to personal identity.[10]

This individual consciousness is characterized by the possibility of developing *self-awareness*, that is, the ability to recognize oneself as an individual distinct from the world, the sense of the individual self in space and time.[11]

For psychoanalysis, self-consciousness emerges from a dialogue between conscious and unconscious processes, mediated by language and the relationship with the Other. Self-consciousness includes personal awareness.[12]

3.2.2 Conditioned consciousness: The Ego

Ordinary human consciousness is often described as a reduced state of consciousness, of a "Sleep" of consciousness.[13] *The Ego is conditioned, tainted, by the principle of separation.*

The cause of the sleep of consciousness seems *inherent in the dual manifestation*: as mentioned above, *there is a function of* cosmic consciousness *in creation*, which is to emanate reality by forgetting itself as creative consciousness: a tendency to *remain in* apparent *separation*, to identify with creation, necessary for the maintenance of creation itself: an illusion of reality, in the reality of Being.

This urge to forget and sleep would operate as a tendency to oppose the return to the One, to remain in the *separation*: it would constitute a *principle of separation.* In the Judaeo-Christian tradition, it is *dia-ballo*, root of the word *devil.*[14]

At the same time, sapiential texts speak of *Awakening* as the *way to salvation*, from suffering; a "way" to Paradise, to return to our true nature, of union (Yoga, Tantra).[15] They explain to us the aspiration latent in the sleeping consciousness in general, and in each of us, for reunion with its higher, realized state, the drive behind the myth of the eternal return. They speak to us of the "*Ultimate Healing Health*" to which we aspire (see Divine Comedy), of the *Resurrection*; Buddhism speaks to us of the "Great Liberation" (from the wheel of reincarnation), of the original state of mind, of *Buddhahood*.[16]

As we can see, the universal, archetypal symbols in every tradition guide us from suffering to peace, from darkness to light, to the promised land.

They therefore speak to us of Sleep and Awakening, of an internal, intrinsic drive of consciousness to awaken to itself, to remember itself.

There would thus exist a *tendency in creation in general and in man in particular not only to remain in illusion, in forgetfulness, but also to return* to pure consciousness: a *reunifying* drive in creation and in man, to return to the One.[17]

Between these two polarities, *forgetting and remembering*, the creature navigates in a *tension* that has perhaps the sole purpose of "waking up."

3.2.3 Consciousness

A more general reflection that concerns us is the fundamental question of *whether consciousness is an emergent product of the brain or possesses an autonomous reality* that manifests itself through the body. There are two perspectives:

- *The first* perspective *holds that consciousness is a product of brain activity*[18]; this view, dominant in modern neuroscience, holds that consciousness *requires* physical support, and sees consciousness as a *biological phenomenon rooted in evolution*, an adaptation useful for interpreting the environment and making complex decisions.
- *The second postulates that consciousness would be a fundamental property of the universe*, not generated by the brain *but existing* "upstream" *of physical reality*.[19]

In support of the first thesis, there is plenty of *neuroscientific evidence*: for example, brain injury, anesthesia, neurodegenerative diseases, and stimulation of specific brain areas modify or nullify consciousness, suggesting a close dependence on neuronal activity. Indeed, modern neuroscience tends to explain mental functions as a result of brain plasticity and synaptic connections. Several *scientific theories* have been proposed to attempt to explain how consciousness emerges from these processes.[20]

Supporting the second thesis *is the difficulty of explaining* from a purely neuroscientific perspective the *subjective experience*, i.e., how physical processes give rise to the inner experience, the "qualia."[21] Qualia are the "bridge between brain and consciousness."[22] The brain processes physical signals, but it is consciousness, through the qualia, that transforms them into subjective experiences with meaning.

Consciousness cannot in fact be reduced simply to neuronal activity: there is a difference between the neural representation of a mental state (e.g., happiness) and the subjective experience of that state. Neuroscience may correlate certain patterns of brain activity with states of consciousness, but it does not explain why and how these patterns produce the subjective experience itself.[23] This philosophical perspective holds that consciousness is a reality distinct from the brain, not reducible to matter.[24]

Since *Descartes*, many philosophers have argued that consciousness (*res cogitans*) is separate from matter (*res extensa*) and possesses its own reality independent of the body. Consciousness according to this view could exist independently of the physical medium, although the brain may serve as the instrument through which it manifests itself in the physical world. NDEs (near-death experiences), and OBEs *(out-of-body* experiences, i.e., perceptual experiences in the absence of detectable brain activity, subjectively confirmed by many) are brought to support this view.[25]

Quantum and spiritualist hypotheses have been proposed.[26] According to the "Quantum Theory of Consciousness," consciousness would be linked to a universal vibratory field that transcends the brain itself, and would be associated with large-scale *entanglement and synchronization* phenomena that could potentially be accessed by systems other than the human brain.

From this perspective, consciousness could be a fundamental property of the universe, *existing* "upstream" *of physical reality*, in line with some Eastern traditions or conceptions of universal consciousness. *Universal/ Cosmic consciousness* postulates a consciousness that is immanent to the whole of reality, not tied to individual organisms. In this view, every entity (atoms, plants, stars) possesses an elementary form of consciousness (panpsychism).[27]

Transpersonal psychology, in contrast to Cartesian-Newtonian models that consider the mind contained in the brain, is based on a unified view of reality. Spiritual traditions describe multiple "bodies of different densities" (vital or etheric, astral, or of knowledge, mental, causa, terms depending on the traditions) and suggest that it is not only the brain that is the device for connecting with the divine, but *the whole body becomes the sensory organ and field of expression of consciousness.*[28]

The main criticism of this view is the *lack of objective empirical* evidence for the existence of consciousness independent of the brain; for neuroscience all observable manifestations of consciousness are linked to brain structures.

3.3 Energy (Shakti)

3.3.1 The map of the microcosm: The subtle body

The terms *macrocosm* and its correlative *microcosm* were used by ancient philosophers (e.g., Plato Pythagoras) to indicate that the external world is like an animate entity analogous to man, and composed, as such, of soul and body. There would exist a relationship linking macrocosm and microcosm, a relationship of analogy.

We will describe *the map of the microcosm, of the subtle body of man,* as conveyed by *Tantra*, in *the map of Astrology*, and finally as represented in the *Divine Comedy.*

These maps all help us to *understand* the structure (anatomy) and the circulation of energy (Physiology) in the subtle body.

This knowledge will be extremely useful and clearer when we examine the relationship between energy and psyche in mental disorders.

3.3.1.1 The map of Tantra and Yoga: Chakras *and* Kundalini

The *concept of Kundalini* has its origins in ancient Indian spiritual traditions, particularly Yoga and Tantra, and denotes that form of divine power that ordinarily lies dormant in the body. This powerful energy or force is described as a *coiled serpent*, representing unexplored potential energy, located at the first *Chakra* at the base of the spine, in the the sacrum region.[29]

Kundalini Shakti, called the "coiled-up," in its quiescent form in the human body is that which maintains life, the "form" of incarnation, and all physical and mental ordinary movements. Once awakened, it can lead to profound spiritual experiences and transformative changes. *Kundalini* awakening is often associated with the activation and harmonization of the *Chakras*. The ultimate goal of *Kundalini* awakening is spiritual evolution, self-realization, and union with the divine.[30]

In *Eastern literature* there are many descriptions of the subtle body, and its structure, described as a set of energy centers (called wheels, or *Chakras*), connected by channels (*Nadis*).[31] They are represented as an ordered whole, organized anatomically and functionally, in *a map, or mandala.*[32]

In the *West*, knowledge of the *Chakras* has existed for several centuries.[33]

However, the diffusion of the doctrine of *the Chakras* in the West came mainly as a result of the translation of an Indian text, the *Ṣat Cakra Nirūpaṇa*, by the British Orientalist *Sir John Woodroffe*[34], alias *Arthur Avalon*, in his *The Serpent Power* (1919).[35]

The Chakra systems find their earliest descriptions in the texts of the *Kaula traditions*, Tantric religious traditions that date back to the 11th century and originated in Kashmir and adjacent regions.

The oldest text in which the system of the six *Chakras* is described, the one most widely used today, is the *Kubjikamata Tantra.*[36] It is named after the term *Kubjika*, which stands for the *Goddess*, described as "humped," or "curved," or "coiled," and which is associated with *Kundalini.* Here is how the text describes it:

> *Between the anus and the virile organ lies the basic center, Muladhara, which is like a matrix, a yoni (female organ). There is the bulb-shaped* "root" *and it is there that the fundamental energy Kuṇḍalinī is wound three and a half times around itself.*
>
> *Like a snake, it encircles the starting point of the three main arteries, holding its tail in its mouth just in front of the opening of the central artery.*[37]

The "arteries" referred to in the text *are the Nadis* (a term that can be translated as "tube," "channel"), in which energy flows. In this map of the subtle body *Sushumna* is the *central axis*, corresponding to the astral spine, running vertically from the coccyx to the crown.[38]

Ida (lunar, left) and *Pingala* (solar, right) are the two *lateral channel,* represented as two *snakes.*[39]

These channels in their spiral ascent *intersect the central axis* at certain points, forming subtle centers called *Chakras,* which in Sanskrit means "wheel," centers, or wheels of life, because of their energetic activity.

Seven *Chakras* are therefore depicted along the vertical axis of the central tree; these represent cardinal stations along the earth–sky pathway, *energy powerhouses, centers of consciousness*, which are the elements of the subtle body in which divine energy is believed to reside latently, sustaining the life of body and soul.

It is in the *Chakras* that the *Karma* of previous lives is stored, or, put another way, it is in the *Chakras* that we find deposited the "*Vrittis*", that is the thought-forms that condition the flow and its obstruction along the channels.[40]

Life energy (*Prana Shakti*, the Shakti in a quiescent state) flows through the channels in the form of *breath*.[41] *Nadis* and *Chakras*, together with the *Prana* (corresponding to "breath" or "life energy") circulating through them, are the main "anatomical" *constituent components* of the "subtle body."

Kundalini awakening manifests in a syndrome called *Kundalini Syndrome*, as we shall see shortly; this expresses as various sensations (e.g., heat, energy, vibrations moving up the spine), with symtoms on the physical level (like unexplained pains, digestive issues, nervous system sensitivities), psychological level (like anxiety, depression, insomnia, depersonalization, derealization), and at the perceptual level (like visual or auditory hallucinations, energy sensations).

It is crucial to differentiate *Kundalini* experiences from *psychiatric disorders*; *in fact, in the KS* a more supportive and holistic approach is often recommended.[42]

3.3.1.2 The map of astrology

Astrology in the modern world is considered little more than a curiosity of the past, an anti-scientific and derisive superstition, a conversational fad.

However, it was once considered a sacred science and with good reason.[43] This ancient science deals with the knowledge of the world and man, his diverse energy and the consciousness that generates and perceives all this, and makes it an organized system at different levels, adapted to the different levels of the men who question it.

It tells us about consciousness and the world, the macrocosm and especially the *microcosm*; it tells us about the *Unus Mundus*,[44] and about time in manifestation.

Astrology presents us with a map better known (but less recognized) in the West than that of yoga concerning the anatomy and physiology of the subtle body.

The horoscope describes the position of the planets in the outer zodiac, the *macrocosm*, but also the inner sky, the *subtle body of man*, the microcosm. Astrology therefore deals with the circulation of energy, of light in the subtle body.

It describes the psychic and outer manifestations of the movement of the planets propelled by the divine energy-breath. *The planets (the* "Sun and the other stars" *in the Divine Comedy)* are *moved by the One*[45] and are also *the way back to the One*: they are personifications of the divine, of the different qualities of energy, divinities themselves,[46] circulating in the *inner zodiac*.[47]

This circulation of energy, which in the tantra map we saw described as traveling along a caduceus (lateral and central channels), is now represented here in the form of circulation along a *circular track*, or two semicircles extending into each other, like an *uroboros,* a single snake eating its own tail, recirculating within itself. The astrological and tantric maps clearly correspond.[48]

The planets (the *Sun and the other stars*) are differentiated, qualified energies, *emanating from the individual Chakras and representing them*: they are "the stars within," they are their *ambassadors*. They move along a path divided into sections (star fields) with different qualities (twelve signs, actually six double stations).

We can trace a clear *correspondence between the Chakras* that follow one another along the central axis in the tantra map, and *the planets* of the solar system, which circulate along the circular track of the *zodiac.* Let us take a closer look at these *correspondences* in the chart in Figure 3.1, in particular:

- *Saturn*, rules both Aquarius and Capricorn, and corresponds to the first *chakra*
- *Jupiter*, rules Sagittarius and Pisces, and corresponds to the second *chakra*
- *Mars*, rules Aries and Scorpio, and corresponds to the third *chakra*
- *Venus*, rules Libra and Taurus, and corresponds to the fourth *chakra*
- *Mercury*, rules Gemini and Virgo, and corresponds to the fifth *chakra,*
- *Moon and Sun*, each ruling one sign (Cancer for the Moon and Leo for the Sun); the two luminaries, givers of light, correspond to the posterior and anterior poles of the sixth *chakra.*[49]

These Chakra planets are symbols of differentiated energies, on the physical[50] *and psychic levels.*

Let us take a closer look: the seventh *Chakra, Sahasrara chakra,* corresponds to the eternal, and in this sense also to empty consciousness where everything happens; the sixth, *Ajna Chakra* is connected to conscious vision. The fifth, *Visuddha chakra,* corresponds to the thinking function; the fourth, *Anahata chakra,* corresponds to the affectivity function, sensitivity. The third, *Manipura chakra,* corresponds to the function of self-affirmative will, action, and the second, *Svadishtana chakra*, corresponds to creativity, expansion, and sensation. The first *Chakra*, *Muladhara chakra*, or root *Chakra* (*Mula*), corresponds to the function of survival (if threatened, to the sense of alarm), to concreteness, to solidity, to where to ground oneself; in short, it corresponds to the base, to inner certainties, to solid points of reference.[51]

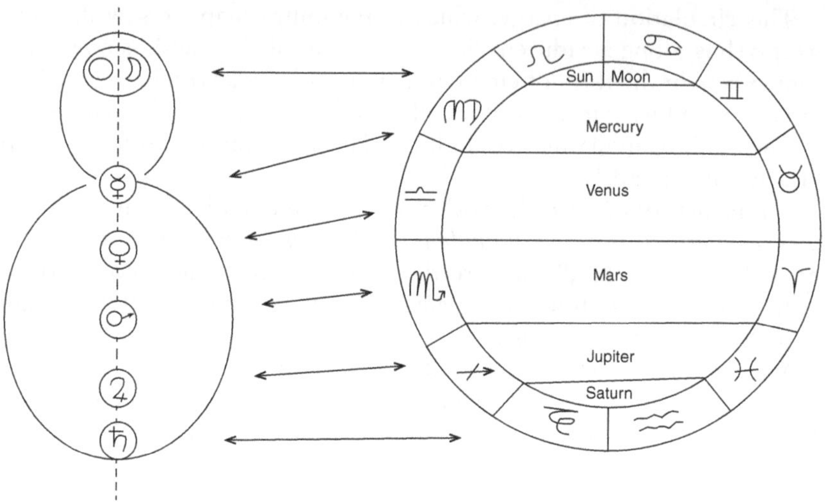

Figure 3.1 Correspondence of *Chakras*, Planets, and Zodiac Signs

3.3.1.3 The map of the Divine Comedy

Dante Alighieri's Divine Comedy can be read as a detailed map of the evolution of human consciousness, guided by an energetic process that mirrors the awakening of the *Kundalini*.[52] In the Commedia, Beatrice represents *Kundalini* energy, the ascending and purifying feminine force that drawls Dante through the three realms.

Dante's journeys through Inferno and Purgatory are described as spiral movements. These represent the process of "unwinding" the *Kundalini* (which was dormant in egoic identification), a *preparatory purification* of the "medium" (Dante's individual consciousness and subtle body).

In *Inferno*, the movement is spirally left-handed, descending (Hell is a downward-pointing cone, hollowed out by Lucifer (the ego), representing the downward pull of gravity, identification with the separate "me").

The path traverses seven circles closer and closer to the attractive lower pole, corresponding to the seven *Chakras*. Dante and Virgil's 180-degree inversion of Lucifer reverses the downward spiral, symbolizing a "baptism" and a "death of the ego."

In *Purgatory*, the movement is still a spiral, but now an ascending one, composed of a vertical vector (the stairs followed by the angels of the beatitudes) and a horizontal one (the seven terraces, where vices and virtues are confronted).

The seven terraces again represent the seven Chakras. This path symbolizes the integration and purification of consciousness through the Kundalini that "pushes up."

In the first and second realms, a rectification of the descending and ascending spiral takes place, to return to the center, to the straight path that was lost.

Rectified Kundalini will then travel in the third realm through all the planetary skies, penetrate at their center all the seven planets-Chakra.[53]

In Paradise, in fact, Kundalini ascends in Sushumna: having completed purification, Beatrice (who represents the Kundalini driving force) moves in Paradise in a direct, rectified, ascending mode. Here ascent is similar to a "lightning bolt" or a "fire" returning to its origin, the ascent through the heavens ending in the "Candid Rose" (the Sahasrara chakra).

Beatrice here is no longer an external guide, but the Kundalini within Dante: his divine love for her transcends all separation, symbolizing the reunion of Shakti and Shiva.

As we see, there is a transparent analogy in the Comedy's structure with the Chakra system: in these energies one is, when asleep, identified and imprisoned (Inferno); from these one gradually gets liberated through abandoning ego attachment (Purgatory). Through these, finally, one gets enlightened and enlivened, transcending all earthly limitations, able to experience and enjoy the specific light-energy of each one of them in the ascent (Paradise).[54]

A crucial aspect emphasized is the *readiness of the disciple*: "When the disciple is ready, the master appears", *as we know*; but, conversely, once the disciple is fully ready and free from separation, the *master* "disappears" because the *Kundalini* energy has become one with the individual and they both go back home. The *Kundalini* knows the way, and governs the process, and the path is much easier for those who are prepared to let go and accept the transformation.

3.3.2 Subtle perception of the Chakras

We have mentioned, for now only on a theoretical level, that these energy centers and the circulation of energy are fundamental to comprehend the TP approach in psychiatry and TPP.

Recognizing and treating these diversified energies requires a knowledge of the nature of the subtle body, which we are now expounding only on a theoretical level, and which we will revisit later on from a clinical and therapeutic point of view; only then will we see how operative they are.

The maps briefly indicated here, from yoga, astrology, and the Divine Comedy, allow us to symbolically identify regions, and specify operative modalities in relation to these, for TP diagnostic or healing purposes.[55]

The individual *Chakras* furthermore provide us with indications of the psychic functions connected to them. For example, examining the fourth *Chakra* in the map will give us indications as to the affective life of the patient. Upon examination of the third chakra, we will have indications on the capacity or inhibition of self-affirmation, or regards expression of anger. We will have an idea on the expansion and openness or blockages in the area of pleasure and sexuality, just by examining the second *Chakra*; in this case, the first *Chakra* will give us indications as to problems related to insecurity, or basic security, and fear.

For Buddhism, man is a *sentient being*; the consciousness within us, the consciousness that we are, perceives the external and internal world. Planetary energies and *Chakras* are clearly perceptible in meditation, as well as in the therapeutic field.

However, we can go a step further, and become able to perceive and identify the energetic conditions in the *Chakra* regions, observing the correlation with the related psychic functions. This can have a diagnostic and therapeutic TP side, as we shall see in the clinical example of TP therapy, for we can recognize and sustain guided energy transformations.

These energies are perceivable by the therapist with one's subtle senses, *directly with* one's "antennae," i.e., one's *Chakra*-planets, once he is aware and trained for that, as we shall see further on.[56] Thus, in a psychotherapy session, this knowledge which now still seems theoretical, will actually prove to be very useful for the diagnosis and therapy of these energies.

3.3.3 Chakras *and karma*

According to universal law, *every action corresponds in the dualistic world to an equal and opposite reaction*: the concept of *karma* is closely linked to the law of cause and effect that characterizes every action in God's world.

Karma, whether individual or collective, corresponds *to the sum of the conditions of consciousness that have accrued in the course of evolution*, in this life or in many previous lives. It represents the action we set in motion and its return, the consequence of it. The *actions, thoughts, and omissions* we set in motion in this life are indeed the cause of consequences, positive and negative, for the future, in this and future lives. In turn, however, they are also the result of actions performed in previous lives or in this life; and so on, in an unceasing chain.[57]

According to *Patanjali*, the memories of the subtle body are deposited in the *Chakras* in the form of small vortices of energy, called *Vritti*. Thus, in the *Chakras* of the astral body we find our history, our memory; there we find crystallized, deposited, our *karma*, our desires, our fears.

These *energy vortexes* are desires (attachment and aversion), ego-attachments, which alter the flow of energy in the *Chakras*: they are energy spirals that are generated as a consequence of *thought-forms* that we still carry with us, that we inherit karmically, and re-produce or produce in this life.

Since *energy follows thought,* every past and still present thought or action generates an energy movement, spiralling, descending or ascending, a *vritti.*[58]

Vrittis thus interfere with the functioning of the subtle centers and channels, with the functioning and flow of energy between the inner earth and sky.[59]

The karma we will encounter in this life is not the entire karma we have accumulated in all our previous lives, but only a portion of it, which we would have chosen to face in this life; moreover, by making the right choices during this life, we can change future karma, either by reducing negative karma or by accumulating positive karma.[60]

Notes

1 The passages of consciousness, the mode of operation of the guide, the transformation of the lead of suffering into the gold of clear consciousness and peace, described in detail, will not be understood by those who read these texts with an ordinary level of consciousness; for them the text will only indicate indirect operations, it will not be medicine.

2 Other traditions, including Christianity, also use similar language (Christ-Mary) to represent the same general issues, consciousness and energy. This has nothing to do with religion in the strict sense, with a specific faith; rather, every religion, every wisdom tradition tells us about this.

3 A little girl to her mother: "Mummy, why are there things?"

4 *Shiva* is one of the main gods in the Hindu tradition, part of the Trimurti together with *Brahma* (the creator) and *Vishnu* (the preserver). He is the destroyer and transformer, but also the symbol of supreme consciousness and spiritual asceticism. Shiva in some texts also represents the God before the creation of the world.

5 In the Christian tradition we have similar symbols, such as *God the father*, the male principle (the Pantocrator, the Christ consciousness), and the *Mother* (divine feminine principle)

6 *Shakti* as the divine feminine principle manifests itself in various forms of Goddesses; for example, in Hinduism as *Parvati*, *Durga*, and *Kali.*

7 Just as fire in essence cannot be separated from its power to burn, so *Shiva* cannot be separated from *Shakti.* One way of representing this intimate constant

connection is the continuous sexual conjunction between the two, depicted in Hindu and Buddhist temples (*Yab-Yum*).

Another iconographic representation of this union is *Ardhanarishvara*, a deity who is *half Shiva and half Shakti*, symbolizing their inseparability.

Jesus or God crowning Mary assumed into heaven is a similar symbol.

8 Shankara: "Brahman is real, the world is illusion, the individual soul is nothing but Brahman." The concept of *sunyata (emptiness)* and the teaching of *non-duality* (e.g., in Zen or Dzogchen) emphasize the absence of separation between observer and observed. Master Longchenpa writes: "*The mind is empty, but everything arises from it.*" Meister Eckhart speaks of the "bottom of the soul" where "God and man are one."

9 A radical non-dualist view denies there is anything outside absolute consciousness, a division between absolute and relative; the world and the Self are forms in which the One appears. From this point of view, the "I" keeps itself separate from the whole through consciousness, knowing, or awareness, which consists in knowing natural reality, which functions perfectly without the need to be known: everything that happens is totally without consciousness or awareness. Consciousness and awareness only emerge in the dream for the dreamer. (Tony Parsons).

10 Self-consciousness would emerge between 5–9 months as a sense of a bodily "I" separate from the world, and would consolidate with the acquisition of language and the internalization of social norms (identification with the body and mind, the person); the child goes through the phase of "I" and "mine," goes through the phase of *wanting to understand*, through the oppositional phase of "no." (V. M. Mead)

11 From a neuroscientific perspective, Damasio distinguishes nuclear consciousness (bodily self) and extended consciousness (autobiographical narrative). Nuclear consciousness, rooted in the body, precedes the development of extended consciousness, linked to the construction of a narrative identity.

12 That is, alertness and attention to internal or external stimuli. It can be primary (immediate perception, e.g., hearing a noise) or secondary/metacognitive (reflective awareness, e.g., "I know I heard a noise" or "I know I don't remember"). Personal awareness, however, goes further, embracing subjectivity, intentionality, and deep self-reflection. For example, an individual may be aware of external stimuli but not necessarily have full consciousness of self or the meaning of one's experiences.

13 A deep sleep, like that of a *sleeping beauty in the* wood. Throughout history, this concept has been expressed many times in different forms. In Christianity as 'original' *sin*, as a fundamental disconnect. In the Bible, it is said that *God put man into a sleep*; and only God can awaken him from sleep, and from dreaming, from the enchantment. We have already mentioned Plato and the Neo-Platonists: *Plotinus*, in the Enneads, often speaks of the condition of the incarnate soul as a state of sleep or spiritual torpor: ordinary man lives "asleep," immersed in the corporeal dimension and unaware of his true divine nature. He writes: "either one is here in consciousness, or one is not here, that is, one is asleep," and describes ordinary life as a state of dreaming or forgetting the true home of the soul. The metaphor of "sleepers" referring to ordinary people is found, even earlier, in Plato and Heraclitus, and is later taken up by Porphyry. Buddhism speaks of illusion, of *impure vision*. Jesus speaks of "people who have eyes and do not see." Dante says that he entered the dark inner forest, (that is, he entered in the state of clouded consciousness)

"so full of sleep was he on that point / that the straight path I abandoned"; but then there is awakening.

14 In Genesis, this is recounted as a consequence of having taken within oneself (that is, of having eaten), the "fruit" of the garden tree, (the tree of division, of the polarity good/evil), that is, separation; hence the birth of suffering, but also of individuation.

15 As we can see, knowledge about how the world is made (the big one, the macrocosm, and the human one, the microcosm), about how consciousness can evolve and overcome suffering, has always been transmitted in all traditions. If we think about it, this is exactly what transpersonal psychiatry is about, the painful difficulty of consciousness waking up and the methods to help it in the birth of the new being.

16 The teaching for realization, the awakening, takes place for example in the Tantric tradition in the form of a loving dialogue, where *Shakti*, the Goddess, sitting on *Shiva*'s lap, *questions* him *and gets answers about the nature of reality*, and about the *method*, i.e. about the way to Awakening, how to "come home."

For example, in the VBT (*Vigyana Bhairava Tantra*, Knowledge of the Tremendous), a very important text in the classical Tantric tradition, 112 methods of meditation are described. The exact dating of the VBT is uncertain, probably between 600 and 1100 CE; Osho claims the oral tradition dates back 5000 years.

According to tradition, the Vigyana Bhairava Tantra has no human author. The text is considered to be of divine origin, attributed directly to Shiva (in the form of Bhairava).

17 "He is that sea to which everything moves," says Dante. "Anima naturaliter religiosa (est)," it was said (a concept already present in the Platonic and Stoic tradition, and later in Tertullian and Scholasticism). This tendency towards reunification is referred to by the term "*symbol*," from *sum ballo*. This is the sense of the many spiritual paths, of the clear consciousness of the Buddha, of Jesus who says he is One with the Father, of Shakti, the Goddess, who wants to be reunited with her beloved Shiva, that is, with the cosmic consciousness that emanated her, the world of forms. This process of transformation of consciousness in its awakening has been the main point of interest of all cultures, philosophies, the history of the world, of economics as well as of art, the way back to the One of every lover, of every knowledge, action: Jung's own process of individuation speaks of this.

18 This view is called monistic, in the sense that consciousness and brain are one. Leading neuroscientific theories (such as the *Integrated Information Theory* (ITT) and the Global Workspace Theory) seek to *explain consciousness as emerging from complex neural networks*, and that consciousness emerges from the complex integration of information and electrochemical processes in the brain. Consciousness is seen by some as an evolutionary adaptation rooted in biology.

19 This is a dualistic view, as far as consciousness as a *reality distinct from the brain is* concerned. Since Descartes, it has been assumed that consciousness (*res cogitans*) is separate from matter (*res extensa*) and has its own reality independent of the body. However, there is no definitive objective empirical evidence for the existence of consciousness independent of the brain.

20 For example, Giulio Tononi's *Integrated Information Theory* (IIT) proposes that consciousness emerges from the integration of information between

neurons. The *Global Workspace Theory* of Bernard Baars and Stanislas Dehaene, on the other hand, suggests that consciousness results from the diffusion of information between different brain areas. Neuroscience explains absolute consciousness as hyper-synchronization of brain networks (DMN, default mode network).

21 This is the so-called "hard *problem*" of consciousness. *The Qualia problem* is at the heart of the challenge to physical explanation. This term (derived from the Latin quale, "quality") refers to the *intrinsic experience of a sensation, emotion or mental state, i.e.,* "what it feels like" *to experience something. Qualia are the qualitative and subjective properties of conscious experiences.* For example, in experiencing a sunset we do not only refer to the stimulation of the neurons of red, but to the subjective experience of that "red," which differs from person to person observing the same sunset. Another example is that the suffering one feels from an injury varies from person to person, given the same nociceptive stimuli. In short, mental phenomena are only knowable in the first person, immediately.

See https://neurosciencenews.com/physics-consciousness-21222/.

22 V. Federico Faggin.

23 Neuroimaging techniques, for example, show *that specific mental states and levels of consciousness are associated with well-defined brain circuits* (particularly in the cerebral cortex and thalamocortical system).

24 With the development of *artificial intelligences* and *robots*, the question arises as to whether they are conscious or not; in fact, they are functional entities with no inner experience, incapable of experiencing joy, pain, or wonder. The neurobiological explanation of consciousness does not seem able to account for this fundamental of being or not being conscious.

25 *NDEs* and *OBEs*, as well as *mystical phenomena*, feed the hypothesis of an autonomous consciousness, or at least one that is not totally dependent on the normal functioning of the brain. Indeed, many people who experience near-death experiences report sensations of detachment from the body, the vision of an intense light and the perception of a spiritual reality, which are interpreted in religious terms as indications of a survival of consciousness after death. In Tibetan Buddhism, NDEs are compared to the intermediate states of the *bardo*, experienced by the soul between one life and the next. Scientific hypotheses explain these phenomena as due to the cerebral hypoxia of the coma state. The "non-individual consciousness" is a metaphysical concept that cannot be falsified.

26 For example, those of Federico Faggin or Penrose and Hameroff.

27 Traditions such as the Indian Advaita Vedanta speak of "Brahman" as pure consciousness that permeates everything, while some quantum theories assume that consciousness is linked to universal quantum phenomena. This view overcomes mind-body dualism by proposing a single substance or field in which consciousness and matter are interconnected aspects.

28 In transpersonal psychology, "consciousness" can refer to ordinary self-perception, while "awareness" indicates the non-conceptual state of presence.

The distinction between individual consciousness (ego-bound) and non-dual awareness (beyond the ego) is central in authors such as Wilber and Grof, but some schools (e.g., Advaita) even deny the existence of a separate "individual."

29 See Gavin Flood, British historian of religions.

30 Some speak of *Shakti Kundalini* referring only to the active, ascending phase.

31 An example is the Kabbalistic *sefirot tree*, or even the Jewish *Menorah*.

32 See also Mircea Eliade, *Yoga. Immortality and Freedom* (1954), BUR, 2010. This text is based on his doctoral thesis in philosophy, based on a four-year stay in India. As a boy, Eliade had written a short story at the age of 14 entitled "How I Discovered the Philosopher's Stone."

33 One of the color plates in Gichtel's *Theosophia Practica* (1696) illustrates the seven secret energy centers of the human body, already known in Indian literature as *Chakras*.

Subsequently, other Western authors wrote about the *Chakras*, albeit from very different experiential and philosophical bases, such as the bishop and clairvoyant C. W. Leadbeater who published a book containing his own studies and observations on the centers of force in the text *The Chakras* (1927). Also Rudolf Steiner, founder of anthroposophy, talks about the development of the *Chakras* in his book *Initiation and Its Results* (1909), as does Tommaso Palamidessi, founder of archaeosophy, who sees them in the light of Judeo-Christian esotericism.

34 The author (1865–1936) moved to India at the age of 25, where he was a judge and from 1915 president of the English high court in Calcutta, as well as a Sanskrit and Tantra scholar; he translated and published some 20 texts on Tantra, as two volumes with this title which spoke of the *Kundalini* and its awakening.

35 "The Power of the Serpent," by Avalon, (pseudonym for Sir Woodroffe,) Ed. Mediterranee, 1983. The book, published posthumously in 1919, was and still is a source of interest for Westerners interested in *Kundalini* yoga; for example, this text was the focus of the seminar held in Zurich in 1932 by Jung, *The Psychology of Kundalini-yoga*. Two texts are translated in the book, one of which, *Sat Chakra Nirupana* or "Description of the Six Chakras," constitutes chapter six of *Śrī Tattva Cintāmani* written by Swami Purnananda in 1526.

This text describes the *Chakras* in the Tantric system and is still the main source of dissemination of these concepts in the West. Examples of these authors include the American academic David Gordon White, the Romanian historian of religions Mircea Eliade, and the French Indologist Jean Varenne.

36 Previous texts mention different numbers of *Chakras* variously and differently located in the subtle body.

37 *Śiva Saṃhitā*, text from the 16th–18th centuries; quoted in Alain Daniélou, Śiva *and Dionysus*, translation by Augusto Menzio, Ubaldini Editore, 1980, p. 131.

38 This in turn would be composed of three layers, for within the central channel we first find *Vajra nadi*, then *Brahma nadi*, and within it again we find *Citrini nadi*, thin as a hair; "this is the path taken by yogis to enlightenment."

39 Symbolically, in all traditions, the three channels ascending are represented as a *tree* placed in the center of Paradise, or the subtle body. It is to this central axis of the human world that the symbols of conjunction in all traditions refer: *the rainbow, the pillar, the celestial ladder*, *the tree of life* in Genesis. In the Divine Comedy this axis is the lost "straight path."

40 Classical tantra flourished in Asia between 500 and 1200 CE, profoundly influencing the continent's spiritual traditions. It preceded yogic literature, which developed later, starting in the 15th century.

In the yogic texts, the *Chakra* system was enriched and complexified, sometimes losing touch with its Tantric roots. For example, *the Chakra system of*

Kubjika Tantra became a standard model only after the 13th century, and influenced later Hatha Yoga *texts.* There are several Tantric traditions with different *Chakra* systems. For example, the *Srividya* tradition has *nine*, while the *Kaulajnananirnaya* describes *eleven*. Each school and master had its own *Chakra* system, making it difficult to define a standard model. The *Chakras* are often represented as lotus flowers with coloured petals, each associated with a deity and specific symbolic energies. These representations symbolize the emanation of the cosmos and the process of reabsorption.

41 For example, *Krishna playing the flute* represents how the divine breath passing through the seven holes manifests the divine music, the world. *Anemos*, from which soul, is an equivalent concept, and indicates precisely this invisible force, the wind, the divine breath in man; see for example in Genesis, when God blew his breath into Adam. The term prana refers to energy in its dormant state, keeping the organism alive, and regulating its physical and emotional movements; there would be five types of pranas.

In the psychological field, *Freud* spoke of libido, making it coincide with sexual energy. *Reich* spoke of it as Orgone. *Jung* spoke of libido in a broader sense, as vital energy, which animates and sustains all psychic life: one of his very first works was an extensive and in-depth reflection on this libido and its symbols and transformations. (*Transformations and Symbols of the Libido* (*Wandlungen und Symbole der Libido*), published between 1911 and 1912); Jung revised the text profoundly in the following years: in 1952 he published a final, revised and expanded version under the title *Symbols of Transformation* (*Symbole der Wandlung*).

42 For example: Mind-Body Practices: Yoga, meditation, and deep breathing exercises can help regulate energy flow and promote relaxation. Psychotherapy: Therapy can address emotional challenges and help individuals integrate their experiences. Medication: in some cases, medication may be necessary to manage severe anxiety or other symptoms.

43 See my book *Astrology and Yoga*, Chiara celeste ed. (2023), where these concepts are set out much more clearly and in greater detail.

44 The concept of *Unus Mundus* (meaning "one world" in Latin) is an alchemical idea that refers to the fundamental unity of reality. Alchemists, along with mystics and philosophers, used this term to describe a condition of existence where all things are interconnected and derive from a single original source. The concept was also adopted by C. G. Jung, who interpreted it as the basis of the collective unconscious, a kind of archetypal field shared by all humanity. From this point of view, the fact that there are celestial bodies in the sky outside corresponding to these stars inside does not come as a surprise, since it responds instead to the concept of a *Uni verse*, of a *single macrocosmic and microcosmic reality*, coincidental, co-essential, contemporary, analogous, univocal, universal.

45 Dante: God is "the Love that moves the Sun and the other stars," as well as "He is that sea to which everything moves."

46 Mythology, like astrology, tells us of the movement and interaction of these qualified energies, these "gods." The gods of Greek mythology are expressions of the one God, (and not a polytheistic antithesis to the one God), the *Elohim* through whom God-consciousness creates manifestation (energy-form).

47 The planets of the outer solar system, and those of the inner solar system are two aspects of the same reality: the distant stars in the celestial constellations, and those of the inner zodiac are the expression, the mobile and different

reality of consciousness, they are the *Great Shakti* and the *Shakti Kundalini* present in the human body, in different degrees of sleep or awakening.

48 The map of yoga and tantra represent our hermetic caduceus, a central axis with the two serpents that wrap around it; they thus describe the heaven–earth circulation in the subtle body of man. In astrology, energy in the form of planets (the stars within) flows along a circumference, the inner zodiac. However, a closer look reveals the correspondence: the *caduceus is none other than the wrapped zodiac*; or if you like, *the zodiac is none other than the caduceus (Shushumna and Ida and Pingala) unfolded.*

49 In the inner zodiac, the signs correspond and are matched to the planets two by two: *each planet-Chakra represents two signs*, one with masculine polarity (odd signs, *Yang*) and the other feminine (even signs, *Yin*) *for a total of twelve. The earth is not counted* in the sequence of planets because it is where we stand, our base of support. In a sense it is what stands still while the rest moves. It is as if we were inside the sphere of the earth, and its inner surface corresponds to the vault of heaven within which the energies we are considering circulate.

50 *Melothesia* is the astrological science that studies the equivalences that exist between the Seven Planets and Signs of the Zodiac with the individual parts of the human body. "The Egyptians set Aries as the origin of the circle of signs, defining each sign by analogy with the parts of the human body." Hyginus – De Astronomia.

Therefore, this science studies the correspondence of the zodiac with the parts of the body and with the endocrine glands, which is useful in *medical astrology* here we see how the seventh *Chakra* corresponds to the *epiphysis*, the sixth (anterior and posterior) to the two lobes *of the pituitary gland*, the fifth to the *thyroid*, the fourth to the *thymus*, the third to the *pancreas*, the second to *the male and female gonads*, and the first to the *adrenals*. For example, an energetic disturbance in the physical region and organ of the heart pertains to the fourth *chakra*, a physical disturbance in the throat to the fifth *chakra*, etc.

51 In this table of correspondences, the relationship between *Chakras* and elements of creation is crucial. Each *Chakra* corresponds to a subtle element, which in turn corresponds to a material element. The first *Chakra* corresponds to the earth element, the second to water, the third to fire, the fourth to air, the fifth to ether, and the sixth to super ether.

52 See my book *The Divine Comedy as a Map to Awakening* in the bibliography.

53 The poem provides operative indications for transmutation in the present, both in Paradise but more generally throughout the work, The Divine Comedy is a veritable encyclopedia of psychological, therapeutic, and spiritual techniques to help the patient in his spiritual rebirth. For example, at the beginning of Paradise Dante indicates the technique of 'breath of fire' *(kapalabhati pranayama)*; again, the technique in which he imitates Beatrice gazing at the Sun as the eagle does, as a way for attuning consciousness to the divine light for *transhumanation*.

54 In the Divine Comedy and in life, *Inferno (Hell)* consists of the conscious re-examination of separation from the Self, that is, of the adversary, the shadow, the force opposed to union with the Self. The happy ending, *Paradise*, on the other hand, consists in the conscious revisiting of higher, harmonious, and progressive states of consciousness, a condition only possible after this travail and the re-alignment and integration at the individual level, i.e. *Purgatory*.

55 People know these centers intuitively, from experience, even if they are not usually aware of them. In everyday language we often refer to specific *Chakras*, without realising, when naming the regions in which they are located and which they govern: the *Chakras* suggest symbols, images, paths that we also find in the language of everyday life. For example, we give the greatest importance to the *seventh Chakra,* as indicated by the symbolism of *the crown, the magician's hat (full of stars...), the Kippah (Jewish papal tiara), the pope's tiara, the areola of the saints.* For the sixth: *casting/having the evil eye, seeing with a good eye, envying (seeing negatively), having a clinical eye, not seeing clearly.* For the fifth: "I have a knot in my throat," "I don't feel up or down," feeling "caught by the neck." For the fourth *Chakra*, of the heart: "my heart is broken," "I have a weight here on my chest," "when I saw you my heart leapt for joy," "speaking from the heart in my hand," speaking "core to core." For the third *Chakra*: "I have my stomach in my mouth," "I have a hole in my stomach"; *rejecting something is expressed as* "rejecting," "vomiting," *e.g.*, "he vomited a lot of insults at me." For the second *Chakra* we should not have many doubts, because of the numerous references to the sexual organs; e.g., "this relationship is castrating..." For the first one: "Out of fear I felt the ground beneath my feet disapperaing..." etc.

56 For example, the perception of an energetic contraction on the patient's fourth *Chakra* will have something to do with an obstacle to letting one's affective energies, and feelings, flow, since the fourth *Chakra* and the heart is the center of the affections; in fact, we do not say "I have a feeling in my elbow," but "in my heart,"

57 The term *Karma* comes from the Sanskrit root *kr*, to do, (hence *Kryia*, meaning "action, accomplishment, ritual, production, activity, work"). *You reap what you sow.* Dante also calls it the *Law of Retribution*, although there are subtle differences in the two concepts. The concept of reincarnation was almost universal in pre-industrial cultures.

It is well known that the concept of karma underlies numerous Eastern spiritual systems, such as Hinduism, Buddhism, Jainism, the Sikh religion, and Tibetan Vajrayana Buddhism. The broad spectrum of other cultures and groups that have shared the belief in past lives is very rich, including the ancient Egyptians, American Indians, Parsis, Polynesian cultures, and the Orphic cult of ancient Greece.

It is not commonly known that similar concepts also existed in Christianity before 553 CE, when they were banned by a special council held in Constantinople under the emperor Justinian, against the teachings of the bishop Origen. (From Gianfranco Bertagni, "In Quiet" website.)

58 When thought is more inspired and directed upwards, to the transcendence of the ego, towards what uplifts and towards love. If, instead, the tendency is to cling to what pulls downwards, a descending energetic flow is generated. This can be so frequent and massive that the entire stream of consciousness could be drawn downwards, magnetized to descend, and this will cause the *Kundalini* energy to descend as well.

59 *Patanjali* was a great sage who summarized the entire science of yoga in an important book, the "Yoga Aphorisms." The text summarizes the Yoga path to self realization. Patanjali's compilation can be traced back to a time between 400 and 200 BCE. The *Vrittis* or *vortices* are found in the *Chakras*.

60 Traditionally, several types of karma are distinguished. We speak of *Sanchita karma* to refer to all the accumulated actions of past lives that have not yet

produced effects. This karma represents our "reservoir" of actions that may manifest in future lives. Then there is *Prarabdha karma*, as in the set of actions ready to bear fruit in this life, which is seen in the horoscope. On this we can act, this is the *KriYamana karma*, (also called *Agami* or *Vartamana Karma*) which refers to the actions we are doing at this time and the consequences that will produce in the future.

Chapter 4

Psychiatry and awakening

4.1 The psychiatric crisis

Let us start with the crisis.

The psychiatric crisis (PC) can be seen as the basic constitutive element of any more complex psychiatric clinical picture. Let us see what characterizes it.

In a book written by an American psychiatrist in the 1970s, Dr Lee Sannella, entitled *The Kundalini Experience*, we find a preface that begins as follows:

> *Tissues torn, blood vessels severed, blood spurting and a flood of bodily humours; the heart gallops and the blood pressure soars. Moaning, crying and screaming. A serious injury? No, just a rather normal human birth.*
>
> *The description sounds pathological because the symptoms are not being considered in relation to the outcome: a new human being.*
>
> *In a dark room there is a man sitting, alone. His body is shaken by muscle spasms: indescribable sensations and sharp pains run through him from his feet to his legs and rise from his back to his neck. His skull feels as if it were about to explode and inside his head he hears strange roaring and high-pitched whistles. His hands burn and his body feels as if it is being torn apart froom the inside. Then suddenly he bursts into laughter and is overcome with bliss.*
>
> *A psychotic episode? No, this is a psychophysiological transformation, a rebirth process as natural as a physical birth. It seems pathological only because the symptoms are not understood in relation to the outcome: a psychically transformed human being.*
>
> *When completed, this process can end with a deep psychological balance, inner strength and emotional maturity. However, its initial stages often present the violence, bewilderment and imbalance that are common to the birth of extra-uterine human life.*[1]

DOI: 10.4324/9781003676461-4

In this passage, it is argued that the birth of the new state of consciousness can be compared by analogy to the physical birth of a child, to childbirth.

The psychiatric crisis, in this view, is seen as a process of transformation, that is, of death-rebirth, of the birth of a new being.

It is said that in that condition it is crucial to understand what the process is.

From this understanding comes an appropriate response: one of obstetric assistance (i.e., organizing around this dramatic but positive and sacred process), rather than an inadequate reaction of alarm—an intervention aimed only at eliminating the problem and reducing the symptoms of distress.

Childbirth can become complicated, and qualified assistance is certainly appropriate and necessary to help, but it is not an illness: it is a natural process of the emergence of new life, a birth that is all the more difficult to sustain the more resistance there is to the newborn's passage into the light. Symptomatic intervention is meant to help birth, not suppress it.

Proper assistance in childbirth involves understanding the nature of the process, and possessing the technical know-how—the understanding of how to help.

This allows for guidance on when and how to act (e.g., when to push and how to breathe), and for containment within an atmosphere that usually leads to a happy ending, rather than tragedy.

If, on the other hand, the woman herself and her carers often do not understand what it is all about, then the subjective reactions of pain, drama, fear, become the focus of attention, the main problem.

In this case, the swelling of the belly could be interpreted as evidence of a pathology (e.g., of a tumor), and the cyclic repetition of the contractions of childbirth as indicators of subsequent relapses into disease (e.g., spastic symptoms of a neurological pathology or something worse), and the spilled blood as a sign of grave danger, which must be stopped.[2]

In psychiatry, unfortunately, we are still usually faced with this second type of situation. In a psychiatric crisis, neither the patients, nor those who intervene (doctors, family members) understand what the nature of the crisis is, its genesis, nor the way it evolves, nor the possible transformative solutions.

Let us elaborate a little on this analogy between Psychiatric Crisis (PC) and childbirth.

4.1.1 The physical birth

When the time comes for birth, labor unfolds naturally. Mild contractions gradually become stronger, more regular, and propulsive, to prepare for and support the expulsion of the fetus.

Interestingly, it is the fetus itself that signals its readiness for birth through chemical signals transmitted to the mother.[3] It is therefore the maturity of the fetus more than that of the mother, that ultimately determines the right moment for the birth of the child.

The "rupture of membranes" ("water breaking"), i.e. the opening of the membranes that kept the intrauterine environment sealed, usually occurs at the beginning of labor in a natural way. Symbolically, this rupture and opening to the outside world corresponds to the beginning of the separation between fetus and mother: an irreversible, immediate, definitive process.[4]

The rupture of membranes thus symbolically corresponds, in this analogy, to a first and total separation from the mother, from the matrix that has generated and nourished it up to that moment. At that point the period of the one-all-ness ends, and the physical differentiation from the mother begins. The end of intrauterine life, that "death," the separation, *corresponds at the same time to* the beginning of *life, to birth.*

At this stage everything is still invisible, included in the womb; the first separation, which determines the end of the previous condition (of quiescence, of pregnancy), is the fundamental factor.

In a physiological birth, the rupture of membranes marks the beginning of the expulsive phase, of *contractions*. The fetus must overcome the resistance that the tissues of the cervix and birth canal and pelvis offer to the expulsive thrust.

Uterine contractions are generally perceived as *painful*. They are unusual activity, extra-ordinary compared to the milder contractions of the quiescent phase.

The pain of childbirth varies greatly from woman to woman: for some the pain is intense and agonizing, while others experience little or almost no pain. The pain depends on several factors.

On the one hand, it depends on the physical conditions of childbirth, *the set*: for example, the size and conformation of the fetus, and of the pelvis, the number of previous births, the presentation of the fetus, the woman's beta-endorphin levels, her individual pain threshold, and even the position in which she gives birth.

On the other hand, other factors intervene, such as psychological and cultural conditions (e.g., fear, certain cultural ideas about childbirth) as well as external conditions, *the setting* (e.g., the support received during labor).

These conditions influence the pain threshold, and affect tolerance to more or less intense pain.

The child makes its way forward, the passage opens, and *thus comes into the light*, bringing the labor of birth and suffering to an end. Suffering ends with the birth of the child, for both mother and fetus; the two are part of the same and only one process.

4.1.2 The psychic birth

Let us now return to *psychiatry*. Dr. Sannella argues that psychiatric crises are characterized by a fundamental *separation from the original identity* (comparable to the fundamental separation from the prenatal mother–child unity).

The identity of those who had not yet passed through an awakening, before coming into the light, was the identity with the mind–body, with the "me". it was a state of consciousness unaware of its true nature, an inner clouding of which one was not even aware; the state of the "sleeper."[5] That identity corresponded to the sleep of consciousness with respect to itself, a kind of '*Sleeping Beauty*' state.

In this condition, the energy related to this state of consciousness is also in a quiescent, sleeping state, traditionally represented by a snake coiled on itself for three and a half coils, while keeping the basic functions of physical and psychic life alive.

In the analogy with the physical birth, which passes from fetus to infant, from darkness to light, the awakening of consciousness to itself corresponds to a psychic birth, the birth of a new being. One goes from "unconscious," to "coming into the light," i.e. to clear consciousness, to awakening: and this involves an *identity crisis.*

From the point of view of the me, this process of awakening, of healing from darkness, appears as *a split,* a schizoid *state*, a dissociation from the old identity.

A death-rebirth, that is, a transformation.

PC would correspond in this analogy *to a transition from a state of inclusion*, to a coming out of the darkness, out of sleep in the womb, to "come into the light", an *awakening.*[6]

This identity crisis is also characterized by an *intense activation of the energy-affective system*, by the activation of the dormant *Kundalini* energy which begins to circulate at a much more sustained regime in the *lateral channels,* and flow, when the system is sufficiently clean, into the central channel, to ascend up to the seventh *Chakra*. This energy is the true driving force that propels the system towards change and death-rebirth, until the process is complete.

The purpose of this activation is to bring about this shift, to bring about the birth of a new being:

the identity crisis triggers this energetic activation, which in turn further drives the process and sustains the awakening in a circular fashion.

As in childbirth, this new identity condition and this strong energetic activation are the cause of intense *psychic suffering*, due to the difficulty the person encounters in the process of awakening.

Supportin PC (seen as a psychic birth) *requires adequate* (calm and competent) *physical, psychic, and spiritual care* by personnel qualified in this regard. This assistance is essential, given the intensity and danger of the process, which can be unbearable, go awry, *complicate*, and result in dramatic and even tragic conditions.

4.2 Clinical features of psychiatric crisis (PC)

As we have seen, PC is characterized by an energetic activation of the *Kundalini* and the concomitant identity crisis due to Awakening.

The intensity of the crisis will depend on the intensity of the energetic movements in that specific system (i.e. how much *Kundalini* has been activated and is ascending), which gives rise to an *energetic syndrome*; also, it will depend on, how strong and sudden the dislocation from the old to the new identity will be; this will give rise to an identity crisis syndrome, which we will now examine.

However, in addition to the aforementioned specific Awakening-related symptoms, there is always a third *"reactive syndrome"*, interfering with the ongoing process, triggered by the ego in crisis.

The destabilizing thrust of awakening in fact clashes with the difficulty on the part of the ego to accommodate the process, and reacts with alarm and the tendency to maintain the old homeostatic equilibrium, to oppose the process with escape defense mechanisms, or control. This egoic resistance and interference is a source of additional suffering, and is of great importance for prognosis, i.e. in determining the favorable or tragic outcome of the process.[7] Let us take a closer look at these *three clusters of symptoms.*

4.2.1 *Identity crisis*

On the level of individual consciousness, Awakening involves *a fundamental and irreversible shift of consciousness from the me to the Self, an identity crisis.*

It is a separation, a *disconnection*, of what was previously united, identified, unconsciously taken for stable, a losing of the ground on which one's feet previously stood.

Psychiatry speaks of a *shizoid* condition, as if it were negative to go to pieces, to split into parts, or rather as a part from the whole; however, one could see this process not only as a death of the old regime, but also as a reconnection to a new, original, total condition, i.e. as a rebirth. Perceived death corresponds to the end of the illusion of separation, of identity with the separated part, the "me." No one dies, only the someone dies.[8] With this move we dissociate from the dissociative state normally present in us, that is, from the identification with the person, with the body–mind.

It is therefore a dissociation that marks to the beginning of *healing* andoning the illusion of being a separate someone or something, (and thus experiencing things from that point of view). This major, central crisis of identity, this disconnection, is *ego-dystonic*, unwelcome to the "me," and is experienced as a pathology. For the "old regime" it is overall a "calamity", (as *U. G. Krishnamurti* calls it, who describes it in detail), or as an overwhelming flood of energy (as *Gopi Krishna* puts it).

C.G. Jung also described in his own way in his *liber novus* (The Red Book) his *dark night of the soul*, which is difficult to bear.

This process is *irreversible, irrevocable, unacceptable, unbearable.*

The psychological consequences of the awakening are a *first cluster of disturbances,* relating to this loss of the sense of the old identity of the individual ego, which will later be "re-inhabited" by the awakened consciousness.

The identity crisis is thus characterized by the *disappearance of the familiar world, and of certainties about self and reality:*

Thus, the subject will feel that he is no longer in the right place, he will feel and believe that the world collapses on him, that everything collapses, and he too will feel lost, destroyed, in crisis.

The specific symptoms of this phase include *depersonalization, derealization, demotivation, disorientation, a sense of emptiness, of being lost, no longer finding oneself as an identity...* etc. *Confusion, difficulty in thinking, remembering, participating and belonging* are also often present. *A profound upheaval.*[9]

In psychiatry, this first type of alteration manifests itself in every disturbance of consciousness, it is "the" disturbing factor of the previous calm, it is the basis of the disturbance of constituted balances, of personal development.

Mainstream psychiatry deals mainly with this crisis (of derealization, depersonalization, confusional psychosis, schizophrenia), trying to counteract it, to reconstitute the old identity.

From the point of view of TP psychiatry, on the other hand, this loss of the old equilibrium is the starting condition, *the beginning of the troubled journey of the healing of the Self.*

The crisis condition we are describing manifests not only as a *collapse of certainties, of meanings, of the motivation linked to identity,* but also as a *nullification of the tasks* and *social role* connected to the old identity. The crisis leaves one without direction or strength, *as if there were no longer any meaning, motivation, orientation and goal, connection.*

In the PC there is no longer anything or anyone: the prevailing experience is one of lack, absence, loss of that person with whom we identified ourselves, and through whom we were previously recognized; it is an experience of deprivation, of collapse, of catastrophe and post-catastrophe, of *desert*.[10]

4.2.2 Energetic symptoms

Concurrently with the awakening, a *second cluster of symptoms* almost always occurs, *related to the energetic change in the system.*

PC involves in fact a concomitant necessary libidinal energetic disinvestment from the old regime of the individual ego (from the ego complex, from defenses, from relations) passing through an intermediate phase of free energy, which precedes its re-investment in a new equilibrium.[11]

We witness the *awakening* of *the Kundalini, its activation and ascent (in varying degrees) in the central channel, along the axis of the Chakras*; this entails a consequent purification and transformation of energy and consciousness at the level of the individual *Chakras*, and of the more general energy circulation, and the emergence of thought forms, emotions, and sensations due to their activation.

The energetic syndrome manifest themselves on a local and general level as a result of this *energy overflow or imbalance at the level of* the *Chakras* and organs and apparatuses or functions connected to them, or as *alterations in the quantity and quality and direction of the* energy *flow* in the subtle system.

We will distinguish different types of energetic alteration shortly, but for now it is enough to note that such energetic symptoms are always present in conjunction with identity crisis.

This process can be highly destabilizing, difficult to bear. This is especially true when there is a more complete ascent into the central channel, which can be fulminating, a true revolution: on the one hand, in fact, we will have a flow of energy that is too strong, and on the other, the perception that this force is something utterly unfamiliar, never previously experienced, almost alien, since the subject does not recognize it as his or her own.

Consequently, these phenomena are usually perceived as worrying, as an imminent death (a psychological death), and are almost always accompanied by intense fear.

4.2.3 Egoic reactions

A *third cluster of* symptoms does not arise from the process itself, from the identity crisis or the energy drive, *but rather from the differentiated resistance to these two processes*, and is due to the still persistent egoic identification.

The crucial issue lies here in the *evolutionary level of the ego*, or rather the degree of purification of the subtle body at all levels, in all *Chakras*.

Awakening will in fact manifest in people with different levels of consciousness: some with an evolved level of consciousness, capable of not to oppose change too strongly and to allow their individual consciousness to expand; others, instead, remain anchored in a strong and rigid residual egoic identification, unwilling to accept the transormative process.

It is precisely this third set of reactive symptoms that usually drives those going through these crises to consult psychologists and psychiatrists. This *residual* ego (or rather this *residual identification of the ego with the principle of separation*) is in fact the one who protests, is alarmed, does not admit, does not recognize, does not collaborate with the process itself, opposing transformation through two fundamental strategies: *flight and control.*

It is the ego that suffers, and it is also the ego that makes one suffer.

In cases where the loss of identity is only partial, or rather to the extent that the old identity partially remains active during the process (which is almost always the case), over time a *defensive organization of the remaining part of the identity* develops, giving rise to different syndromes in terms of characteristics, prognosis, and treatment; for example, panic disorder and obsessive compulsive disorder.

This position of contrariety, of interference, can be maintained over time,[12] and is the main reason for the *chronicization* of psychiatric conditions.[13]

4.2.4 The desert

As we have seen, the ego's reaction during a crisis is usually to reject the process. In the initial stages, and sometimes afterwards, much more weight is given to what is being lost than to what is being presented and achieved, and one reacts by considering the process as negative, *ego-dystonic*.

As the crisis progresses, it brings with it a state of *emptiness, both outwardly and inwardly:* a power vacuum, a desert. In this desert *the real trial* begins; that psychological death, that *desert of life* must necessarily be endured, traversed in order to reach the possible subsequent blossoming of the Self. This trial is what makes this phase so fruitful in penetrating deeply into the transforming consciousness.

It has been called *the dark night of the soul.*[14] It is as if one were without guidance, *blind*; but it is precisely at this stage that one begins to see with other eyes, from within. Precisely because *what is essential is not visible to the eyes*, it is necessary to pass through a phase of obscurity and loss, a *no-man's-land.*[15]

4.2.4.1 The dark night of the soul

The "dark night of the soul" is a process of profound spiritual transformation, characterized by a sense of inner darkness and loss of reference points, in which faith operates in uncertainty and in the absence of knowledge of the final goal. The entire journey, often painful and devoid of certainty, leads to deeper knowledge and love, where mystical wisdom is always accompanied by the love that infuses it.

Indeed, with the loss of perception of any kind, in the absence even of self-perception (one feels lost, as if vanished), spontaneous attention is much closer to *returning to the original observer, home, in the Self.*[16]

4.2.4.2 "Residual states"

The desert condition may continue over time. A part of the desert remains barren even when the desert begins to bloom.

Once the surprise and bewilderment of the new condition has been reduced or exhausted, what emerges is a *residual state*, which does not vanish: an awareness of not being what one was before, of not regaining motivation, feelings, identity similar to those preceding the PC, usually persists even after the acute phase of the process, and remains as long as some egoic identification endures.

In the post-acute phase the residual ego reaction then presents itself with other symptoms (more *defective* than productive, as it is called in psychiatry), such as *demoralization, despair, social withdrawal, anhedonia,* emotional blunting (that is, the feeling of no longer experiencing emotions as before, or of no longer having any feelings at all).

This state is often ego_dystonic. This condition generally evolves over time into an integration into the new condition, but sometimes it does not recede altogether; one grows accustomed to it.

That sense of "missing what once was" turns into an acceptance of the change, a quieter and more resigned painful awareness, a "being without."

In psychiatry, the residual state is viewed only in a negative light, and never as the stabilization of the new state of consciousness in the presence of the persistent egoic rejection, though weakened and powerless.[17]

Thus, for example, demotivation, confusion, memory and attention deficits, social withdrawal, are not interpreted in connection with the identity crisis; likewise, irritability, anxiety, low energy which result from the energetic reorganisation of the evolving system.

However, it is undeniable that syndromes that evolve "badly," in a defective sense, can actually produce over time a significant reduction in the quality of life, difficulties in social and occupational adaptation, increased vulnerability to relapse, and the need for ongoing treatment and support.

4.2.5 Summarizing

The clinical severity of PC will therefore depend on this combination of factors, to which we must add the effects of therapy.

- It will depend first of all *on the intensity of the awakening,* whether it is more or less prolonged and definitive.
- *It will also depend on the intensity of the activation of the Kundalini, which may be more or less activated and circulating in the lateral* channels, more or less ascending in the central one (ascension which may in turn be more or less complete and definitive).
- *It will also depend on the egoic resistance,* almost never absent, especially after the acute phase; the intensity of the reaction in turn depends on the degree of illusion of being separate, on the degree of sleep still persisting and dominant in that individual consciousness. This may lead to conditions of greater or lesser splitting of the reactive nucleus from the central ego, favoring dissociative syndromes.
- Finally, the severity of the crisis will depend on the specific characteristics of the individual consciousness,[18] and on the pharmacological and psychotherapeutic therapy, in short, on the specific help put in place to accompany the ongoing process.

The *PC* (the identity crisis, the energetic manifestations accompanying it, and the egoic resistance reactions), taken together, are *the way in which the transformation takes place, the way.*

Almost always the first two sets of symptoms mentioned, identity and energy, are co-present, but in varying proportions; they compete for the same purpose, without really being able to say which is the cause of the other.

The energetic component (KS) as we shall see shortly can sometimes constitute, almost on its own, the initial presentation of a PC. Usually, however, it is *associated* and concomitant with the identity crisis and the defensive reactions of the ego in crisis, manifesting an accessory and not predominant symptomatology.

The reactive component, by contrast, is almost never absent; it accounts for the subjective evaluation of the crisis as negative, as evil, as mental illness (i.e. *in* and *of* the mind). Seen in this light, the suffering that psychiatric patients present prompts reflection, allowing one to *reconsider psychic distress in a different light,* as a conflictual expansion of consciousness.

4.2.6 Suffering and healing

Awakening entails the dissociation from the identification that characterizes the ordinary psychological functioning. On the one side there is a "finding oneself" on the side of the "Self," and a "losing oneself" on the side of the "me,".

However, if things were that simple, awakening would always be a fairy tale with a happy ending, a Divine Comedy populated only by the blessed; instead, sometimes those who go through these experiences live a life of Hell, sometimes they suffer as in Purgatory, and only a few fly in joy to Paradise.

Most often, in fact, patients experience all three of these states, albeit at different times and in different proportions, *and this makes all the difference.*

Sometimes the patient is at the same time in Hell and in Paradise and in Purgatory; sometimes they have hellish phases, and sink, then paradisiacal phases, and fly towards the Sun; sometimes, like Icarus, they burn their wings and precipitate, or transcend.

In the process of awakening and its integration, things very often become complicated.

This depends on many factors: sometimes the impetus for awakening is hesitant, sometimes excessive; sometimes resistance is enormous and long-lasting, sometimes less drastic and only temporary. And then it depends on the imponderable; and on Grace.

In any case, suffering characterizes the awakening in most cases; and part of this suffering is inevitable, as in labor; another part, often the main one, depends on resistance.

It is a general law: *Suffering equals resistance.*[19]

In order to speak of mental suffering and its resolution, we will take the map of the Divine Comedy as a trace, since it is exhaustive and clear.

I refer to the famous tripartition of the spiritual realms in Dante Alighieri's *Divine Comedy*, already mentioned, an unsurpassed fresco of *human conditions and of the path to overcome suffering.*[20]

Suffering during awakening always depends on being still under the limiting, separating influence of *Lucifer*, the force that pulls one down, towards the center of one's (inner) earth.

Those who abandon this identificazion, they get rid of suffering; so they can pass through the first two earthly realms, and experience a condition of Paradise on earth (Earthly Paradise) or fly free into the heavens of life (Heavenly Paradise). Some even go beyond all limits, and attain "the *Ultimate Salvation,*" the "*Great Liberation*" of the Buddhists.

Dante explains in detail how one can help this process of liberation from suffering, how one can accompany (through transpersonal psychotherapy) these suffering souls, depending on where we meet them on their inner journey.

4.2.6.1 Hell

In this world, many "suffer the torments of Hell"; and thus impose this darkness on others. They are those who have lost "the light of reason". All those who do not recognize the identificaton with the principle of separation as the cause of their suffering, or choose it, are under its influence.

Some of our patients suffer in this way, without hope of ever coming out of their inner hell, without knowing or without the will to come out; some patients with OCD, paranoid, split and disconnected, are poor devils who nevertheless despite suffering do not choose the light.

*Suffering here depends on being caught, imprisoned, captive (*in italian "cattivi," has the same root, meaning *bad,* i.e. separated from the good) in that hell, in that lower level of light, of love, of common sense, of union with the divine. Hell corresponds to the condition of a consciousness that experiences separation, dissociation from God, from the One. *One is a prisoner of that darkening* force, the dark side of God: a power split from love.

This separating, divisive, diabolical force (from *dia ballein,* to separate), in the *Divine Comedy* is depicted by *Lucifer*, which literally means "the bringer of light."

In the Commedia, *however, it is said that one can get out of Hell*, that the door is open; but *two conditions* are required to get out.

The first condition is *discrimination* (distinguishing good from evil), which comes from *Awakening*. From the very first lines in the Comedy it is said that it is this that brings one out of the dark forest, in which one had been sleeping for a long time.[21]

Awakening thus is the essential condition that enables us to see and recognize that we are not what we thought we were, that we are light and consciousness.

Jesus says "It is the truth that will make you free."[22]

The second condition is *the choice, the intention.*[23] This too is made clear from the beginning, in the second canto of Hell. Dante must make a choice: to save himself not for egoic reasons, but for the love of heaven. He does not choose for himself, egocentrically, but for love, of Beatrice specifically.

It is therefore a matter of choosing to renounce Satan and all his temptations.[24]

Hell and the devil, however, have an important function; walking between good and evil, man can wake up and choose.[25] *If one overcomes Lucifer, one obtains light.*

To get out of Hell, it is necessary to take responsibility for one's own liberation, to choose not to persevere in evil.[26]

4.2.6.2 Purgatory

Suffering is present in Purgatory, with a different modality (corrective and not retributive punishment), with hope of what lies ahead.

Suffering here wanes as one moves away from Lucifer by active distancing, ascending the *Chakras* of the holy mountain.

Once the direction of *Kundalini* has been reversed with right intention, then a gradual purification takes place in every single terrace, in every single *Chakra*, through discernment: all residual identification with that specific *vice,* which is to be abandoned, will be rectified with the corresponding corrective *virtue*.

One thus reaches the end of suffering, to Paradise on Earth, to Eartly Paradise.

In psychotherapy, when the patient chooses to heal and is committed in this direction, the path always proceeds towards the best, within the limits of what it is given to the therapeutic couple to do, in order to support the process of death and rebirth, of transformation.[27]

4.2.6.3 Paradise

Here there is no more suffering, because consciousness is completely disidentified from the principle of separation, of opposition; it is totally aligned, transparent to the will of the Self, there are no more "two" who struggle: "in His will is our peace," say the blessed in Paradise; "and what He wills, we will." So we will not talk about that here.

Sometimes one accompanies patients who fly free and blissful.

I am not referring here to those patients in the manic phase, where the ego is still quite present, and is flying because it is inflamed by the energetic overflow, and attached to this euphoric state, only to be equally unhappy when it then recedes.

Nor am I referring specifically to those ecstatic states induced by the traditional techniques of the sacred, such as meditation, dance, enteogenous medicine, which (when used in people who seek to align their lives with the spirit) often do not involve conditions of suffering, but only of temporary experimentation of these ecstatic states, which can therefore also be a guide, a comfort, a support on the path.

I am speaking here above all of those ecstatic states (*ex stasis*, meaning outside of oneself), which sometimes occur *spontaneously* after awakening but in a phase in which the ego didn't yet vanish completely, but nevertheless does disappear for a while, and everything goes as it should.

In short, sometimes patients suffer the torments of hell, sometimes they transmute in the fire while accepting it, but sometimes fly into the light of the shining fire.

In all these situations, we are dealing with non-ordinary states of consciousness, more or less obstructed; *Kundalini* has awakened, the identity crisis is ongoing and irreversible: the individual's preparation and reactions make the difference.

4.3 Factors favoring PC

Let us now examine the triggers of PC.

The crisis often arises spontaneously, on the basis of a predisposition, which will be genetic for biologically oriented medicine, subtle for TP psychiatry.

It is assumed in these cases that there is a predisposition in the physical or subtle constitution, to which the most diverse factors could contribute: intrauterine psychic experiences, reactions learned in childhood, family genetics, and even memories of previous lives, who knows.

From this point of view, PC would not develop as a result of identifiable causal or con-causal situations: in other words, no relevant childhood causes, traumas, can be traced to explain the present crisis; not even important present-day triggers can be identified.

The crisis, in these cases, would therefore be unexplained, idiopathic, *endogenous*.

One might ask in such cases then why the PC is triggered at a particular moment. Perhaps crises follow an inner clock, a moment in life that can be identified in the person's horoscope, for example, a "right time" (*kairos*) that matures at a certain moment.

Other times, however, *external triggers or determinants*, or at least *concomitant causes, can* be identified, such as:

- *The use or abuse of psychoactive substances*, especially if used regularly, such as cannabis, cocaine, synthetic hallucinogens like LSD, or DMT, or, less often, the use of hallucinogenic mushrooms, Ayawasca and others.
- *A psychological bereavement*, such as the death of a loved one, a parent or child, a friend, i.e. a psychological encounter with death.

- *Other times it is a close encounter with death on a physical level*, such as a car accident, with coma, the discovery of an incurable or otherwise potentially fatal disease, or any situation in which we came close to death such as a driving or plane crash, etc.
- *Having gone through specific traumas in the past* (including sexual abuse, which activates the *Kundalini* at a still immature age),[28] *or recently*.
- *Crises that have matured over a long period of time due to meditation practices*, in which one tries to force the energy system in an inappropriate way (this could happen, but more rarely, even in the case of more balanced meditation practices).[29]

  Other factors may favor this activation, such as *sleep deprivation, fasting, isolation*, and others.[30]
- *However, the main factor most often remains mysterious, and perhaps we could call it "Grace".*

We could summarize what has been said by saying that the activation of energy is observed in conjunction with all situations in which one encounters death, when one sees death in the face, up close; most often, as in psychiatry, it is a *psychological death*.

In the history of a psychiatric case it is very common to find that the first PC followed an encounter with death at some level.

Every time the ephemeral security of our continuity, of our identity, is seriously questioned; every time we find ourselves in a vacuum, there is an identity crisis.[31]

And then what happens is what happens when you close your eyes: *you, as a person, are no longer there.*

4.4 The *Kundalini* syndrome[32]

When in a PC the energetic component is acute and prevalent over the other two sets of symptoms, we speak of *Kundalini Syndrome* (henceforth KS).

It is *characterized* by a *series of characteristic signs and symptoms*, which depend on the *awakening and activation in varying degrees of the Kundalini from its dormant state*. They reflect the intensification of circulatory activity, an hyper afflux at first in the lateral channels, and then its ascension in a more or less complete form in the central channel, stimulating each Chakra.

This circulation and ascent encounters in its evolution blockages and difficulties in the subtle system, which resist the flow and lead to various *reactive and ego dystonic symptoms*. From the point of view of the old "*me*," these symptoms are often very disturbing and unusual, and therefore feared and controlled. These tend to emerge and organize themselves into structured defensive forms as time goes by.

The activation and rising of *Kundalini* is the cause of the *symptomatology*, which we will see later in detail, and is characterised by symptoms at various levels: strange postures, sounds, powerful waves of emotions, anxiety, anger, sadness, joy, fear of imminent death, fear of madness, paradoxical manifestations such as weeping and laughter, a sense of ecstatic rapture, visions, a sense of connection with the whole, a state of expanded consciousness. Memories and reactivation of psychological and physical traumas, perinatal sequences, archetypal experiences in the form of physical and emotional manifestations may emerge.[33]

Symptoms manifest at the level of the subtle body, and change over time. It is not at all uncommon to see a PC open up with a KS, which over time changes in intensity, receding into the background; the energetic syndrome also tend to become more and more inextricably mixed with the other two syndromes, identity and reactive, while at the same time there is an underlying rearrangement of the individual personality.

Identifying its presence and course in PC is essential in TP psychiatry.

KS usually *activates* between the ages of 18 and 25. The process may be temporary, incomplete or complete, and its duration varies greatly, with the most intense manifestations in the early stages. The energetic activation presents itself as a dynamic process that can manifest itself in various ways, from gradual to explosive, generally not as a single, static event

The syndrome has a *cyclical course*, both in the sense that it gradually rises and falls, but also that it tends to recur over time. The energy cycle can last for months or years, with *phases of activity and quiescence*, with intervals that can also extend over many years. Its activation or reactivation is often linked with the seasonal cycle (spring and autumn), but may also depend on concomitant triggering factors.

Triggers include intense spiritual practices (meditation, tantric yoga), deep emotional events (love, grief, trauma), near-death experiences, the use of psycho-active substances, childbirth, or encounters in high-energy places. As with PC in general, an indefinable factor, "grace," is also considered an integral part of the process.

There is a tendency to go through a phase of *repetition* and *deepening* around mid-life, at about 35 years of age. Further phases of activation or reactivation of this cycle are also observed in the period of menopause and retirement, post-partum or post-abortion. *Kundalini* activity is preferably present during moments of relaxation and sleep, when egoic control is lowered.

The KS is ubiquitous: all cultures of all times have spoken of the activation of the *Kundalini* as a fundamental phenomenon in transformation.

The awakening of the *Kundalini* has always been the path to the transformation of consciousness. When the *Kundalini* awakens, the journey has irreversibly begun.

In the past, this awakening was described as a relatively rare occurrence; nowadays, however, it seems to be much more frequent, especially in the Western world.[34]

However, it is often misunderstood, and especially in the West it is almost invariably interpreted as pathological.[35]

4.5 Phases of *Kundalini* activation and ascent[36]

In its dormant state, the *Kundalini* (*Prana Kundalini*, in this form) is not a dull, absent energy, but rather *the life force that keeps the body system alive and evolving*. It is responsible for physical as well as psychic functions (emotional movements, thought, sensations, sexual energy, excretory functions, etc.).

The activation and rising of the *Kundalini* is a vast and complex process.

It is difficult to study the process and come to a conclusion, due to the difficulty of comparing the different stages of the cycle, some of which occur simultaneously; moreover, there are inter-individual differences that complicate the picture.

The symptoms as we shall see can be many and varied, and often surprising to those who experience them without adequate preparation.

They range from imperceptible sensations to rapid and powerful movements.

Kundalini activation can be gradual or sudden, and its intensity and effect vary depending on the individual's development, constitution and temperament.

For Greenwell, *the stages* that appear along the way in this understanding of self *are never predictable or linear*, and the journey is *never what one expects*.[37]

4.5.1 Kundalini awakening can manifest in very different ways

The ascent of Kundalini can proceed in very different ways: it might *rise partially and then "withdraw"*, once or several times. In some it might rise in a *specific area*, in a certain *Chakra*, where it might stop and seem to be stuck for months, or it might even go all the way up to the last *Chakra*, in a few days or years, or it may even be propelled suddenly and explosively *throughout* the whole body. The process of ascent may be *temporary and incomplete, or complete*, and will depend not only on the process itself, but also on the state prior to the beginning of the crisis, the balance, and the evolutionary level of the person, and the person's lifestyle, history, and practice.[38]

a. Awakening can manifest *Positive Experiences*: *pleasant physical sensations* (energy flows, vibrations), *positive emotional experiences* (joy, peace, love, gratitude, ecstasy, unexplained bliss), and *altered states of consciousness* (expanded consciousness, visions, sense of connection with the whole). Bonnie Greenwell, for example, describes her awakening as an entirely positive phenomenon, with intense joy and bliss.

   It can also involve the development of *psychic abilities* such as clairvoyance, aura perception, precognition and mind-reading, or even unexplained healings.
b. Awakening can manifest *Negative Experiences and Psychiatric Challenges:* The *Kundalini* can manifest with *dramatic and destabilizing symptoms,* which are often misunderstood and interpreted solely as pathological in psychiatry.

   Disturbing Physical Sensations: Intense cold-warmth, tingling, pains that appear and disappear, uncontrollable shaking, and feelings of "electric shocks".

   Negative Emotional States: Fear, anxiety, anger, sadness, depression (often described as part of the purification process), and a deep sense of loneliness. Fear of dying or going mad is common.

   Mental and Behavioral Alterations: Accelerated or inhibited thinking, mental confusion, disorientation, memory and concentration difficulties, depersonalization and derealization. Paradoxical behavior may occur, such as involuntary crying and laughing.

In the case of an excessively powerful or sudden rising of Kundalini, one can be swept away, overwhelmed and traumatized; this is what happens to many psychiatric patients, unprepared to manage this condition[39].

Mythology and religion speak of people who are 'struck by lightning', for example by Jupiter's thunderbolt, which kills, knocks to the ground and can bring about an instantaneous conversion, a spiritual conversion. This was the case with St. Paul, who was struck by God on the road to Damascus.

4.5.2 Initial phase

The awakening of the *Kundalini* usually begins with a very intense movement of energy along the spine, or from the feet upwards, sometimes ascending up to the head; however, this flow often stops in the heart or throat.

The *upward movement* may *occur continuously*, fluidly, and slowly, or instead *intermittently*.

It can also manifest itself as a *sudden and brief* phenomenon. In this case, the symptomatology may overlap with that of a panic attack.

It usually begins with a *shaking*, with an internal *vibration* (sometimes also visible externally), as an internal tremor of varying intensity (sometimes intense) accompanied most often by *fear,* sometimes by an *ecstatic feeling* (or even both).

It is initially perceived as a *pressure,* a pain, a blow, localized at the affected *Chakras*.

Not infrequently, "somatoform" *symptoms* appear, characterized by subjective functional disturbances. These are bodily functional symptoms (in the absence of any underlying physical illness), related to the altered circulation of energy. Often this is accompanied by psychological discomfort, which biological psychiatry considers to be the cause of the psyche-body short-circuit.[40]

In any case, one will perceive something unfamiliar happening.

It constitutes an *initiation* into the encounter with psychic death, and may be remembered as a traumatic experience.

Being unfamiliar, this symptomatology usually frightens, and induces interpretations on the somatic level, and adopting avoidance-based defensive strategies for the future.

4.5.3 Evolution of the process

After the initial experience of the awakening of the *Kundalini*, there may follow a period, even a prolonged one, in which one may experience or observe *various phenomena*: high energy, or lack of energy, movements of energies that may also be rather chaotic, with internal and external *tremors* at times, blockages in the body, *streams* of energy *flowing* through the body, which may be perceived as disturbing or perceived as pleasant, or flows of *hot and cold sensations*.[41]

Local and general symptoms stabilize or exacerbate, *evolve*.

All kinds of intermediate conditions manifest between the initial awakening and the complete activation and ascent of the *Kundalini* in *Shushumna*.

In the *initial phase of* activation, the energy circulates more or less intensively in the lateral channels, without having yet begun its ascent in the central channel.

In this condition, one may observe an *anxious, diffuse state of prewarning or alarm*, fearing that it may become more activated and go out of control.

The clinical picture resulting from a *partial or total ascent in the central channel* is relatively characteristic. Let us now look at the full spectrum of symptoms (*i.e. subjective descriptions*) and signs (*i.e. objective data*) of the fully developed KS.

We can place signs and symptoms into *four basic categories*[42]; some phenomena are just different aspects of a whole complex integrated experience, while others manifest only in one of the following categories.

1 Motor phenomena

- *Spontaneous and automatic body movements and postures*, such as *Kryia* (sometimes smooth and sinuous, or spasmodic or vibratory): these range from muscular contractions to prolonged trembling to yoga postures. *Tics and Mudras* fall into this category, as does *rolling the eyes* backwards and upwards.
- Motor phenomena may also include spontaneous *crying, laughing, shouting and whistling.*
- *Unusual types of breathing* may occur (let's remember that prana is closely related to breathing, which is the mechanism by which the life force enters and leaves the body).
- Finally, *paralysis or paresis* (i.e. partial paralysis), or blocking of the body in specific positions (as was seen in classical catatonia) may occur.

2 Somato-sensory symptoms or sensory manifestations

- Spontaneous *vibrations or tingling* (e.g., shivering).
- Spontaneous *orgasmic sensations.*
- *Progressive sensations rising* from the legs up the back and up to the head.
- *Itching* sensations, of the skin or of the whole body.
- *Heat or cold* sensations throughout the body, or in isolated areas of the body; sensation of a *flow* of heat along the body. These may also have objective manifestations. (e.g., prolonged basal fever).
- *Pains* that come and go suddenly, in various locations in the body (e.g., in the lower back, or pains in the head, or in the eyes).
- *Interior lights and colors* that are seen from the inside (sometimes also from the outside), *visions.*
- *Sounds* (e.g., whistles and hisses, flute notes), inner voices, and other inner sounds.

3 Psychological and interpretative phenomena

- *Abnormal or excessive emotionality,* like feelings of great gratitude, peace, love and devotion, joy, harmony; sudden sense of ecstasy and unexplained bliss.

Yet other feelings may also arise: sudden unexplained anxiety or depression, anguish, fear; feeling of deep loneliness.

- *Alteration of mental processes:* the thought process may be accelerated, slowed down, inhibited altogether; disharmonious, strange or irrational thoughts.
- Spontaneous *states of trance, confusion, feeling alienated, detached* (as if observing one's own body, thoughts, feelings, and sensations from a distance, called "witness consciousness").
- *Sensation* of *expansion beyond the body* (*experience of the big body*, like feeling several meters taller). Out-of-body experiences.[43]

4 Non-physiological symptoms

- Emergence *of psychic abilities and experiences* (phenomena that are a consequence of the awakened *Kundalini*, although they often precede the awakening), like heightened intuition and sudden insights into oneself or others (sometimes described as "knowing" things without normal inference.
- In the initial stages of *Kundalini* awakening, there is a risk *of ego inflation, i.e. of identifying with this sense of expansion, as being produced by one's own ego*. Some do not experience this risk, others get caught up in it (as in many psychiatric psychotic cases).
- Another risk of these phenomena due to the *Kundalini* is *spiritual bypass*; in such cases one avoids processing the shadow of the ego, and prematurely believes that one has already transcended; here we are dealing with a higher level of denial.[44]

4.6 *Kundalini* Syndrome and *Chakras*

There are specific energetic symptoms, arising in specific regions, which are linked to hyper-activation, to energy hyper-inflow into specific *Chakras* or in the *channels* that connect them. If we recall the psychic connections of the *Chakra* with psychic manifestations, we can observe:

First Chakra: we will have, for example, phenomena related to fear, with a sense of extreme alarm, disorientation. This can stimulate at the neuroendocrine level an overactivity of the adrenals, or a malfunctioning of other endocrine glands, resulting in hypertension, contractures, prostate and rectal disorders such as hemorrhoids, etc. The first chakra is associated with our fundamental survival attachments to reality and our world of interpreting the world, hence the alarm.

Second Chakra: this energy can block or on the contrary intensify sexual functions, and even whole-body orgasms can occur; we may have symptoms of *erotic expansive hyper-activity*, with promiscuous or compulsive sexual activity, excessive masturbation, even inappropriate adventures, driven by an unspecific drive, falling in love. *Disorders of the abdominal region related to the gonads* may also occur on a physical level, including the possibility of cystitis, urethritis, miscarriages.

Third Chakra: *anger, aggressiveness, impulses for self-assertion* that are too intense and difficult to contain, poor impulse control, grudges; feeling of "blows" in the abdomen will be observed.

On the physical level, we may observe *irritative*, disharmonic, or excessive *activity* in the gastric region, such as gastritis, nausea and vomiting, contractions, gastrointestinal disorders.

Fourth Chakra: we may have a sense of pressure, a great weight on the chest, or even intense *pain* in the chest, with a fear of dying of a heart attack, *labile and alternating affectivity,* excessive opening and closing of affects.

On the physical level, we can frequently observe alterations in the *heart rhythm*, such as tachycardia (even intense and persistent), *blood pressure* disturbances. [45]

Fifth Chakra: one may observe *a sense of suffocation, loss of the ability to articulate words, or to swallow,* an uncontrollable wheezing *cough*, vomiting and stomach closure (anorexia and bulimia have a more complex genesis but we can observe symptoms at this level).

Sixth Chakra: activation here can manifest as *light, heat, sounds and lights, visions,* or even real *hallucinations* (i.e. perceptions that arise from this internal activation, and not from a real external objective support).

One may observe *blurred vision, disorientation, dizziness, tinnitus* (mistaken for ENT disorders), *unusual smells, unusual tastes; frequent headaches or migraines, intense nuchal pain, a feeling of a bursting head*, etc. [46]

An example of hyper-afflux with engagement of specific *Chakras* is generally present in the first panic attacks, with extreme tachycardia, feeling of suffocation, dizziness, etc.

Sensations tend to be interpreted negatively, dramatically, amplifying them, and thus triggering a reaction of alarm (generating a vicious circle between sensations and alarm).

4.7 *Kundalini* as therapy

Spiritual and philosophical traditions have always emphasized that the awakening and ascent of the *Kundalini* can bring *great benefits,* and important (although not always easy) transformations. However, they have also always warned about *potential risks*, and danger about the misuse of this energy by people who are spiritually unprepared to receive it.

In this regard, the outcome of the process is closely linked to the alignment (i.e., the acceptance, positive interpretation of the process), or vice versa to the opposition to the process itself (i.e., the rejection, fear, negative interpretation of the crisis and the disorganization it entails) of the individual or societies in which it occurs.[47]

According to some, the significance of KS is spiritual.

In ancient Tantric texts, the activation or awakening of *Kundalini* energy is responsible for mystical experiences. Gopi Krishna, for example, goes so far as to say that *every spiritual change has this basis*. Some speak of this event as an intervention of the divine, of the Goddess who loves us and sweeps us along the path of light.[48] For Ramakrishna, "the spiritual consciousness of a human being is not awakened until Kundalini has risen."

Transpersonal psychology regards *spiritual awakening as a natural evolutionary tendency towards a new level of human consciousness*. The KS represents the *beginning of the end, and signals a new beginning*; it is she who stands at the base, and who initiates every psychiatric condition. The KS, among all PCs, is the most frequent, obvious, dramatic, worrying clinical syndrome, the one that most likely will bring the patient to visit a psychiatrist.

Hence the importance of recognizing the syndrome, in order not to misdiagnose it, and accompany it in the best way possible.

Stanislav and Christina Grof coined the term "spiritual emergency" to describe these intense experiences which, although dramatic, are not pathological but indicate a process of transformation. The energy activation and restructuring of the subtle body lead to the dissolution of conditioning and to the liberation of consciousness.

For Greenwell, KS is a *consequence of man's profound desire to know the nature of God or himself*. It corresponds to a spiritual quest, aimed at understanding energy and consciousness, which activates transformation when the soul is ready; as in the analogy with childbirth, when the child is ready it signals the mother to begin the great change.

Kundalini awakening involves a shift from a purely physical perception of self to a more energetic one. The ultimate goal of the process is transcendence of the ego and union with the higher consciousness, or "cosmic consciousness." This state, according to yogic tradition, is achieved when the *Kundalini* ascends to the *Sahasrara Chakra* at the top of the head, leading to supreme bliss, the superconscious state and the highest knowledge.

Others argue, however, that the activation of the Kundalini is not always associated with spiritual awakening, and that *one should not confuse the KS with complete spiritual awakening*. For some authors[49] it is only a stage of awakening, which can be a prelude to further development, while for others it is a by-product of awakening and only indicates a certain degree of resistance and need for purification.

Caution is needed both in assisting the process and in prognosis. *Sannella considers the Kundalini process intrinsically therapeutic*, and capable of leading to a higher level of functioning. However, he cautioned that the *Kundalini* process can also be destructive if left to itself. One could be overwhelmed by doubts and fears, and therefore it is very important that there be an understanding environment (e.g., a spiritual abode or monastery) where the side effects of awakening are properly interpreted, accepted, and even welcomed.

Without this understanding, this force could act in many undesirable ways.

Some might interpret the experience as a sign that they have lost their sanity.

Sannella also points out that much of the agitation in these cases can be attributed to misunderstanding and lack of knowledge about the process. Therapists should instill knowledge and confidence to allow the process to progress at as smooth and natural a pace as possible, and be able to recognize the *Kundalini* phenomenon as a non-psychotic process.

Still others finally give the KS a neurophysiological explanation, and believe that it is merely a psycho-physiological mechanism. Along these lines, the research of Bentov and Sannella tried to provide biomechanical and clinical explanations for the phenomena associated with *Kundalini* awakening.

Dr. Sannella introduced the term "physioKundalini" to describe specifically the bodily and psychological manifestations of *Kundalini* awakening, its circulation and ascent. In particular, he hypothesized that the typical symptomatology of the activation sequence of the ascending sensations along the spine, with the symptoms of the stimulated *Chakras*, could have a neuro-psychological explanation.[50]

4.8 The Bentov model

The activation of parts of the body corresponding to the progressive ascent of the *Kundalini* along the corresponding *Chakras* follows a characteristic sequence.

The activation sensation often starts at the toes, then moves and ascends along the legs, back, head, then descends again to the eyes, face, down to the throat, ending in the abdominal area.

Itzack Bentov[51] observed how along the sensory cortex of the brain the order of the represented areas corresponds precisely to the sensory innervation of those body regions. He therefore created a *neurophysiological model* to explain the phenomenology of *Kundalini* activation and ascent described in the ancient spiritual texts of many cultures.[52]

He observed how an energy ascending from the groove separating the two hemispheres, continuing radially outwards, would activate the very areas affected by the symptomatology of KS.

He, therefore, *hypothesized that KS would be due to an electric current that is activated in the central region of the brain and travels radially through the cerebral cortex (thus activating these innervation areas in sequence); a sensory activation would then be perceived and interpreted by the subject as a sequential ascent of a current, of different sensations, in the body areas described.*

In his model, he also hypothesized that *the activation of the abovementioned sensory areas could depend on the pressure wave generated under certain conditions by the aortic resonators, then transmitted through the cerebrospinal fluid to the cerebral ventricles, to finally activate the neurons of the central commissure, and then spread radially in the sensory cortex*, generating the illusion of an ascent of perceptions.[53] Moreover, an *involvement of the motor area* could explain the Kryia and tics. This process could explain the *experience of Kundalini* awakening and the related mystical phenomena.

Sannella considered Bentov's model to be the best explanation available in Western scientific terms to study the physiological dimension of the Kundalini experience.[54]

However, the model shows obvious *limitations*; for example, it excludes all spiritual and evolutionary aspects that go beyond mere physiology.[55]

This type of study nevertheless opens an interesting and fascinating chapter by proposing to re-examine clinical evidence, historically documented in all spiritual literature, from the neurophysiological point of view.[56]

4.9 KS and psychopathology: Psychosis or transcendence?

Kundalini awakening represents a *critical bridge between spirituality and psychopathology*. As we have seen, *Kundalini* awakening experiences can manifest with symptoms that mimic psychiatric disorders, creating diagnostic and therapeutic challenges.

There is still no general consensus on how to *distinguish a spiritual emergency from a psychotic episode*. Much depends on the experience of the psychiatrist, who should know how to recognize the signs of a mature integration or a psychic fragmentation underway in KS.

The diagnostic challenge lies in distinguishing between a genuine spiritual experience and a pathological manifestation. The symptoms of *Kundalini* awakening often do not allow one to distinguish which KS will evolve into a spiritual emergence and which into a frank psychosis.

An accurate diagnosis requires *avoiding both indiscriminate medicalization (*in the West, spiritual experiences are wrongly pathologized leading to inappropriate interventions) *and romanticization of real risks.*

The difficulty of distinguishing psychosis from transcendence (see Sannella's book, see Grof's work on spiritual) is part of a debate that is still open.

4.9.1 How to differentiate Kundalini experiences from pathological crises

The most widely accepted thesis in the literature holds that there is a *substantial difference between psychoses* and those conditions that evolve positively towards awakening, called *spiritual emergencies.* An alternative thesis sees these syndromes placed in a complex continuum, in which several dimensions converge and intersect; in this continuum, a common genesis and substantial nature is recognized: the evolution of individual consciousness.[57]

Let us see what arguments are put forward in favor of the thesis that these are very different phenomena, and the criteria proposed for distinguishing them.

- *Origin:* When analyzing the differences between psychosis and spiritual emergencies, it is essential to start with their origins. Psychoses are generally considered to be organically based disorders[58]: often, a single cause cannot be identified, but predisposing factors such as a personal or family psychiatric history, substance abuse, or other elements may contribute to the onset of the illness. In contrast, spiritual emergencies have their roots in spiritual experiences: they can be triggered by intense meditative practices, deeply transformative life events such as bereavement, or sudden mystical experiences. In these cases, the triggering factor is often clearly identifiable and connected to a process of personal growth or inner exploration.
- *The nature of the symptoms* is another distinguishing element. In psychosis, typical symptoms include fragmented delusions, threatening hallucinations, social withdrawal, fear of death or disappearance, and a general lack of spiritual content. Those experiencing psychosis often suffer from a loss of contact with reality, accompanied by feelings of anguish and confusion. On the other hand, spiritual emergencies may

also involve unusual perceptions or even delusional experiences, but these are often accompanied by non-distressing mystical experiences and specific energetic symptoms, such as a sensation of warmth along the spine or bodily vibrations.[59]

- *The way the crisis is experienced and interpreted* by the individual is also profoundly different in the two cases. A psychotic crisis is generally perceived as a tragic event, a loss of control over one's life, and a real threat to physical and psychological integrity. In contrast, those going through a spiritual emergency tend to maintain a certain awareness of the transformative nature of the experience: people often describe a "light at the end of the tunnel," a psychological rebirth, or a passage through the symbolic death of the old self towards a new integration. In this context, the presence of insight is a key element: in psychosis, the individual often shows little or no insight ("The voices are real, I am not ill"), whereas in spiritual emergencies there is more frequently an awareness of the process taking place ("I am going through a change").
- *The evolution over time* also helps to distinguish between the two conditions. Psychoses tend to worsen and become chronic if not properly treated, while spiritual emergencies develop in a more dynamic way, alternating phases of acute crisis with moments of integration and personal growth, often leading to progressive improvement over time. Consequently, the response to pharmacological treatment also differs: in psychosis, medication is often necessary and produces clear effects, while in spiritual emergencies it may be less effective or sometimes even unnecessary, leaving more room for targeted psychospiritual support.

Summarizing, Spiritual Emergencies vs Psychoses: see Table 4.1[60]

Table 4.1 Differential Diagnosis: *Kundalini* Syndrome (KS) vs. Psychosis

Criteria	*Kundalini Syndrome (KS)*	*Psychosis*
Onset	Often sudden or develops after intense spiritual practice, meditation, or energy work.	Often acute, sometimes linked to stress, substance use, or spontaneously without clear trigger.
Nature of Experience	Sensations of energy moving in the spine (heat, vibrations, tingling), expanded consciousness, feelings of bliss or unity; also anxiety, confusion, sometimes fear or loss of control.	Chaotic or bizarre experiences, persecutory or threatening themes, thought disorder, fragmentation of self.

(Continued)

Table 4.1 (Continued)

Criteria	*Kundalini Syndrome (KS)*	*Psychosis*
Physical Symptoms	Strong somatic phenomena: shaking, spasms, heat, waves of energy, spontaneous body movements, altered breathing, sensory intensification.	Occasionally agitation or catatonia, but rarely energetic phenomena or precise bodily sensations typical of KS.
Hallucinations	Vivid inner visions (lights, mandalas, archetypal symbols), sometimes voices interpreted as guidance; typically structured and meaningful.	Hallucinations are usually threatening, disorganized, or command-like (e.g., hostile voices); lack structured meaning.
Emotional Tone	Alternates between ecstasy, awe, confusion, anxiety, or fear; often oscillates with periods of calm and insight.	Predominantly anxiety, panic, agitation, confusion, or blunted affect; emotions often destabilizing.
Insight	Partially maintained: experiences may be questioned or explored symbolically; some awareness of the internal process.	Insight is absent; delusions and hallucinations believed to be 100% real.
Relation to Reality	Preserved ego boundaries, able to reflect symbolically on experiences; usually does not lose touch with reality.	Loss of ego boundaries, perceptions externalized, attributed to agencies or forces outside the self.
Functioning	Generally preserved or only temporarily affected; possible to maintain therapeutic alliance.	Marked and persistent impairment of social and functional domains; severe disorganization.
Energetic Symptoms	Prominent and specific: sense of energy rising along the spine, heat, spontaneous postures, "*Kundalini* phenomena."	Absent or nonspecific: physical symptoms usually due to medication, anxiety, or agitation.
Prognosis	Typically transient if integrated well (weeks to months); strong potential for personal growth and transformation.	Often chronic without treatment; risk of cognitive decline and social isolation if untreated.
Treatment Approach	Supportive, containment, symbolic integration (e.g., journaling, art); pharmacotherapy rarely indicated.	Requires stabilization, antipsychotic medication, restoration of boundaries.

The symptoms of *Kundalini* Syndrome (KS) differ in important ways from general Spiritual Emergencies. KS is characterized by unique somatic and energetic phenomena, as well as transformations in consciousness, which are not typically present in standard psychosis or even in other types of spiritual crises.

4.10 Clinical example

In the case we present, the components of the identity crisis, the accompanying energetic symptoms, and the reactive symptoms linked to egoic resistance are clearly visible. It concerns a 28-year-old young man,

---

The PC had started gradually before the acute phase for which he consulted me.

For some time, the patient had felt very strange, weak, as if he was not completely in control of his body; for example, he could not hold shopping bags, and always had a sense of death.

He could no longer masturbate, that energy was no longer available; no matter how hard he tried, he could not get an erection, or an orgasm, or little sperm came out. This was in great contrast to a short time before, when he was practicing masturbation a lot and had a very strong sexual appetite.[61]

However, the patient on the whole was somehow "functioning," and had managed in despondency and depression to finish his degree course.

Then at the age of about 25, he fell in love. It was love at first sight, for a foreign girl, who was also already engaged. Their affair lasted only a few months, always with this betrayal controversy; he was very much in love, but then she left him.

The patient attributes the beginning of the crisis to this abandonment.

The crisis had started in an obvious form in June; he had been feeling "strange" for a few days, but did not know what was wrong.

During a meal with family members, he had to leave the table due to an unspecified and intense illness, saying that he went to lie down on the bed, that he could not stand upright.

In bed he thought "I am dying."

He could no longer feel his legs, and he began to feel something move from the sacrum towards his belly: he felt pulsations, blows, in the region of his genitals. It was as if the energy in that region had withdrawn: he could see his genitals shrinking, as when one has a fever, and his penis had become very very small. Then the blows and the sensations began to rise; he felt very strong blows at the level of his stomach, and then his arms, his hands, his head began to move, to shake, and everything inside his body pulsed, as if air were coming out of him.

It was as if he was emitting the air of a hair dryer from his skin; the sensation, which he said was also objectively noticeable, was that he was vibrating as if he were a sheet of paper close to the air escaping from his skin. In reality it was an internal feeling of trembling, accompanied by an intense sense of fear.

His mother came into the room to see how he was. He told her that he was dying.

The process continued for days afterwards. Because of the numbness of certain parts of his body, he began to think he had multiple sclerosis; he did not sleep at all, he was dizzy, he struggled to do everything, and there was always this internal trembling all over his body. The process continued, always changing form.

In the following months he had more panic attacks. Once he was with his father, and it felt as if his heart stopped; he had a strong tachycardia. At that time he still had the strong blows, for months; he felt these blows in his stomach, and beyond the blows he felt a sense of blockage in his belly, he had diarrhea and couldn't eat well.

His energy soared, and twice he even had nosebleeds. He had "clicks" in his jaw, i.e. the temporomandibular joint made a clicking sound when he moved it, and a small sound could be heard; this "click" was (and still is) fixated on, as if it were a sign that something was wrong inside him. He had a pain in his teeth, he had difficulty chewing; he had a cough, which he interpreted as if through the cough he wanted to remove something, some blockage inside, like when one has food stuck in their throat.

He had an itchy feeling in his throat, and coughing, and fear of choking or swallowing food, accompanied by "wormy" thoughts ("what if you are gay, or trans," "what if you wants to wear heels?"), doubts (e.g., whether he was attracted to children; every child who came, the thought came up). He felt strong knocks in his head, in the middle of his forehead.

At that time he woke up one day with this clicking in his jaw and the feeling that he was no longer totally in his body. It was as if he was somewhere else, a feeling of bodily non-presence, a feeling still present today.

This continued until the moment he came to me for his first consultation.

On that occasion I prescribed a mood regulator, which, however, he took sporadically, and we had a few sessions.

He was receptive, the climax passed, he returned to his home country, recovered, and then went to work in the North.

After a few years, I happened to resume talks with the patient for a similar symptomatologic reactivation; this time, however, the patient experienced it differently: he was more conscious, the symptomatology more manageable, and yet still characterized by great intensity and energetic activity.

He had many dreams per night, he had a lot of anxiety and many thoughts, the symptomatological picture tended to grow.

The movement of energy in his belly had become reactivated, and it bothered him, and could be felt also in his arms and in other parts of his body; particularly in the sacrum, where there was continuous "work," and where he felt a "plug," a blockage, which he usually interpreted as proof that something was wrong there.

Moreover, when the activity increased in that region, it also increased in his face, and he felt in these cases a greater discomfort in feeling the crack in his jaw, the stiffness in his neck.

And when it pulsed more, he felt again that the genitals withdrew, although not as before; sometimes now that turned into sperm, or went into the body as vapor, and rose like waves: but now he recognized it, it was that same energy.

Notes

1 From the book by Dr. Lee Sannella (1916–2010), *The Kundalini Experience: Psychosis or Transcendence*,

Sannella was an American physician, psychiatrist, ophthalmologist, writer, and *Kundalini* researcher; he worked in San Francisco and the Bay area; he ran his own psychiatric clinic in Berkeley from 1962 to 1972 and an in-patient service for substance abuse problems. In 1974, he co-founded the *Kundalini Clinic* in San Francisco.

He has been consulting and giving lectures and seminars all over the world, from Iceland to Brazil, for several decades.

He was a student of the American spiritual teacher *Adi Da*, whom he considered his main spiritual guide.

2 There is a joke that *calmness is the virtue of those who do not really understand the situation;* conversely, we could say that *agitation is the vice of those who do not really understand the situation.*

3 In recent years, numerous studies have shown that, during a full-term pregnancy, the maturation of fetal organs—particularly the lungs—leads to the production and release of specific molecules (such as the *surfactant protein SP-A and platelet-activating factor, PAF*) in the amniotic fluid. These signals "alert" the maternal body that the fetus is ready to survive outside the womb, triggering a cascade of inflammatory responses that culminate in the onset of labor and delivery (see *Fetal-to-maternal signaling to initiate parturition*, Erin L. Reinl , Sarah K England , in PMC).

4 Contractions usually trigger at a later time; however, they can sometimes precede this.
5 See Plotinus, and later Porphyry, a view that would later be taken up by Plato as well.
6 The fetus is no longer there, a newborn is present now. It is a different state of the same being: a true transformation, of one into the other; different, yet the same. Since the newborn is born from the fetus (in the sense that it derives from him), which instead dies (is no more), we could say that birth is also a death-rebirth. In religious terms, one speaks of the *Resurrection*, one speaks of the birth of the "son of man," since he is born from what was before but is something else entirely. From the point of view of the collapsing "me," this process of splitting from sleep, in other words awakening, appears as a tragedy: the world collapses, and the character around which that world revolved collapses as well.
7 It is no coincidence that Dante considers the death-rebirth process of the journey a *Comedy*, that is a drama that ends well, and not a *tragedy*; it is nevertheless true that for the old ego it is the end.
8 That is perhaps why Hippocrates, in his treatise on the "Regime of Acute Diseases," said: "To be born and to die is the same thing;/ to be born and to separate is the same thing;/ to perish, to decrease, to separate is the same thing."
9 An hospitalized psychiatric patient told me: "*I need to make a revolution that will restore my equilibrium*"
10 I believe this is the reason why many narrative forms take the desert as their setting, from the *temptations of Christ*, to the "deserted plain" of *Dante's dark forest*, to the desert of "Roadrunner and Wile E.Coyote."
11 See Jung, *Psychic Energetics.*
12 This residual identification, this "residual ego," however, gradually dissolves and will become less and less troublesome as time passes, as the *Kundalini* continues its work of purifying the consciousness of residual identifications. For this reason, the second crisis is usually handled better and with more awareness than the first, is often less ego-dystonic, and allows for greater adherence to pharmacological indications.
13 Of course, part of the prolonged suffering belongs to the process itself; some bipolar forms can remain active for years, although they change in intensity and quality over time; the same is true of severe dissociative forms. Here, however, we are insisting on complications due to defensive interference, which also prolong subjective suffering indefinitely.
14 St John of the Cross deals explicitly and in depth with the dark night of the soul in his writings "Dark Night" and "Ascent of Mount Carmel," fundamental works of Christian mysticism and Carmelite spirituality.
15 This is the reason for Jesus' passage into the desert, for the monks' retreat to the convent or the caves. It is only in the absence of everything, in fact, that one can perhaps rediscover what was always there, the awareness that forms the backdrop to life. There is a saying: *Close your eyes and you will see.*
16 The dark night of the soul for St John of the Cross is divided into three main stages:

Beginner: This is the stage of purification, where one progressively loses attachments to the senses and psychic faculties (thought, imagination, desire). The subject experiences aridity, dissatisfaction, and loss of pleasure even in spiritual practices, learning to accept the present as it is, without ascetic heroism.

Proficient: Here detachment deepens, involving the subtler faculties (intellect, memory, will). The "dark night of the spirit" manifests itself with even more intense dryness, inner suffering, and often even physical discomfort, a sign of the body's difficulty in supporting the strength of the spirit.

Perfect: In this phase the mind is empty of content and the spiritual light no longer finds anything to reflect on, appearing as "luminous darkness." The person does not perceive particular states, but when the light is reflected on something, understanding is immediate and profound. The heart is pervaded by an infused, passive love that grows like fire in wood: the only action required of the soul is consent to this transformation.

This happens when PC happens in people who are more prepared for transformation, who sense (even if confusedly) the potential contained in the crisis, that is, a process of restructuring and change.

Speaking of the dark forest, after narrating the great difficulty of finding oneself in this condition, Dante wants to emphasize the positive potential of the crisis, saying that it is in that darkness he found the light; in these cases, the crisis can lead to a new life , to a new state of consciousness in life.

17 A *residual state* in psychiatry refers to a phase in which, after the remission of acute symptoms (such as delusions, hallucinations, manic or intense depressive episodes), certain "residual" or deficit symptoms persist that do not reach the severity of the acute phase but continue to negatively influence the person's overall functioning and prognosis. *Residual* symptoms are attenuated elements of acute symptomatology that persist after remission. The *residual syndrome*, on the other hand, represents a stable set of symptoms and deficits (especially negative and cognitive) that persist over time, independent of the active phases of the disease, and often require specific interventions.

18 Secondary conditioning factors also include the characteristics of the individual's consciousness, whether it is more rational or emotional, more attentive to the body or more abstract from the world; the person will also react in one way or another depending on how formal their mind is, and thus produces forms and monsters; and on how much they believe it, what their mind says.

19 *It is the law of karma:* you reap what you sow; if you are not happy, it is only your own fault, as a tibetan proverb goes. The *law of contrapasso* almost replicates this concept; in Hell the punishment is retributive to the moral nature of their wrongdoing, but in Purgatory it is corrective.

20 It is not a matter of medieval fantastic images, to be interpreted on a literal level (characters reported and who really existed with their illustrative stories), or on a symbolic or allegorical level (the psychological vicissitudes of the soul, the metaphor of psychotherapy as an accompaniment), but rather of the description of alchemical operations, described in detail, therefore to be interpreted on an anagogical level. The text explains what happens to the consciousness in its obscuration and its resurrection from death, what the transformative steps are, how to accompany them in a transpersonal psychotherapy.

21 "Io non so ben ridir com'io v'intrai /tant'era pien di sonno in su quel punto / che la diritta via abbandonai" Inf I, vv 10–12.

22 "You will know the truth and the truth will make you free" (John 8:32). This knowledge of who one really is, "who I am", is an essential condition; in fact, this is the first question that Cato, the guardian of Purgatory, addresses to the two who have emerged from the Inferno (Hell): "Who are you?". Pur, I, vv 40–48.

23 The saying "giving up smoking is the easiest thing in the world. I know because I've done it thousands of times" is often attributed, without evidence, to O. *Wilde* or M. *Twain.*

24 On a symbolic level, it is the sacrament of the sacrament of *Baptism*, i.e. a ritual death and rebirth, a washing away of the stain.

25 This dark polarity, *the emperor of the painful realm, the prince of this world,* the power without love is, according to Jung, *the greatest factor of individuation*: it represents and is in the dualistic consciousness the polarity that pulls down, that narrows the light, that obscures: it is the downward-facing *Kundalini*, the opposing force, personified as "the Adversary." Within us is the unconsciously separative ego-centric force, at least until consciousness is still identified with the principle of separation.

Proverb: "If you have never seen the devil, look at your ego!"

26 *And the choice of the good is free, there is free will*: as long as there is ego as long as we are on earth (first two canticles) we can choose, or at least desire the good. This philosophical and clinical issue is of paramount importance, and Dante articulates his discourse well: consciousness is more or less free depending on its evolutionary level, on its purification from ego attachment. At the level of Hell and Purgatory, as long as there is identification with evil, freedom is only relatively free, or more or less impeded: after awakening, however, the faculty to choose ripens, becomes complete, having finally seen what our true nature is. Even in the harshest prison, it is always possible to choose to become free; the jailers will then prevent it, but freedom is saved. Virgil explains to Cato, to justify his exit from Hell, that Dante values freedom more than life. Even in therapy, when one succeeds in showing the patient the way, and he chooses not to recognize it, he takes it upon himself to deny healing. In heaven, on the other hand (third canticle), our will is entirely "sound, rectified, and free," and coincides with that of God himself, because there is no longer any participation (identification) with the principle of opposition (*in his will is our peace).*

27 The purification process ends when our consciousness becomes spotless (the Immaculate), and can thus ascend to heaven (the Assumed). In Purgatory, suffering decreases as one renounces Satan and all his temptations (Renunciation of Evil: Baptism), which allows one to no longer move backwards, but only forwards (Pursuit of Good: Confirmation); purifying and uplifting coincide in the symbolic geography of the inner journey. Suffering thus becomes tolerable, and during therapy it decreases; consciousness is centered and Kundalini spiral is inverted and rectified, and peace on earth is achieved (Earthly Paradise).

28 Childhood trauma also partly falls under the previous point, as when, for example, in a childhood trauma the parent was unable to protect the child, who felt betrayed and orphaned, as in bereavement Traumatic events can destabilize the energy balance, creating a state of prolonged stress that facilitates the sudden opening of energy centers (*Chakras*) and the rising of latent energy along the spinal column.

29 E.g., with *yogic breathing practices,* or intense pranayama (like Kapalabhati, Bhastrika pranayama, fire breathing), *Kryia* (specific movements to release emotions), *mantras,* used especially in *Kundalini* yoga. The fire-breathing technique is mentioned in the Divine Comedy, in the first canto of Paradise, in the invocation to Apollo, as activating the ascent to heaven.

30 *Asceticism and austerity* (tapas), such as exposure to extreme climatic conditions, *Prolonged fasting or specific dietary restrictions, Repetition of specific mantras* (e.g., Soham, Om Namah Shivaya), *Deep meditation practices* (e.g.,

Dhyana on the spine*), Use of specific sounds and vibrations* (e.g., tibetan bells nada yoga), specific *Visualization techniques* for the energy rising up the spine, such as a *chakra*-by-*chakra* visualization (imagining each energy center "lighting up" or glowing in a certain color, proceeding from the bottom up). Other visualization techniques are Global Visualization (perceiving a beam of light or a flow of light rising up the spine, then radiating throughout the body); also, representation of Symbols or archetypes (some traditions invite specific visualization of deities or symbols. Finally, *contact with a spiritual master* (guru) who confers activation (*Shaktipath*). This last situation is the direct transmission of energy (Shakti) from an accomplished master to a disciple. Transmission can take place through gaze, touch (e.g., a touch on the third eye or the top of the head) or even at a distance by focusing the master's consciousness.

31 An interesting hypothesis is the one put forward by Dr. Yvonne Kason in which it is claimed that every time the *Kundalini* is awakened, the consciousness goes through an NDE, which is then the cause of CP.

32 As we saw in the chapter on energy, the *Kundalini* is a vibratory, pervasive, and active force, inseparable from Shiva (the primordial cosmic consciousness).

The *Kundalini* itself is considered a manifestation of the "Self," the "Pure Consciousness" (*Chit-Kundalini*) that underlies various states of consciousness. It embodies *the intentionality of consciousness* that manifests the world.

33 See Greenwell, *The Kundalini Guide* in bibliography

34 This could be due to a much faster and more radical collective and individual transformation, the increased attention and ability to recognize these processes, perhaps even the the growth of the world's population.

35 However, there is interest in studying the phenomenon; for example, Sanches, L., & Daniels, M., in 2008, developed a psychometric instrument to assess the experience of *Kundalini* awakening, the *Kundalini Awakening Scale (KAS)*, drawing on symptoms and descriptions from the *Kundalini* literature (Krishna, Sannella, Bentov, Grof) and clinical cases. The final version of the scale includes 76 items, divided into five subscales: Changes, Negative Experiences, Positive Experiences, Involuntary Postures, and Physical Symptoms. The scale has demonstrated excellent internal reliability. There are also other scales, such as that of B. Greyson (*Physio Kundalini Syndrome Index* with 19 items), of Thalbourne, or of Prosnik & Evans (the PhysioKundalini Syndrome Index 7 (PKSI-7))

36 See B. Greenwell who gives a clear exposition.

37 *The Kundalini Guide* already cited. In the case of Greenwell, who recounts her own experience of awakening, for example, it was an entirely positive phenomenon: energetically, she felt an intense spasm of energy that began to flow up her spine, reaching her head; she perceived strong shaking in her body, as if it was being traversed by electric discharges, perceived as joy. The phenomenon was repeated cyclically, pushing higher and higher.

Her state of consciousness was transformed: her mind was unclear, empty, she no longer felt in her body or in the room; the sensation was of being in a vast open space, acutely aware, almost floating. For her, the sensation was very pleasant, a feeling of pure pleasure in meditation the state of bliss intensified. This condition lasted several weeks in her case.

38 "Sometimes the Spiritual Current goes up the spine, advancing like an ant. Sometimes in samadhi the soul swims joyfully in the ocean of divine ecstasy, like a fish. Sometimes again when I lie on my side, I feel the Spiritual Current pushing me like a monkey and wanting to play with me merrily, I remain still. Still like a monkey, the Current reaches Sahasrara with a leap. That is why

sometimes you see me take a leap. Sometimes again the Spiritual Current hops like a bird going up from branch to branch; and in the place where it rests it seems a fire is burning there ... At other times still the Spiritual Current rises moving like a serpent, advancing in a zigzag until it finally reaches the head and I enter the Samahdi" M. (Mahendranath Gupta), *The Gospel of Sri Ramakrishna*, translated by Swami Nikhilananda, New York, Ramakrishna-Vivekananda Center, 19.

39 One of my patients did not have time to get up from his chair to reach his bed, almost as if in an epileptic fit; for years afterwards, he remembered the intense tachycardia, disorientation, fear of dying, marveling that he was nevertheless still alive.

40 An example would be *migraines*, which could represent an energetic imbalance in the channels, perceived as pressure or lateralized pain. Sometimes the energy could channel into the *more superficial network of channels* (acupuncture channels) acutely or chronically disturbing the functioning of organs and apparatuses, uni- or bilaterally; for example, *fibromyalgia* could have such a component.

In Freud's time, these conditions were referred to as *somatic conversions* in hysterical neuroses, which were probably closely connected with *Kundalini* revelations, and which in the Freudian method were then interpreted in a psychogenetic sense.

Somatoform disorders are not to be confused with *psychosomatic disorders*, which are instead real physical illnesses (such as gastritis, asthma, dermatitis, hypertension), in which there is an objective organic damage, in which psychological factors (stress, anxiety, negative emotions) act as a *concomitant or triggering factor* of an already existing or predisposed organic illness.

41 *Greenwell* emphasizes how people going through a spiritual transformation are surprised at the impact on the body's energy; however, if we consider that the energy blocks that the energy encounters in its progress are there from early childhood, due to conditioning, we can understand how the intense stress can lead to great difficulty in accepting them and the need for a prolonged period of adaptation. However, this adaptation and purification of the system is an essential part of the preparation of a new consciousness.

42 See the book of Lee Sannella when he talks about the *physio Kundalini*, adapted; see also *Characteristics of Kundalini- Related Sensory, Motor, and Affective Experiences During Tantric Yoga Meditation*, Richard W Maxwell, Sucharit Katyal in Pub Med.

43 On the psychic risks of *Kundalini* activation see also www.sciencedirect.com/science/article/abs/pii/S1744388120311609?via%3Dihub.

44 For example, one usually perceives an increased identification with one's ego, which is strengthened and structured into the form of a spiritual ego, and which one believes to be superior to other ordinary mortals, rather than moving towards a progressive dis-identification. Examples of this defensive process of denial are talking about rebirth without being changed at all, focusing only on the bright side of things as happens in some spiritual sects, developing a specific attachment to a guru or technique. These people may tend towards spiritual control, trying to control themselves or others, denying spiritual spontaneity and richness; they tend towards an "all or nothing" way of thinking, the same for behavior. They may still experience feelings of fear of shame and confusion. They are too willing to tolerate inappropriate behavior of themselves, feel easily frustrated, or have addictions or compulsions, and still have unnecessary pain.

45 Greenwell reports that it is believed that when the *Kundalini* rises above the level of the *heart*, the progress becomes irreversible, and one is necessarily propelled on an evolving inner path, which may be more or less short, or with more or less deviations.

46 Sudden intestinal movements, or even chronic inflammation, in the intestines, such as Crohn's disease, or pain in the reproductive system can express an acute symptomatology that goes beyond the inflammatory objectivity and can also be sustained by these energetic movements that do not find their way and maintain tension, heat, and irritation in the region of the lower *Chakras*. Fibromyalgia is another syndrome that is poorly understood and only interpreted as a physical disorder with a component of "*stress*," a term for tension that is not motivated by specific reasons, but is nevertheless recognized as an operating agent in the condition.

47 This misalignment is more evident in technologically advanced societies, where separation and control are more pronounced, and where spiritual behavior is repressed, so that people are much less prepared to accept the process.

Other cultures are far ahead of us in this regard. In Bali, for example, the trance state serves an important adaptation function for children; in African Bushmen, trance is experienced with a ritual that is central to promoting social cohesion. In the Himalayas, the trance medium plays an important social function; and so on.

48 Many books talk about it; in this section I will refer mainly to Lee Sannella's book (Lee Sannella: *Kundalini: Psychosis or Transcendence?*, where he focuses on energetic phenomena at the level of the subtle body and the *Chakras*, and another, that of Bonnie Greenwell, a transpersonal psychologist active in the USA (Bonnie Greenwell, *Guide to the Kundalini: An Accompaniment for the Inner Journey*. This is a short, valuable and comprehensive work that provides a better understanding of energetic phenomena that are often categorized as psychiatric, pathological, and disturbing).

49 Also Greenwell.

50 According to Greyson, however, this phase would only correspond to the onset of the KS picture, i.e. an activation but not an ascent of K.

51 Itzach Bentov, 1923–1979, born in Czechoslovakia, was a Jewish scientist naturalized in the USA, author of several inventions including a seismographic device to record the heartbeat and in particular the resonances of the aorta. He was one of the pioneers in trying to explain spiritual phenomena such as the *Kundalini* through a scientific lens. See for example his book *Stalking the Wild Pendulum: On the Mechanics of Consciousness* (1977). In this book, Bentov explores his ideas on *Kundalini* and consciousness, combining scientific knowledge with mystical concepts. He was convinced that consciousness permeates everything and practiced meditation.

52 "During normal breathing, the reverberations in the aorta are out of phase with the heartbeat and the system is disharmonious. However, during meditation and when holding the breath, the echo coming out of the bifurcation of the aorta at the pelvic level resonates with the heartbeat and the system synchronizes, thus using a minimal amount of energy. This resonant beat is about seven cycles per second, which corresponds to the magnetic pulsations of the Earth, (which is about seven cycles per second, known as the Schumann resonance), but also to the alpha rhythm of the brain." Bentov, in his work on spiritual phenomena and consciousness, theorized a possible link between the Earth's natural frequencies and mystical experiences, such as the awakening of the *Kundalini*. (From Wikipedia).

53 In the context of the human body, vibrations or pressure waves, if strong enough, can theoretically create mechanical deformations in piezoelectric tissues. *Piezoelectric transduction* refers to the ability of certain materials to generate an electrical charge in response to mechanical stress. It a known phenomenon in some biological tissues, but its direct application to neurons in the sensory cortex requires further study and scientific evidence. Piezoelectric transduction could potentially generate electrical signals that stimulate neighboring neurons, which would in turn generate an activation wave that would propagate.

54 A more recent author, Kieffer, argues like Bentov that *Kundalini* is not just an energy, but a *biological mechanism* that regulates the evolution of human consciousness and affects all the cells of the body, particularly those of the nervous and brain systems. For Kieffer, the *Kundalini* process is observable and potentially scientifically explainable as an evolutionary and biological mechanism, not just a mystical experience. Psychophysical preparation and a complete understanding of the cycle are essential to avoid imbalances or negative effects after awakening. See *Understanding the Kundalini Process* by Gene Kieffer (2013).

55 Some of the sensations of the KS could be explained by central stimulation of other areas: for example, the hypothalamus is thought of for heat and cold sensations, while the phenomena of light and sound could correspond to simulation near the lateral and medial geniculate regions, as well as to permanent waves generated by the ventricles. *Other phenomena, however, are not as well explained by Bentov's model*; if for the visions and voices one can think of a spread of stimulation of the adjacent areas connected with language sound and vision, and perhaps detachment and dissociation may result from stimulation of area 39 of the cortex, no explanations are provided in the model for the mechanisms underlying emotions or for altered forms of thought.

56 Greyson, for example, showed that *Kundalini* arousal is accompanied by a distinctive neurophysiological profile, but admitted it was impossible to say whether *Kundalini* experiences cause or facilitate these neurophysiological traits, or whether persons with these traits are more prone to *Kundalini* arousal.

57 We will return to the discussion of awakening symptoms as KS or Spiritual Emergency (SE) in more depth there; here we just want to emphasize how the energetic activation of the KS can lead to spiritual emergence but is not identical with it.

58 This is, after all, a different presentation of the dualism between body and spirit, of Cartesian origin, which arises from a materialist view seeing spirit also as matter overcomes this dichotomy.

59 If we look closely, Kraepelin's old classification of mental disorders (essentially *mood* (affective) disorders and *thought* disorders) reflected this understanding that it is important to distinguish between the energetic and identity components in a psychiatric syndrome, giving the thought disorders component a more negative prognostic value.

60 Integrated with: "Psychosis or Spiritual Emergency: The Potential of Developmental Psychopathology for Differential Diagnosis, St. Arnaud & Cormier, 2017." *International Journal of Transpersonal Studies*, 36(2), pp. 44–59.

61 Probably that earlier high energy condition was part of a recent euphoric springtime excitatory phase, which had now shifted into a dysphoric state.

Chapter 5

Classification

We will now examine the psychiatric conditions that most frequently occur after the onset of a PC. What do these so-called "mental illnesses" look *like*? How do they arise and take shape, what symptoms do they present, how can they be recognized? How many are there? We will also see how a transpersonal approach can make a difference in understanding, treating, accompanying, and alieviating them: how could we meaningfully group them according to a CP criterion?

These conditions rarely present as single, separate entities, but most often overlap with each other to varying degrees.

We will first present the individual pictures as presented by *mainstream psychiatry*, but then provide a *TP reading of* them.

5.1 Classification according to DSM-5

In the DSM-5[1], published by the *American Psychiatric Association (APA)*, 297 disorders or true diagnostic formal "syndromes" are listed, organized into approximately 20–22 chapters (macro-areas). These chapters reflect the main symptom dimensions or areas, such as schizophrenia spectrum disorders and other psychotic disorders, mood disorders (divided into depressive disorders and bipolar disorders), anxiety disorders, obsessive-compulsive and related disorders, personality disorders, neurocognitive disorders, and others.

Roughly speaking, the structure of the DSM-5 still reflects—at least in part—the dichotomy introduced by Emil Kraepelin between so-called schizophrenic "psychoses" (early dementia, schizophrenia, with their thought disorders), and mood disorders (manic-depressive, bipolar and depressive disorders).[2]

5.2 TP classification

In the TP perspective, it is Awakening and its clinical evolution that must be the main criterion for classification. As we have seen, Awakening is

DOI: 10.4324/9781003676461-5

the prime mover in the opening of CP, which very soon expresses different characteristics as it is characterized more by the first or second series of symptoms, in different proportions. Very soon, however, the third cluster of symptoms intervenes, complicating the picture, leading to chronicity and making the symptoms of the two previous clusters often recede into the background, thus conditioning the diagnosis, prognosis, and therapy.[3]

CPs thus differ and evolve differently, to the point that often when confronted with a specific clinical situation one hardly recognizes the common origin of mental suffering, and the forces that characterize these different evolutions.

What makes the psychiatric picture so specific depends fundamentally on two interacting factors.

On the one hand, the intensity of the awakening phenomenon and the accompanying energetic activation.

Here all possible variables are observed.[4] There are cases of awakening with *lightning intensity*, such that no one would be able to accommodate such brutal and shocking phenomena; at other times things are *more moderate,* leaving the subject time to adjust; these return in cycles that fade or are spaced further apart from each other, and things go differently. Still others have such moderate and gradual awakening and activation phenomena that they appear almost asymptomatic. There are also cases where the *Kundalini* is awakened since birth, perhaps already in utero.

On the other hand, the crucial factor is always the subject's unconscious or conscious resistance to the process.

The intensity of the process often leaves no alternative; not being ready for "death," one has no choice but to try to control the process resisting it, or to avoid it,[5] or finally even to escape but leaving a part behind, as in the forms of splitting.

This resistance is often reinforced by the resistance of the patient's social environment, family, society, psychiatrists, who manage these crises by trying to abate them, in order to normalize the situation.

When Awakening occurs in unprepared people, where ego-identification is still strong in the individual consciousness, the process usually ends up as a *medicalized psychiatric problem,* and will easily have an abortive course.[6]

5.3 Classification criteria

We too will partly follow Kraepelin's and MS psychiatry's proposal, that is, to recognize in the different clinical conditions *two prevailing tendencies,* different forms of presentation of Awakening, occurring in *persons differently unprepared* to integrate the transformation.

In the classification we will now propose, we will distinguish the syndromes according to the following criteria

- *Predominance of a series of symptoms* (*energetic or identity*, the first two components of CP).
- *Intensity of the process*, which will push the picture in the identity or energetic direction to different extremes, allowing us to distinguish milder syndromes from more severe syndromes, manifesting pictures with different characteristics.
- *The differentiated type and intensity of the third set of symptoms*, the ego in crisis reactions, which modifies the clinical symptomatology with the defense mechanisms of control or avoidance,[7] conditioning the PC evolution towards chronicity.

This way of proceeding *is useful both for diagnostic purposes*, i.e. for recognizing the type of process and its stage of maturation, *and for prognostic and therapeutic purposes*.

We will thus be able to examine and describe the specific features of the individual disorders in their various stages.

5.4 Classification

In this new classification we will therefore proceed according to the described criteria; *we will first identify the different types of PC* in the energetic or dissociative group, *at their onset*.

Then, in the same context, we will show (in the two series) the evolution of these syndromes once the *defensive organization comes into play, sometimes in a heavvy way (as in OCD): this resistance is a main factor in chronicization*, and appears to be present in virtually in all psychiatric conditions, but neurosis in particular.[8]

The individual conditions will then be catalogued *in the acute phase* (when the reactive component has not yet manifested itself or is not yet significantly organized), according to the criterion of the type of component giving rise to symptoms, that is, depending on whether the symptoms of the identity or energy crisis prevail: in the first case we will have *Depersonalization and Dissociative syndrome (DD), and Psychosis*; in the second we will have *Panic Attacks (PA),*[9] *and Bipolar Syndrome* (BD) when the intensity of the energetic activation increases. There are also pictures in which both components are involved, as in *schizoaffective disorders*.

In their evolution, the reactive component may prevail, causing the acute identity and energetic symptomatological series to take a *back* seat (or interact and somehow *merge* with the symptomatology resulting from the intense and organized egoic reaction).

In this evolution, when the clinical picture is dominated by the energetic activation, we will have the "avoidance disorder" of the energetic component: the Panic disorder (PD), on the one hand, or the obsessive "control disorder, which is more linked to the identity crisis (i.e., the *OCPD* and *OCD*), and the *Paranoias,* when the dissociation and fragmentation of identity is greater.

To sum up (see Table 5.1):

1. **Disorders with a predominantly energetic-affective component:**
   - SK, *Kundalini* syndrome, perceived as AP (panic attacks).
   - DAP (panic attack disorder), and other organized forms of anxiety disorder.
   - The BD (bipolar syndromes).
2. **Disorders with a predominantly identity crisis basis, or dissociative disorders**
   - Personality disorders.
   - Depersonalization and derealization syndrome.
   - OCD (obsessive compulsive disorder).
   - Dissociative psychosis.

There are some other clinically significant conditions that are not included in this list and that may nevertheless fit as *mixed conditions* into the general scheme just proposed.[10]

I will present some *clinical examples* to clarify the described syndromes. Finally, after presenting the symptomatology of each syndrome, *we will outline the therapy.*

This expository scheme can be summarized in Figure 5.1, where the three axes will correspond to the three components of PC: identity disorder, energetic disorder, reaction to these two; we will thus have a *three-dimensional* representation using *Cartesian axes.*

On the x-axis and y-axis we can represent the intensity of each clinicalpicture, acute or chronic, according to the greater expression of energy activation (on the x-axis) or identity crisis (y-axis), i.e. the two constituent components of PC.

On the z-axis we will represent the intensity of the egoic reaction.

We will thus have an idea at a glance *of the relative weight of each individual* component.

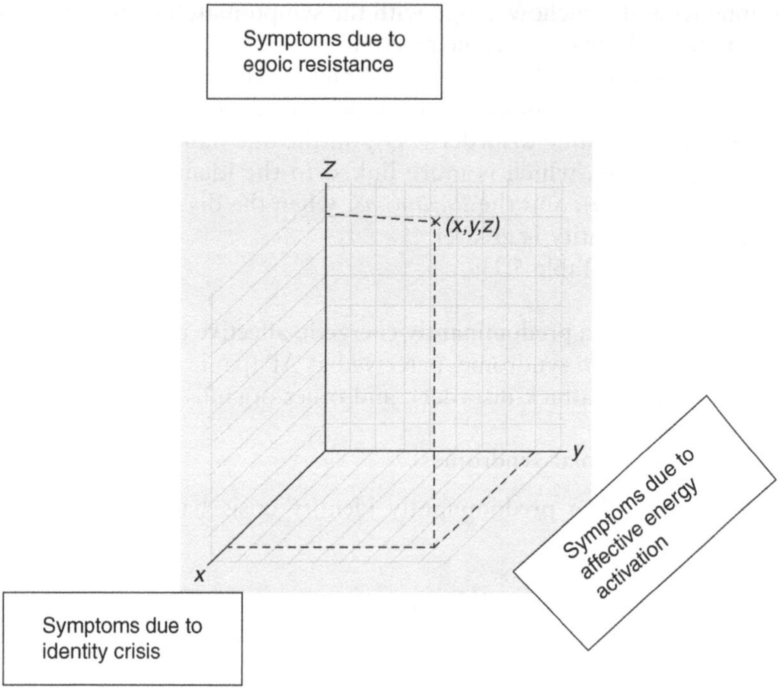

Figure 5.1 Components of the Psychiatric Crisis.

Notes

1 DSM, the *Diagnostic and Statistical Manual*, is the most widespread and widely followed classification of mental disorders, now in its 5th edition.
2 This also applies to the previous DSM-IV; it too listed 297 syndromes/formal disorders, and was organized into five axes (multiaxial system), where Axis I included most clinical disorders. We should note, however, that DSM-IV and DSM-5 also classify many other groups of disorders that do not fit neatly into either thought or mood disorders, with clinical overlaps between these large groups, leading to a more nuanced classification.
3 "I don't know, what do you think, Doc, does insanity have a measure? For example ... the way you can measure one's height, or fever?"
4 We could say that the Self, or God, does as it pleases, in awakening in its children: it awakens as and when it pleases, beyond the fact that one may be more or less prepared for it. See also James, "The Varieties of Religious Experience: A Study in Human Nature," from the Gifford Lectures given at Edinburgh University between 1901 and 1902.
5 Proverb: "Fleeing is not shameful, but life-saving." But Jesus also said: "Whoever loses his life will save it!"
6 *The ideal condition would be to be without opposition*, with nothing to save. When the consciousness is purified (*pure)*, unblemished (the obscuration due

to the separation principle that defiles the ego, immaculate), it is also "willing" for this ascent of energy towards Paradise. In such cases we can witness the birth of a new being, a birth of joy, a transformation from caterpillar to butterfly. Birth is not always painless, but neither is it always a pathology. In the Divine Comedy, Dante explains this point well, in the conclusion of Purgatory, which is precisely about purification, saying that at that point he has completed the process, and is thus *pure and willing to ascend to the stars*, where the stars are the stars within, the *Chakras*. Conversely, if "impure" and "unwilling" when this force is activated, things can go wrong.

7 Almost always, however, one can observe clinical pictures in which both control and avoidance strategies are present: control is in fact a form of avoidance, and systematic avoidance, on the other hand, provides a form of control.

8 *Neurosis is not always a less demanding condition than psychosis.* In fact, neurosis is often characterized by a more fierce resistance, perhaps due to a greater identification and strength of the ego, and/or a lesser intensity of the process; greater subjective suffering is often observed, although it seems less disruptive to the person's life (which is actually true, since the process is not fully activated).

Neurosis can sometimes heal in the form of *remission*; however, a true definitive healing will only be possible by overcoming the egoic defenses, with its surrender; therefore, it may sometimes be necessary to go through a temporarily heightened, sometimes even psychotic, condition of destructuration.

9 In the DSM, DAP is described at length. In DSM-IV Anxiety and Related Disorders, ODD and Stress Disorders were part of Anxiety Disorders, whereas in DSM-5 Anxiety Disorders, ODD and Related Disorders, and Disorders Related to Traumatic or Stressful Events are three separate categories. Furthermore, whereas in DSM-IV Panic Attack Disorder is found WITH and WITHOUT Agoraphobia, in DSM-5 Agoraphobia is now a comorbidity of DAP, and Agoraphobia is part of the Phobias and a separate category.

10 For example, *eating disorders,* which may fall under obsessive disorders, but have a strong anxiety component, *as is the case with anorexia*, but also *bulimia.*

Among these syndromes we also find energy-based *impulse dyscontrol* (similar to PA), such as *impulsive personality disorders*, which detect an unstable energetic-affective component, or *substance abuse disorders*, where an attempt is made to actively modify the energetic and consciential condition for egoic, defensive reasons, (hence energy disorders, but also identity disorders, and above all neurotic reactive disorders). These and other conditions will not be dealt with in detail yet, as here it is of interest to indicate a different way of framing cynicism, and not an exhaustive list of every condition of psychic distress.

Chapter 6

Disorders with a predominantly energetic-affective component

An initial symptomatic manifestation of energetic activation in the system is a state of *anxiety*. We could define anxiety as the subjective perception of an *unpleasant (ego distonic)* inner *tension.*

Tension actually occurs in the *subtle body* but is generally not recognized occurring at the energetic level. Being unconscious, it is often projected into the inner theatre of the mind (where emotions of conflict and danger are represented with thoughts and images), or onto the physical body (as somatization of tension), or interpersonally (as if it were something in the outside world generating anxiety or alarm)[1]

Tension arises from the conflict between the system's homeostasis—maintaining the *old regime* of activity and energy circulation (in the subtle channels and centers)—and a *new, higher-level energy* regime which requires change and adaptation, triggering defensive reactions to maintain previous homeostasis.

We can imagine it as a situation within us where a force is pushing against a resistance: as a consequence we perceive this conflict as the dust raised by the two fighting knights, i.e., anxiety.

Anxiety disorders are very common.[2] There are different psychiatric syndromes in which anxiety predominate: *here is how they* are *classified* in the most recent diagnostic manuals:

Generalized Anxiety Disorder,
Panic Disorder and Agoraphobia,
Social Phobia and Other Phobias,
Post-Traumatic Stress Disorder, and
OCD (Obsessive-Compulsive Disorder).[3]

Anxiety disorders are often associated with each other[4] and we shall rarely encounter them without the intervention of ego defenses.[5]

DOI: 10.4324/9781003676461-6

Anxiety disorders manifest with a series of *associated symptoms*, which vary according to the specific disorder, including:

> ***Physical symptoms*** *such as accelerated heartbeat, dizziness, hypervigilance, shortness of breath, and a feeling of air hunger. Nausea and stomach tension, diarrhea, irritable bowel syndrome. Sometimes associated with muscle tension, tremors, twitching, feeling of pain* or *muscle soreness, and other symptoms such as easy fatigability, sweating, headaches.*
>
> ***Psychic symptoms*** *such as difficulty sleeping, fear, agitation, tachycardia, mental confusion; restlessness, nervousness, irritability, difficulty in concentrating or a sense of mental emptiness are often present*

All anxiety disorders share characteristics of excessive *fear and anxiety.*[6] Panic is characterized by a sudden feeling of dread and imminent danger, in addition to a series of unpleasant and distressing physical sensations already mentioned.[7]

Anxiety sometimes presents itself in a more free-floating form, as "generalized anxiety," *at other times linked to* "specific" *situations,* or *more organized as a syndrome* (e.g., social phobia).

6.1 Generalized anxiety

Generalized anxiety disorder is characterized by "excessive anxiety and worry that occurs almost every day for at least six months," with respect to a series of events or activities. Characteristic of this condition is that the *intensity, duration,* or *frequency of anxiety is out of proportion* to the actual likelihood or impact of the expected event: people in these cases exhibit an exaggerated alarm response.

Such worries usually *significantly interfere* with functioning in social, work, or other important areas of life.

A common way of referring to the underlying state of anxiety is the word "stress."

This term refers to a subjective state of tension, worry, unexplained anxiety, usually attributed to external conditions (I am stressed because of work, marriage, etc.).[8]

6.2 Panic attacks (PA)

In the DSM, the description of the panic attack syndrome overlaps with the initial stages of KS, placing greater emphasis on subjective symptoms; or otherwise stated, in the PA the KS is a fundamental component.

The syndrome is characterized by abnormal intensification of energetic-affective symptoms, distinctly separate from generalized anxiety. We read in the DSM:

> *PA corresponds to intense apprehension, fear, or terror, peaking within ten minutes, often associated with feelings of imminent death. During these attacks there are symptoms such as shortness of breath or choking sensations; palpitations, heartbeat, or tachycardia; dyspnea; derealization; and fear of going mad or losing control.*
>
> *Panic attacks may be unplanned (and isolated), and then the onset of the attack is not associated with an environmental trigger, but rather occurs out of the blue; or situation-related, and then the panic attack almost invariably occurs immediately after exposure to or in anticipation of the situational trigger. Finally, they may be situation-sensitive, and then the panic attack is more likely to occur after exposure to a situational trigger, but is not invariably associated with it.*
>
> *The frequency and severity of panic attacks varies widely. For example, some individuals present moderately frequent attacks (e.g., once a week) that occur regularly for months. Others report short series of more frequent attacks (e.g., daily for one week) separated by periods of weeks or months without attacks or with less frequent attacks (e.g., two every month) for many years.*

6.2.1 Clinical examples of KS also described as panic attack

"I wasn't like this before, I was sunny, slowly I got worse. Then work and people started to bother me, I would feel sweaty, cold and hot, and I would and feel hot flashes rising, especially after the menopause. And I often have an internal tremor, in my stomach a discomfort and a feeling of vomiting, a pounding in my heart ... but nothing wrong for the cardiologist. And in my throat, like one unable to breathe, whose breath gets blocked; and when I can't breathe, sometimes my ears ring; and I feel confusion: when this happens, I don't understand anything, I forget things..; it's not that I have dementia ...."

"It's been a while that I'm not well, 'I get strange', that's why then the accident happened to me: basically, I was driving but I wasn't looking at the road, it may be that if there hadn't been the bend I would have just gone straight. This happens to me often, even at work: my head is somewhere else, and I barely even know where I am. The attacks come to me suddenly, I get dizzy, and I get cold, sweaty and panicky."

"I go to bed late, but I don't sleep well, because I don't fall asleep, or then I wake up with a startle and my heart beats faster, like a panic attack, and I'm not quiet and I think about it all the time and I wake up at night ... when I go back inside the house I feel something from inside that rises up inside my head, I don't know what it is, and at times I get these crying bouts again ..."

6.2.1.1 Differences and overlap between PA and KS

A *panic attack* (PA) is a sudden, intense crisis dominated by acute anxiety and strong physical symptoms (palpitations, shortness of breath, sweating, trembling, choking, fear of dying or going mad, derealization and depersonalization). The episode culminates quickly and usually lasts from a few minutes to half an hour. The condition is experienced mainly as a physical or psychic threat and the person only wishes for the crisis to end, often without recognizing a possible transformative dimension.

In a PA, the perceived fear corresponds to this feeling of energetic expansion of the system, seen from the ego's point of view, to which the ego would prefer not be subject to.[9]

The first panic attack manifests in an ego that often has no idea what is happening *feels like it is dying*: more often than not, these are people who are completely unprepared for the massive change that is rapidly unfolding and imposing itself.[10]

In *Kundalini Syndrome* (KS), on the other hand, recurrent and more prolonged energy crises are observed, often linked to intense spiritual

Table 6.1 Differential Diagnosis PA/KS

Aspect	*Panic attack (PA)*	*Kundalini Syndrome (KS)*
Physical symptoms	Acute anxiety, palpitations, sweating, tremors	Tremors, spasms, intense energy sensations along the spine, altered senses
Duration	Short, isolated episode (minutes)	Recurrent, cyclical, often longer episodes
Internal experience	Strong fear, panic, experienced as emergency	Transformative crisis, experienced as "energetic process," sometimes also ecstasy
Origin	Often associated with stress, trauma, partial awakening	Intense spiritual practice, existential crisis, deep energetic awakening
Awareness	Perceived as physical/ psychic threat	Possible symbolic/spiritual insight, experience of growth/ transformation

practices or deep existential crises. Here, anxiety symptoms are accompanied by marked energetic phenomena (tremors, spasms, sensations of heat/energy along the spine, spontaneous movements, altered senses) and changes in the state of consciousness. The crisis is experienced not only with anxiety and confusion, but also as a possible inner transformation or spiritual awakening. There is often a partial ability to reflect on the symbolic meaning of the experience.

One could say that *the PA can be seen as the beginning or prodromal phase of what may become a KS*, but it is distinguished from it by its short duration and reversibility; in the KS the energetic-affective experience is more intense and dominant and can lead to growth. Sometimes, over time and the recurrence of acute crises, *AP evolves into SK* and a more conscious awakening.[11]

6.3 The panic disorder (PD)

PD is a very common disorder nowadays, particularly in Western populations.

It could be estimated that *ten per cent* of the population has had, will have, or has an ongoing PD. Let us see how the official description insists on the chronic nature of the picture:

> *The essential feature of Panic Disorder is the presence of recurrent, unexpected Panic Attacks, followed by at least one month of persistent worry of having another Panic Attack, worry about the possible implications or consequences of the Panic Attacks, or a significant change in behavior related to the attacks (Criterion A).*[12]
>
> *Individuals with Panic Disorder show characteristic concerns or interpretations about the implications or consequences of Panic Attacks. Some fear that the attacks indicate the presence of an undiagnosed, life-threatening illness (e.g. heart disease, epilepsy). Despite repeated medical examinations and reassurance, they may remain fearful and convinced that they have a life-threatening illness. Others fear that panic attacks indicate that they are* "going crazy" *or losing control, or that they are emotionally weak.*
>
> *Some individuals with recurrent Panic Attacks significantly change their behavior (e.g., stop a job) in response to the attacks, but deny the fear of having another attack or worries about the consequences of their Panic Attacks. Worry about the next attack or its implications is often associated with the development of avoidance behavior.* [13]
>
> DMS-5 (2013)

Some individuals are able to expose themselves to feared situations, but endure them with considerable fear. Often the individual is more capable of confronting a feared situation when he or she is with a *companion.*

As we have now made clear, anxiety typically results in *habitual tendency to avoidance* of a variety of situations; for example, *being away from home alone, being in a crowd, traveling in a car, bus, or aeroplane, or being on a bridge or in a lift.*

The individual's avoidance of situations can be a very *disabling* factor in itself; for example, it can impair the ability to go to work or carry out household chores (e.g., shopping, taking children to the doctor).

6.3.1 Psychodynamics of PD

Panic Disorder is dominated by the preventive avoidance of a possible panic attack.

What counts most to the person is being to escape, avoidance. The priority is to save one's life, to maintain egoic equibrium contrasting with that which destabilizes it.[14]

Thus, in a way, *PD* can be regarded as a *control disorder*, in some respects similar to OCD).

Control syndromes are *defensive but also, and above all, offensive strategies*, a preventive activation of egoic defenses, aimed at warding off future threats, a condition that is quite different from the initial assault experienced at the time of the first PA.

We are dealing here with *fear of fear*, i.e. a compulsive mental mechanism of avoidance and manipulation of external or internal situations that may be considered dangerous for the system. Unlike the acute panic attack, panic disorder therefore represents an organized activation of psychic defenses: a massive, intense, long-lasting activation, which becomes an integral part of the personality.

These defenses quickly become a kind of psychic prison, and are quite energy-consuming; yet this condition represents the lesser evil for the ego, which is unwilling to succumb.[15]

As we have seen, *the consequences of a PA depend greatly on the degree of purification of the subject's consciousness*; who may still be unaware of itself, may still—in this sense—be "sleeping," that is, may still be identified with the body-mind complex, with the "me."

In people still very much identified with the ego, PAs are only perceived as a threat, a destabilization whose meaning is not understood, and are therefore ego-dystonic.

We will thus often see these patients engage in a dramatic and extreme *defensive and aggressive policy*, a war of resistance against their own transformational energy: every abnormal energy movement, emotion, or thought is interpreted as dangerous. The patient therefore reacts with alarm, and persists in believing in the reality of the defensive interpretations, produced by the mind, a deception.[16]

This state of alarm is also *self-feeding*: each new symptom or sensation is interpreted as confirmation of danger, reinforcing the erroneous belief and maintaining the disorder.

The physical and psychic reactions, due to the altered energetic condition, can be amplified by the morbid attention of the frightened subject, generating anticipatory anxiety that feeds *the vicious circle of fear of being afraid*, which spirals into ever greater panic.[17]

When, on the other hand, the subject is better prepared to perceive and correctly identify these sensations, they may interpret them as simple energy movements, and not judge them as overly threatening, recognizing their true nature.[18]

6.4 Bipolar disorder (BD) and depression

Bipolar disorder is a condition characterized by a marked alteration in *mood*. Often preceded by one or more PAs, or a KS, this syndrome is a much more challenging and disruptive alteration for the patient's ordinary life, both in terms of intensity, duration, and reactivations (termed "relapses") of the process.

The altered regime of the energetic–affective system[19] lasts several months at each reactivation, and typically tends to occur seasonally.[20]

BD is thus a disorder in which energy phenomena and mood disorders predominate in a cyclic manner.[21]

Kraepelin was the first to distinguish serious psychiatric disorders into two broad categories[22]: that of thought disorders, later called schizophrenias by Bleuler, and that of mood disorders (manic depressive psychoses).[23] Identity disorders in BD are of minor importance and possibly appear later than the most acute phase.

In DSM-5, mood disorders have been divided into two distinct categories according to the type of phase they present: *Depressive Disorders and Bipolar Disorders*.

> The subject presents one or more periods of extreme sadness and loss of interest in life and one or more periods of exaltation, high energy and often irritability, with periods of relatively normal mood between episodes.[24]

In *Major Depression (or Unipolar)*, the person manifests only depressive symptoms and alternates periods of euthymic well-being with depressive phases, without manic aspects.

In the BD, (bipolar), moments of mood depression alternate with moments of mood elevation.

When depressive phases alternate with mania, one speaks of bipolar type I.

When, on the other hand, depressive phases alternate with hypomanic episodes, one speaks of Type II Bipolar Disorder.[25]

The depressive phase alternates, as we have seen, with a (hypo) manic phase that follows or precedes it; sometimes can also have "*mixed*" characteristics, when (hypo) manic and depressive symptoms are present at the same time.[26]

6.4.1 *Major depression*[27]

It corresponds to a depressive episode lasting at least two weeks, with depressed mood nearly all day, nearly every day (or in children/adolescents, irritability), or marked loss of interest or pleasure in nearly all activities. To diagnose major depression, other symptoms, such as agitation, insomnia, or disturbances, must also be present.[28] The syndrome must involve clinically significant distress or impairment in social, occupational, or other important areas of functioning.[29]

6.4.2 *Bipolar disorder*

As we see from the definition, in its typical form BD exhibits an imbalance in the mood pattern of a *sinusoidal* type. In its more typical form, *active episodes* (of depression and mania or hypomania) are followed by a *dysphoric phase* (mixed excitatory and depressive) and a longer *depressive phase*.[30]

An *intercritical asymptomatic phase* follows, generally depending on seasonal reactivation or quiescence of the process.[31] Less often, the intercritical period is very brief or absent, and there is a direct "switching" into the opposite phase.[32]

Manic episodes typically have a rapid onset (hours or days), but may evolve over several weeks.[33] An untreated manic episode lasts on average about three months, with great variability; the depressive phase may last roughly twice as long. In cases with two cycles per year the first episode may overlap with the second. The duration of the overall cycle is very variable, generally months or weeks.

The *restitutio ad integrum*[34] which generally followed the acute phase, was one of the prognostic elements that differentiated these conditions from schizophrenic forms: in the latter, *restitutio* was much less likely and less complete; the identity crisis was in these cases in the foreground from the outset, and the energetic manifestations in the background.[35]

Since BD and depression have the same genesis, that is, a mood disorder, we will discuss these conditions dealing with BD.

6.4.2.1 *Causes*

Generally, BD is activated by *endogenous* causes; a biological cause for MS psychiatry, a spiritual endogenous crisis in the TP view; pyschiatric crisis (PC) activates *Kundalini*, whose activation, intensity, and flow generate this specific oscillating energetic syndrome. The oscillation seems due to *Kundalini* circulating hyperactively in the lateral channels, insisting on the still partially impeded ascent in the central channel.[36]

Given this endogenous predisposition, certain situations are known to easily trigger BD (or promote its reactivation). Let's look at them:

- *External traumatic situations*, and psychological reactions to them; for example, accidents, coma states, surgery (anesthesia may play a part here), moving, retirement, divorce, physical illness, etc.
- Again, attention must be paid to any use of *psychoactive substances* (especially amphetamines, cocaine, and cannabis used on a continuous basis), which often precipitatethe emergence of an endogenous cycle, or instead to the use of *psychoactive drugs* in the course of organic illnesses, such as cortisone, or chemotherapy.
- *Iatrogenic activations*, i.e. due to medical treatment, certainly include the inexpert and untimely use of certain psychoactive drugs, especially the old tricyclic antidepressants.[37]
- *Menopause can trigger a first crisis*, but more often reactivates a BD which had been quiet for some time.
- *Pregnancy or abortions*, or a combination of these: the so-called post pregnancy depression is a typical case of misdiagnosed energy disturbance in the system, due to hormonal imbalances in a predisposed situation or terrain.[38]

After activation, the *process develops in* fairly recognisable and quite different *successive stages*, which we will now describe.

6.4.2.2 *Phases of the process*

1 First phase: Euphoria (flying, rising)

Generally the process begins with an excitatory phase, which must be promptly detected at its onset. Like a tide rising over weeks and months, it is generally co-ordinated with *the spring equinox*, almost like an energetic tide rising rapidly, most often over a few weeks.

This onset of arousal in the spring may show variation: sometimes it starts as early as the winter solstice, when the light grows; other times it appears to manifest itself in the summer, or even autumn; this may be due to several factors, among which are the rate at which the process matures, delayed recognition of the initial signs, double cyclicity in spring and autumn, and/or medication.

As a definition, the excitatory episode is first called *hypomanic then manic*. For the DSM:

> *The manic episode is a defined period of abnormally and persistently elevated, expansive or irritable mood lasting at least 1 week.*

A diagnosis of BD can be made if during the period of mood alteration, *three (or more) of the following symptoms* were persistent and present at a significant level:

- Increased self-esteem or grandiosity.
- Decreased need for sleep (e.g., feeling rested after only 3 hours of sleep).
- Increased talkativeness to usual, or continuous urge to talk.
- Flight of ideas or subjective experience that thoughts follow one another rapidly.
- Distractibility (i.e. attention is too easily diverted by unimportant or irrelevant external siimoles).
- Increased purposeful activity (work, school, sexual) or psychomotor agitation.
- Excessive involvement in playful activities that have a high potential for harmful consequences (e.g., excessive buying, unseemly sexual behavior, reckless business investment).[39]

The *Pre-morbid personality* (i.e. the state prior to the critical episode) is often within the normal range, sometimes with a tendency toward low mood (such as shyness, negative emotionality, lack of fluidity in relationships, poor validity and efficiency). At other times, however, we find a hyperemotional pre-morbid personality, tending towards liveliness, with an above-average ability to perceive emotional subtleties; however, not a pathological or negatively altered personality. Frequently patients regularly used cannabis or other substances for mood regulation, such as alcohol.

Clinical example: Woman, thirty years old, married; active worker, psychiatric familiarity.[40] Lately she started to be hyperactive, justifying this as due to external demands, excessive in her emotional expressions, inflated: she started to open up to increasing social activity, to hang out with more people, go dancing, talk a lot; this condition grew, she started to feel more active energy, to feel as good as she had ever felt. She was over-working, and thought this was responsible for her crisis; but it probably was the other way round, her manic phase made her work too much. She would also think a lot, unstoppably.

She began to sleep less, waking up several times a night, or early in the morning; she'd then sleep only a few hours (very few, even only two hours), or not sleep for days in a row. As the process grew higher, she became very emotional, sensitive, reacting more vividly to the world, feeling very much alive. She started spending money, too much and without good judgement, to write, create, to travel ...

In short, *euphoria grows*, and tends to lead towards an exponential excess, which soon becomes of a different quality, i.e. *dysphoric* as we shall see.

The patient appears to have *inexhaustible energy*, and recharges immediately; *the initially hypo-manic picture quickly* (within hours or days, most often a few weeks) *becomes manic.*

The process is generally ego-syntonic, the patient believes he has finally found his true self, he perceives an improvement in his condition.

It is important to evaluate at the time of diagnosis at what stage of the curve of energy increase the patient is.

At this stage, the patient seldom admits being in an altered state, and desires to remove obstacles (which he believes to be external) to the development of his many activities, refusing all proposals of help or containment.

2 Second phase: Increasing euphoria and dysphoria (*flying too near the Sun, and starting to go off track*)

The process tends to intensify, often over the course of only a few days, or more often weeks (rarely months, but its duration can be considerably reduced if treated promptly and appropriately).

It usually becomes rapidly uncontainable, showing its true nature, i.e. a state of alteration; signs of excess, of *discontrol, of imbalance* begin to appear.

This phase is often still ego syntonic: the patient is happy to have this great energy charge and does not want to reduce it.[41]

In this initial euphoric phase," the patient continues to deny being in an altered state, and refuses remarks and help aimed at protecting him, his family, his work. He considers these concerns exaggerated, inappropriate, or even motivated by bad intentions.

As a result, it becomes increasingly difficult to help the patient; as the process grows, the state of arousal rises beyond the threshold of reasonableness, and it is very difficult to intervene to calm the waters, except by force, when no other options remain.

The patient still retains a residue of control, however; he still manages, for example, to conceal at least in certain situations his alteration; for example, he may behave in an altered manner with family members, but if they then call the police, he then becomes calm, responds adequately and denies any strangeness, and so it is difficult to intervene.

In the meantime, the negative, *dangerous potential grows*, both on the outer and inner side, preparing the next stage.

The process rapidly evolves into a phase in which *control has almost completely disappeared* and can no longer be masked or rationalized; also all those who surround him (family, friends, colleagues) at this stage become aware of the alteration, and try to intervene, proposing medication, which is almost always refused.

Weeks or months may pass since the initial hypomanic phase becomes mature and reaches the dysphoric state, where subjective discomfort becomes stronger.

The new uncontainable phase will at first be evident objectively, through behavior, accidents, quarrels, and confusion. The patient, however, also begins to see what he was refusing to see, to realize he's out of control; he begins to feel *dysphoric*, i.e., restless, uneasy, alarmed, and only at this point the situation begins to *become ego-dystonic.*

This awareness in the patient is fleeting and superficial yet, but at times it makes it possible to gain his cooperation and introduce medication or propose containment in a safer place.

Generally though, it will be difficult for the patient to open to therapy, more likely he will sink further and further in his descent into hell.

In this phase of excess and disharmony, *the patient generally becomes emotionally unstable*, irritable, sometimes explosive, distorts and misinterepts situations out of emotional clouding. He may experiment *emotional states of fear*, or sometimes even real *panic* attacks, which begin to worry him. The excess of mental speed often becomes *mental confusion*, and he cannot focus well on things, he is no longer able to reason normally, coldly, to conclude affairs, to manage personal relationships adequately. He gives himself explanations that are not adequate to reality. He may show excessive sexual behavior, promiscuousness, he may express inadequately his anger, or steal, spend, have car accidents, disturb public authorities.

He becomes frankly dysfunctional compared to the previous euphoric phase. He may come to believe and say that he is severely *depressed,* while the excitatory phase is still in full swing,[42] or he becomes frankly *paranoid,* because of the anxiety, uncoordinatedness, confusion, and interpretations generated by this state. He might believe, for instance, that people who are concerned about his state, who would like to take care of him, to help him, actually do so out of envy, or malice. He might then become suspicious, even fly into a rage with increasing ease, even exaggeratedly, whenever their altered state is mentioned, saying that he is not crazy, it is others who are, or more probably ill-intentioned.

In this more active phase, the patient often starts activating *defensive avoidance strategies* in order to cope with the increasing chaotic and paranoid conditions he experiences in his inner and outer world: he may *isolate* himself, feeling that he has no support and confirmation around him, withdraw from his environment, making intervention even more difficult.

Insomnia, often already present in the initial activation phase, is almost invariably present in the euphoric phase, and often worsens in this later dysphoric phase, becoming an additional risk factor: the patient is always accelerated, but now in a negative sense, putting himself or others in dangerous situations; at night he sometimes has distressing houghts, which he magnifies, and does not exercise lucid criticism on. The patient is rather "out of his mind."[43]

However this second phase unfolds, and becomes more and more evident, it *begins to be regarded as pathological, by the patient's family, friends, and finally, typically, by the patient himself*, and leads to a request for help.

3 Third phase: Psychosis *(from bad to worse)*

A further clinical worsening is observed in some patients in this third and final phase. *There is a further increase in energetic, fire activity*. It is at this stage that the process may veer into psychosis, with *distortions of psychic and sense-perceptual functions* becoming the main disturbance.

Delusions and hallucinations may occur, and there is *marked identity deconstruction*, which in the earlier or moderate intensity phases was scarcely evident.[44]

Individual reactions also escalate here: what was previously ego-dystonic, now turns into terror. The energy flow is such that the ego is overwhelmed, confusion is at its peak; the mind is completely confused and at points completely incapacitated, and the ego responds with extreme reactions, or defenses. Patients at this stage often become suicidal, as the suffering is completely unbearable.[45]

4 Last phase, depression (*landing and sinking*)

After the excitatory phase, there is a generally gradual decline, due to various reasons, including the fact that the active seasonal phase has passed; decrease without medication may require months, but with therapy may be managed in weeks.

Also, if medication was already being used in the previous phase, it may now be experienced as a burden or as causing excessive slowing, and dosages in this phase of decreasing energy should be lowered and re-modulated.

This leads to the true depressive phase, characterized by low energy activity, the opposite phase of the excitatory sinuisodal curve.

The patient is drained, abulic, apathetic, mildly dysphoric, scarcely active; everything seems heavy, slow, and useless to him.

This phase usually lasts longer than the excitatory phase, although there are exceptions; moreover, when the excitatory phase is treated, the subsequent depressive phase is usually shallower and shorter.

5 Evolution

We are all aware that our affective energy system fluctuates physiologically over time, according to the seasons, the time of day. In winter, some animals *hibernate*, and spring is the *mating season.* The world physiologically oscillates between two balanced poles.[46]

The cyclical oscillation of the affective energy system in mental disorders is no exception to the rule, and everyone recognizes the *seasonal variations of nervous disorders*: this applies both to panic attacks and to psychotic crises. Mental disorders follow a cyclical course, an intelligent, predictable alternation.

To help balance these imbalances, we therefore need to take into account how nature moves, to tune in with it and accompany the *vis sanatrix naturae.* As Hippocrates said: "The physician treats, but it is nature that heals."

In bipolar syndrome, the primary disturbance is that the system oscillates in a more evident and specific manner, with a predictable, typical cyclicity: it oscillates in a pathological, altered, dysfunctional, unbalanced manner, thus generating the symptoms of hyper- and hypofunctioning. This is precisely where and when and how we can and should intervene.

The first onset or subsequent relapses of the excitatory phase usually occur in spring, in correlation with the Earth's electromagnetic phase variation, and in nature with the period from the winter solstice to the spring equinox. Some crises begin around Christmas time, most occur in March–April, with the Easter period being the most sensitive period.[47]

Even though the process shows an andogenous disposition to cycle, certain factors favor first crises or relapses, like substance abuse, inadequate psychiatric medication, menopause, abortions, or a combination of these.[48]

Clinical vigilance and experience are needed to recognize properly the beginning of the excitatory phases, which then initiates and maintains the cyclic nature of this syndrome.[49]

As time passes and relapses occur, *the cyclic pattern tends to change:* the most typical form is the one episode per year, generally in spring; frequently reactivation may skip one or more years before reoccurring. Episodes tend to be more distanced though, and eventually the syndrome tends to subside or extinguish.

Also, the excitatory and depressive phases become progressively less clear-cut and distinguishable, and so-called "mixed" states, emerge more prominently, in which excitement and depression are present at the same time, where we have both the active, aggressive, agitative component, and the abulic, negative passive, black, or dull side.[50]

Furthermore, there is a phenomenon of reinforcement or impediment between phases. There are cases with phases that in time reactivate or recur earlier or later in the year, cases in which the oscillation becomes more frequent, with several phases in a year, or even within a single day (*so-called rapid-cycling forms*).

In all this, *drug treatment has a great influence*, since used wisely it is very effective in preventing the reactivation of the active phase. Moreover, medication alters the phase, sometimes flattening and prolonging it, sometimes modifying it in other ways, so that a syndrome under treatment will look different both in the current phase as well as in its further course.

Relapses become in this case more rare, less intense, more blurred, to the point they may possibly even become silent if treated properly at the right time.

This is related also to treating consecutive recurrences so that a treated crisis tends to recurr less often or more mildly, and untreated crises tend to relapse with more probability and intensity.

Phase change sometimes evolves gradually, but sometimes it is *abrupt*, to the point that one needs great clinical experience and intuition to predict it: this possibility and its rapidity is often underestimated. An experienced psychiatrist or psychologist, however, can in most cases *recognize the phase change*. A history of previous episodes will greatly help in predicting possible reactivation and give information on the rapidity of onset of previous relapses.

In the phase in which the mood changes from excitatory to depressive, or from depressive back to normal, an *interlude* is frequently observed in which *symptoms of the OCD spectrum appear*, as thoughts and behaviors centered on control, and the appearance of negative intrusive or self-damaging thoughts, which usually recede over time. This can occur even in the absence of a premorbid obsessive personality, as an attempt to restore an ego-centered control over inner and outer conditions, which were overwhelmed during the excitatory phase.

6.4.3 Clinical observations

6.4.3.1 Diagnosis and illness awareness

An experienced psychiatrist will make an in-depth anamnesis and diagnostic investigation in order to orientate intervention and educational advice to the family. He will begin by gathering informations on how the disorder presented itself in previous seasons, so as to recognize precipitating factors (e.g. substance use), and to have information on the rapidity of the phase change of the sinusoidal wave, in the previous year(s). The psychiatrist will seek information on previous treatment attempts, in the current episode and in earlier ones, so as to know what interventions have been made and with what results. He will try to asses how much the patient is aware and will participate in therapy.

Since the process is endogenous, i.e. it is activated and moves from within, *patients (especially at the beginning) are not aware of it, and lack clear insight into being ill.*

It thus happens that in this phase (but often later as well) the projections that the patient makes on the world around him prevail. Since *what is unconscious is projected,* he generally believes that the destabilizing, anxiogenic stress factors come from outside.[51]

Family and helpers also often attribute the triggering of the active phase to external factors.

However, after the first crisis, the recurrence of the process generally favors an *increasing awareness* on the part of the patient and his *entourage*, who recognize the endogenous and cyclical nature of the process.

6.4.3.2 Comorbidity

Psychiatric comorbidity is extremely common in bipolar disorder. More than half of BD patients have an additional diagnosis, one of the most difficult to manage being obsessive-compulsive disorder (OCD).

The majority of BD-OCD patients experienced the onset of OCD prior to the onset of BD and presented higher prevalence of family history for mood disorders versus non-BD-OCD patients. Moreover, comorbid BD and OCD cycle together, with OC symptoms often remitting during manic/hypomanic episodes.[52]

Treating BD-OCD patients remains a great challenge. Though serotonin reuptake inhibitors (SRIs) are the first-line treatment for OCD, they can induce mood instability in BD, especially if administered at high doses and maintained for a long time.[53]

6.4.3.3 Prognosis and treatment

The predominantly pharmacological treatment of these syndromes *requires early intervention at their onset*, in order to rebalance the affective energy "system," protect the patient in the current phase and modulate the worsening oscillatory course of the phases in the following seasons.

The sooner one is able to intervene on the rising spring wave, for example, the less the risk of getting into out-of-control situations that can be dangerous for oneself and for others. The sooner the intervention, and the modulation of excess fire calms, the sooner the patient can regain control of the situation and return to normal.

If treatment is not instituted in this very first phase, there is *at least* some hope to *propose it in the second, increasingly euphoric* phase, since in this phase the patient generates an impressive amount of problems, for himself and for others, because of the excess of energy that overwhelms him and often makes compulsory treatment necessary.

Finally, it will certainly be even more necessary to *treat the subsequent dysphoric phase*, also because of the risk potential it entails.

In cases treated at an early stage, there is certainly a much greater likelihood, once in pure BD the acute phase has been dealt with, that the patient will be able to resume his ordinary family and social life. The pharmacological rebalancing of these altered waves of energy, often connected to seasonal changes, leads to an objective improvement in mental symptomatology, which often rebalances impressively fundamentally affecting the short-term prognosis.[54]

When, on the contrary, the intervention is delayed, or the intensity of the process very strong, the course may result in an often only partial, slow recovery, leaving after the crisis a residue of alteration, which may even stratify further with each relapse, leading to conditions of permanent disability.[55]

It has been argued that long-term use of high doses of psychotropic drugs could entail significant side effects at the physical, psychological, and relational levels. This may even be considered a factor favoring relapse and, ultimately, an impediment to real recovery from this condition.

Robert Whitaker, for example, reports studies that open a debate on the issue. He argues that the standard clinical practice of administering high doses over a long period of time to patients with acute psychosis may paradoxically worsen long-term outcomes, suggesting that some 40 per cent or more of schizophrenic patients may have a better course without the continued use of such drugs.[56]

6.5 Therapy

6.5.1 Psychotropic drugs

Compliance of the patient with psychotropic drugs is the main obstacle in managing manic phases it is very difficult to help the patient help himself. Compliance tends to improve only when the patient passes from the euphoric phase to the disphoric one, and the subjective condition becomes ego-dystonic, unpleasant, to the point where the person admits that perhaps there is something wrong.

At this point family members often intervene with treatment and pressure, at other times it is the patient himself, due to the increasing overall discomfort within himself and in his world of relationships, who comes to collaborate, manages to undergo treatment, and thus reduces the prolonged state of discomfort. They may turn visit to a neurologist,[57] or to a psychiatrist who will recommend psycho-pharmacological therapy.[58] It is very important that the therapist, the caregiver, the psychiatric service, and family members be prepared to grasp this opening in time and make use of it to initiate treatment, without which things often degenerate.[59]

It is therefore necessary to *inform and educate the patient and the family* - for example in the intercritical phase following the acute phase - about how to manage these situations in the event of relapse. If, in critical phases the patient receives from their environment (partner, workplace, physician, children, friends) a balanced response, neither reactive nor dramatizing but congruent with the situation, he may, as he feels worse and worse, find around him the right terrain to let them institute therapy.

It is in the *third phase,* however, that interventions, required by the surrounding people or the authorities, are most often implemented. In the most intense and severe cases, the intervention of *hospitalization* is sometimes the only best solution: in the best scenario, this could be a voluntary admission, if the patient cooperates, though ambivalently.[60]

In the worst scenario, though, one will have to *forcefully intervene* when things reach extreme, life-threatening limits for the patient or those around them, artificially creating that forced entry into therapy which is compulsory psychiatric admission. The patient, unaware of their illness and uncooperative, must often be forcefully restrained, and this will remain in their memory as a traumatic experience adding to his or her internal disruption.

Pharmacological psychiatric intervention therefore represents the first necessary step to be instituted to change the worsening course of endogenous events. Psychotropic drugs (a major or minor sedative, and a mood stabilizer) can in appropriate proportions and doses calm, attenuate, and stabilise excitatory phases, prevent relapses, and completely - or at least significantly - control the subjective and objective symptoms of distress and alteration with relatively limited side effects if used appropriately.

Pharmacological intervention can reduce and stabilize the out-of-control energy wave, which was impossible before the discovery of these drugs, and must be modulated in relation to the variations in the clinical phases that the patient goes through. One will have to guide, i.e. change the treatment, according to the the course of the process. *In the long term* it is suggested to try to scale down or discontinue neuroleptics when clinically possible to avoid chronification of the condition.

6.5.2 Psychotherapy

Appropriate psychotherapeutic intervention is essential to improve the prognosis of BD.

In the acute phase, it is impossible to intervene with transformational psychotherapy; in this phase, intervention should be limited to supportive therapy and psychoeductive interventions on the patient and his/her environment. However, a TP psychotherapy will have a better chance of being accepted and used by the patient, even in the first stages. Meanwhile, medication will help to contain the picture and allow better conditions for interviews.

There are *two opposing risks* in the psychological approach to a BD:

1. A first risk is under- or over-evaluating the importance of the endogenous
there is the risk of psychologizing the picture, searching for psychological past or present causes for the disturbance, and underestimating the endogenous drive for change. Psychotropic drugs are often seen in a negative light by psychogenetically oriented psychologists but also by current TP psychologists; they maintain that chemicals would restrain the process only to abate it, when it should be understood and accepted.

However, there is also the opposite risk, that of dramatizing, exaggerating the endogenous symptomatology: for example, in relapse phases there is often a tendency to make an elephant out of a mouse. Once a crisis has occurred, one could defensively interpret any minor abnormality as a certain sign of relapse into a major crisis. Every hint of erratic, histrionic behavior, every even moderate excess, even an outburst of joy or crying that would otherwise be considered very normal, is traced back to the most serious and traumatic events already seen in the past. The patient will then live in a sanitary cage, due to the family and sometimes *social stigma*, that remains on him even when the crisis is over and even with a positive outcome.[61]

2. However, a second risk is to do the same with psychotherapy
There is a risk of under evaluating psychotherapy, as sometimes biologically oriented psychiatrists do, considering only the biochemical side of psychiatric syndromes; treating them with chemicals is not the whole job.

-Psychotherapy may be essential to *accompany and sustain and comfort psychologically patients going through a PC,* in the deconstruction and opening up, in their fear of losing their way and falling; this is essential especially in the acute phase, going through their dark night of the soul. It is also fundamental to sustain and clarify the opening up of new opportunities, new horizons, and change.

People going through PC are in fact in a very open and vulnerable condition, and often very open to psychological and psychotherapeutic relationship. They i*nvest a lot in the person who helps them* as a doctor or as a psychologist, even as a guide in their dark night.

Often, even in the pre-crisis phase, they were among the most sensitive people; but during the labor phase of PC they become much more so.[62]

Psychotherapy is *crucial also in clarifying, in sustaining cooperation*, for example pharmacological *compliance*. A good relationship with the patient can also be essential in *diagnosing*, that is in understanding and interpreting symptoms, in evaluating phases.

A good relationship with the patient can help to *manage medication* during the crisis, to gather clues on the cure, on the change of clinical phases, to be able to follow the patient over time, to listen, to respond, to participate in the process. This is of particular importance in the dysphoric phase, in order to intervene and convince the patient that he needs assistance, help, even pharmacological treatment; one can do this explaining to the patient that he is not crazy, that he only needs treatment.

This relationship is also valuable for *educating the patient and family*, providing non-judgemental information about his disorder, giving the tools to identify the stages of his disorder, to detect in time future possible re-activations of the process. This will allow a better cooperation in the treatment, and improve overall compliance.[63]

Notes

1 When people say they are *stressed* by some situation, internal or external, they are referring to the experience of discomfort and tension they feel, which is due to a conflict that they do not recognize as being internal and energetic, before being mental. In this sense, external or internal conflict factors are merely con-causes, acting as projection sites for subjective difficulties and tensions.

2 Globally, it is estimated that, approximately 4.5% of the world's population has experienced an anxiety disorder. In Italy, approximately 14% of the population has suffered from anxiety disorders in the past year. The lifetime prevalence (i.e., the percentage who will experience an anxiety disorder at least once during their lifetime) is between 16% and 34%. They are more common in women than in men (2/1). In Western societies, this figure is significantly higher than in other populations. For phobias, the prevalence is 11.3%.

3 Some consider OCD as as part of the spectrum of anxiety disorders. While acknowledging anxiety as a core symptom underlying the control mechanism in OCD, we would rather classify it among the conditions related to the identity crisis, such as depersonalization and dissociative psychosis, albeit with the reactive component predominating.

4 For example, one study investigated patients with social phobia and found that in 45% of cases there was comorbidity with specific phobia, in 59% with agoraphobia and in 5% with panic disorder. Just as often, in about 50% of cases, those suffering from anxiety disorders are also diagnosed with depression.

5 This generates a more long-lasting syndrome, panic disorders (PD); among patients diagnosed with generalized anxiety disorder, 40% had suffered from it for more than five years and 10% for more than 10 years.

6 *Fear and anxiety are closely related*, and both contain the idea of danger or the possibility of harm. *They* are *two overlapping states, but they also differ*: fear is more often associated with peaks of autonomic activation necessary to fight or flee (attack and flight reaction, ortho- and parasympathetic), and also thoughts of immediate danger, and escape behavior. Anxiety is most often associated with muscle tension and vigilance in preparation for future danger and cautious or avoidant behavior. These symptoms can be traced back to the fear of losing control.

7 *Anxiety* is triggered by the anticipation of a threat, which stimulates the physical-psychological response to *fear* and the perceived threat. This response is an example of operant *conditioning*, an inappropriate and maladaptive *conditioned reflex* (e.g., *false alarm*).

8 Anxiety stems from resistance to the internal or external flow of life; anxiety and stress are therefore indicators of suffering that is not so much due to this succession of life events, but rather to resistance to the fact that things are happening as they are. These conditions are disabling to varying degrees: in these cases we could appropriately say that the remedy is sometimes worse than the evil.
9 Fear in this case, however, while subjectively having a negative, ego-dystonic connotation, also has an objective and real aspect in this view: in other words, it corresponds to the direct perception of the expansion of consciousness, perceived as a massive and overwhelming energetic activation. The dystonic aspect of the ego would be nothing more than the ego's reluctance to expand back into a totality from which the child already came, before learning to identify with a separate identity.
10 The effect in essence and appearance resembles that of a sudden awakening that occurs in a person who is more or less sound asleep; he does not realize what is happening to him, nor does he even recognize any similar episodes in the past.
11 In these cases, in the course of this process the subject wakes up to his or her true being, and sometimes manages to understand and accept that this upheaval comes with a transformative, evolutionary purpose. Let's listen to a TP interpretation of a PA given by a contemporary spiritual master: "Panic attacks are movements of intense energy, calling deep within one's soul for awakening; it is to know the truth about ourselves and the world that they come, that's why we call them. They cease as soon as we stop calling them. In the panic attack you experience that you can witness it: fear is an object within you, and it is not you who are swallowed up by it, overwhelmed by it: you are not the fear, you are the fear. This means that we are greater than fear, which is an object that appears in the 'consciousness of you'; fear is a sensation that protects the 'I', the one who feels separated: if you stay with the sensation, you 'die' in it, it dissolves, because as it came it will have to go. That which instead bears witness to fear, the 'I', will not go away: that is what you really are, that which bears witness. Then you realize that what bears witness cannot die, and you put an end to the ordeal of fear, to panic attacks. Today panic attacks are much more frequent, fifty years ago they were rarer and nobody knew what they were; if at that time an Indian guru had to describe them, he would have said: it's the Kundalini, it's a sign of awakening. And he would have put you in the front row. Although not necessarily everyone who awakens must have panic attacks. The strategies the ego develops to avoid these feelings basically only invite them, and it is because of the lack of understanding that they are pushed away" Avasa (2016).
12 In DSM-5. Furthermore, for the differential diagnosis, Panic Attacks must not be due to the *direct physiological effects of a substance* (e.g., Caffeine Intoxication), or of a *general medical condition* (e.g., hyperthyroidism) (Criterion C). Finally, Panic Attacks *must not be better explained by another mental disorder* (e.g., Specific or Social Phobia, Obsessive-Compulsive Disorder, Post-Traumatic Stress Disorder or Separation Anxiety Disorder) (Criterion D).
13 These *may meet the criteria for Agoraphobia, in which case panic disorder with Agoraphobia is diagnosed.* The essential characteristic of Agoraphobia is anxiety related to being in critical places or situations (e.g., from which it may be difficult (or embarrassing) to move away, or where help may not be available in the event of a panic attack); in addition to anxiety, what characterizes Agoraphobia are panic-like symptoms (e.g., fear of having a sudden attack of dizziness or diarrhea) (Criterion A).

14 A beautiful short poem says: "I am a bird in an eggshell, that is why I speak to you of the shell; when I will be in the sky, I will speak to you about the sky." It states here that the way of thinking, of seeing, is linked to the condition of greater or lesser limitation of consciousness; and so far so good. But in the transitional, intermediate phase, if mother bird notices that the bird is delayed in coming out of the egg, she could with her beak break the shell to free it. Well, PD patients behave as if this liberating action were a death threat; they are convinced that the mother is a murderer, because she wants to kill their old eggshell in order to allow her offspring to fly.

15 The defense mechanism of avoidance control is a healthy egoical defense mechanism, as long as it fulfils its homeostatic, adaptive function; some more and some less, we all operate controls that allow us to remain in our *comfort zone*; moreover, we live in a society of control.

16 In these cases, a central aspect is the *confusion between true and false, believed to be true*. The subject in the grip of a panic attack experiences as absolutely real a threat that, from an objective point of view, does not exist; he may actually believe he is in danger of losing his physical life. The mind mistakes internal reality (fantasies, fears, energy experiences) for external reality, generating a disproportionate defensive response.

17 This catastrophic "virtual reality" ends up dominating the subjective experience, making it difficult to distinguish between what is truly dangerous and what is only perceived as such. The resulting anxiety is managed through pre-emptive avoidance of both real and imagined dangers, *sacrificing truth for safety*.

18 For example, a strong sensation of weight or pain in the chest, instead of being interpreted as a sign of a possible heart attack, causing alarm and a call to the emergency room, could be *recognized* as an energetic opening of the heart *Chakra* and accepted without too much reactive agitation.

19 By the term energetic-affective system, we refer to the underlying emotional tone, basic affectivity, and the overall functioning of the emotional and cognitive mind, observed primarily from the perspective of energy and mood, which is directly and closely associated with it. The term comes from Dr. Attanasio Kukopoulos, who, even more than the professors at my graduate school, was my true mentor in psychiatry when, as a young doctor in the 1980s, I worked with others in the private psychiatric clinic in Rome he directed. He devoted himself primarily to the study of bipolar disorder, which he believed to be the only true mental illness. I owe him a debt of gratitude.

20 In an article by Paola Cavalieri (https://www.atquerivista.it/wp/wp-content/uploads/pdf/atque_17ns.pdf), the author considers the dimension of affectivity as the common denominator underlying psychosis.

21 The clinical interest in this syndrome lies in the fact that it manifests, in a prominent and evident way, a cyclic oscillation of intensity that characterizes all psychiatric disorders. For instance, panic attacks tend to recur seasonally, obsessive disorders follow a cyclical course with phases of worsening, and even psychoses present with periodic relapses. However, in these conditions, a mood disorder is not the predominant feature.

22 Kraepelin exposed this theory in his Compendium, of which several editions were published from 1883 until 1915.

23 As the etiological criterion was somewhat speculative at the time, its classification was essentially based on differences in the development of the disease: inauspicious prognosis for the former, which degenerated into an early form of dementia, while the latter had a more favorable prognosis. Severe mood disorders were originally diagnosed as *manic-depressive psychoses;* in these, although in the more extreme phases a psychotic, delusional and

hallucinatory condition was also observed, the egoic identification was only partially maintained or modified for a short time.

24 www.msdmanuals.com/it-it/casa/disturbi-di-salute-mentale/disturbi-dell-umore/disturbo-bipolare?query=bipolare

25 The hypomanic episode differs from the manic episode in that it is not severe enough to cause marked impairment of social or work functioning, or to require hospitalization, and no psychotic manifestations are present. We may encounter situations with excitatory phases lasting three months and depressions lasting nine months, or situations with two excitatory phases per year and intermittent depressive phases, or situations with more excitatory than depressive phases or vice versa. It is on this basis one distinguishes between bipolar disorder type 1 and bipolar disorder type 2.

26 The definition of *rapid-cyclic* refers to a rapidity of the change to mania or depression in very short time.

27 We should rather speak of "Depressions": in fact, depression in the DSM-5 is not limited to "major depression" alone, but includes various disorders, united by the presence of depressive symptoms but distinguished by duration, severity, course, and age of onset. In addition to major depression, other forms are recognized: chronic forms dysthymia (or PDD , which stands for Persistent Depressive Disorder and is the DSM-5 label that includes dysthymia and other chronic, subsyndromal forms of depression), childhood/adolescent onset forms, forms induced by substances or medical conditions, and sub-threshold conditions ("other specified"), characterized by a variety of specifiers (comorbid anxiety, psychotic features, seasonality, etc.).

28 Here are some of the symptoms that may be present to diagnose major depression: Significant weight loss or gain (without dieting) or changes in appetite, Insomnia or hypersomnia nearly every day, observable psychomotor agitation or retardation, fatigue or loss of energy, feelings of worthlessness or excessive/inappropriate guilt, difficulty concentrating or indecisiveness, recurrent thoughts of death or suicide, suicidal ideation, suicide attempts, or suicide planning.

29 Furthermore, to diagnose major depression, differential diagnosis must be considered: symptoms must not be attributable to substances, medical conditions, or better explained by other serious psychiatric disorders (such as psychotic disorders). To differentiate it from bipolar disorder, there must never have been a manic or hypomanic episode in the patient's history.

30 Generally (but it is not a rule), the longer the active manic phase, the longer the sinusoidal compensatory disphoric and depressive phase ensuing.

31 In reality, the process is almost never typical, since no two cases are the same, due to the intervention of numerous competing factors; for example, drugs, the co-presence of other morbid psychic (co-morbidities) or physical (e.g. thyroid disorders, or neurological disorders, etc., to give but a couple of examples).

32 In bipolar disorder, treatment with antidepressants alone may induce a rapid switch towards (hypo-)manic symptoms. In unipolar depression, on the other hand, there is no such risk.

33 Cyclothymia is a less severe mood disorder than BD. This name is derived from *cyclos*, periodic course, and *thymos*, mood, affective and vital tone. Cyclothymia is therefore a cyclic mood disorder, which oscillates between phases of excess, euphoric, dysphoric, hypomanic and frankly excited manic, and of deficiency, insufficiency, reduction, depression, to the point of slowing down of psychic functions, blocked and negative ideation to the utmost, the desire to extinguish oneself, to switch off, to die. Nowadays, cyclotimia is understood as a "syndrome characterized by episodes of exaltation and sadness that are less intense than in BD, usually lasting only a few days and recurring at

irregular intervals. This disorder can result in BD or persist as extreme mood variability. Suffering from cyclothymic disorder can contribute to success in work, leadership, achievement and artistic creativity." www.msdmanuals.com/it-it/casa/disturbi-di-salute-mentale/disturbi-dell-umore/disturbo-ciclotimico.

34 That is the reconstitution of an integrated personality quite similar to the pre-morbid condition,

35 In 1848 Wilhelm Griesinger (1817–1868) in Germany defined the concept of the "dysthymia (or PDD , which stands for Persistent Depressive Disorder and is the DSM_5 label that includes dysthymia and other chronic, subsyndromal forms of depression), psychosis" (Einheitpsychose), characterized by psychic disorders within a unitary psychopathological continuum.

This concept was later taken up by Karl Menninger, who noted in 1958 that "instead of placing so much emphasis on different types of illness, we should think of mental illness as essentially unique in quality, but rather different in quantity." From www.spiweb.it/la-ricerca/ricerca/psicosi-la/.

In this view, a unique psychopathological process would be present in all forms of mental disturbances, with different levels of severity, and in different ways, would afflict each patient differently. Extremizing the concept, we could say that there would exist as many *forms* of the *unitary mental illness* as there are patients.

36 *Kundalini* would be over-flowing and reversing in the two "serpents," i.e., the two half cycles of the zodiac, preceding the complete ascent, after which no motivation persists for cyclic repetition. It is interesting that in vedic astrology the chart n.2 groups the planets in two signs, that is cancer and Leo, according to their feminine or masculine qualities in that horoscope, giving an idea of the energetic overall balance and flow in the two lateral channels (Ida and PIngala).

37 Antidepressants, especially the earlier, tricyclics, when administered in depressions, easily induce the situation to "switch" into excitement, also because of frequently misdiagnosed depressive symptoms: antidepressants are often, in fact, administered in the presence of anxious and depressive symptoms which are the result of an initial dysphoric activation; thus they can dishinibit a latent euphoric tendency and produce an antidepressant effect.

38 An example of this situation is that of women who, in the pre-pharmacological era, after repeated pregnancies and abortions entered frequently into a self-intensifying cycle that led many of them to hospitalization and chronicity.

39 For a "manic episode" to be diagnosed, the symptoms must not be due to the direct physiological effects of a substance (e.g., a substance of abuse, a drug or other treatment) or a general medical condition (e.g., hyperthyroidism).

40 *Familiarity is not an identical concept to Inheritance*; by "*Familiarity*" we mean a certain prevalence in the family, higher-than-normal presence of mental pathologies (even different from the subject's own), or in any case a sensitive terrain in the normal or pathological psychic world. For example, we could have a depressed patient who has a cousin in the family who is a musician, a grandfather who died in the asylum, a brother who has been in analysis for years, a very religious sister, and a son with artistic tendencies.

41 I remember a patient, treated in this acute phase, coming to me disconsolately complaining: "who stole my incandescent days?!"

42 The intensity of the depressive symptoms reported by the subject also indicates the state of arousal, which some inexperienced people confuse with true depression, a condition in which there is instead a reduction in the activity of the affective energy system.

43 In common speech we use certain expressions that indicate this altered and more or less negatively high states: "to have one's head on fire," "one's head

full," or *empty*; to have "one's head in the air," "one's head like a balloon," *to be* "overthinking," to be "with one's head in the clouds," "to be in a daze," etc.

44 A patient relived her own birth in a deep regression, in a complete deconstruction of identity, passing through all the stages of her own birth with her body movements and perceptions, giving birth to herself.

45 A considerable percentage of *suicide attempts* (and suicides actually carried out) occur at this stage. My personal belief is that suicide rarely occurs if not sustained by a psychiatric condition, taking into account how extremely difficult external conditions normally do not push people to taking their lives; that is not to say we should undervalue their contribution to distress. Being aware of this, it is sometimes appropriate to intervene more decisively at this stage, which can prevent suicide in many cases. Other conditions in which suicide is predictable are the OCDs, where the patient suffers a great deal but does not give up the reasons for his suffering, i.e. resistance; "rather than die, I prefer to kill myself' myself" is their position. Other suicides occur as a secondary effect, they are *praeter intentional* suicides so to speak, and are often however connected to obsessive themes, to the fact of not giving up pathological positions, as is the case with anorexia, drug addiction.

46 Everything in the world of manifestation is bipolar, harmonically oscillatory, and cyclic in nature.

All systems in nature are oscillating, from the energy of the electrons in the atom, to the breath of the galaxies; especially in biological systems the said polarity is evident, with varying degrees of complexity, let us say overdetermination.

47 Psychological or symbolic interpretations of this observable reality are often given; thus, it is said that because people are together at Christmas, those without company will feel worse off. However, the opposite may be true; the festivities of the liturgical calendar (just like the pagan festivities), are coordinated with the cyclical nature and are therefore associated with clinical facts that respond to the same origin. Dante's journey starts off on Easter 1300 because of the particular electromagnetic condition of the Earth at the spring equinox.

48 An example of this situation is that of women who, in the pre-pharmacological era, after repeated pregnancies and abortions entered with a good frequency into a self-intensifying cycle that led these poor people to hospitalization and chronicity.

49 Excitatory relapses can also express themselves in other seasons, because they mature over time at a different pace. A crisis starting at Christmas could be expressed in February, or in April; but if it starts later, it could express itself in the summer, or calm down a little during the summer and manifest itself fully in the autumn, at the next change of season.

50 When this manifests in a less active energetic alteration, this state is what we commonly call an "anxious depressive state."

51 Similarly to someone who rides in a car and thinks it is the trees and the landscape that are moving, so in mental disorder one almost always attributes this alteration to the outside, to the environment, projecting it outwards.

52 This may be because the two syndromes could be *two ways in which a single disturbance manifests*, on a more ego defensive level and on a more activated energetic level. Regarding the treatment of these cases, selective serotonin reuptake inhibitors (SRIs) are often used to treat OCD, but they can induce mood instability in BD, especially when administered at high doses and maintained over a long period. See www.psychiatryinvestigation.org/m/journal/view.php?number=1061

53 Treating patients with bipolar disorder (BD) and obsessive–compulsive disorder (OCD) remains a substantial clinical challenge. Serotonin re-uptake inhibitors (SRIs) are the first-line treatment for OCD, but they can induce mood instability in individuals with BD, particularly when prescribed at high doses and continued for long periods. Mood stabilizers, however, can be valuable during phases of exacerbation in a range of other conditions whose features differ markedly from BD, such as OCD or certain forms of dissociative psychosis—for example, schizo affective disorders—characterized by cyclical reactivations and a fluctuating energetic "background" that contributes more modestly and episodically to secondary bipolarity. So-called spiritual emergencies, as will be discussed, may be less amenable to straightforward medicalization, yet clinical experience suggests that the inner fire is often intrinsically self-regulating; nevertheless, drug dosage and treatment duration should be calibrated to the frequently benign course of the syndrome, so as to avoid unnecessary over-medicalization.

54 However, mood rebalancing drugs in the exacerbation phases can be beneficial to many other syndromes whose features differ markedly from BPD, such as OCD, or certain *forms of dissociative psychosis such as the schizoaffective forms*, which are characterized by cyclical reactivations, characterized by an oscillating energetic "background" (thus participating to a lesser and episodic extent in secondary bipolarity).

Spiritual emergencies, as we shall see, may be less prone to medicalization, but in my experience modulating the fire is always wise, though dosages and duration of medication should certainly take into account of the benign bend of the syndrome and avoid over-medication.

55 The alchemist says: "If you do not know how to regulate the fire regime, you will have to throw away the pot and its contents." He thus advises to pay close attention to the regime of fire, since its excessive action (energy that flares up too long and too thoroughly) can alter the matter in the vessel, leading to its degeneration.

Fire grows and decreases in a natural way. As we know, the fire we are considering here is the light-fire of the Sun, the changes in the activity of the Sun-consciousness, the physiological circulation of energy in the subtle body, and its alterations.

56 Robert Whitaker is an investigative journalist and author of *Mad in America* and other books. In this book, he analyzes the scientific literature of the last 50 years and argues how, despite their short-term efficacy, these drugs may cause more harm than good in many patients when used as continuous therapy. He starts from the seminal study conducted by the National Institute of Mental Health (NIMH) in the 1960s, often cited in support of the efficacy of antipsychotics, which had shown that 75% of patients treated with the drugs had "improved a lot" or "improved very much" after six weeks, compared to 23% of placebo-treated patients. However, this observation was called into question by another study, published three years later, in which researchers published long-term results: placebo-treated patients were less likely to re-hospitalize than those given active phenothiazines. This observation raised the doubt that the drugs, while effective in the short term, might create a greater biological vulnerability to psychosis in the long term. The dopaminergic supersensitivity theory offers a plausible biological explanation for the clinical observations of relapse rates. According to this theory, the prolonged blockade of dopaminergic receptors induces a compensatory increase in their density, creating a vicious circle in which the drug becomes both necessary to control symptoms and the cause of their exacerbation in the event of reduction or withdrawal.

See: www.nopazzia.com/psicofarm/antipsicotici-whitaker.html

57 As mentioned, even today this solution is proposed to avoid going to a psychiatrist, which would already be an admission of insanity, a social stigma.

58 A mistake that is often made at this point is to *look for a psychological solution* to a conflict which is of endogenous origin, and to send the patient to a psychologist. Often psychologists are not very knowledgeable about endogenous and serious psychiatric cases, and it will therefore take some time before they realize that the patient's rapid deterioration is not attributable to psychological or psychodynamic reasons. At that point, a solicitous psychologist might seek the help of a psychiatrist; however, psychologists often consider psychiatric pharmacological intervention a sign of failure of their work. On their side, psychiatrists tend to treat patients only pharmacologically, and tend to devaluate the importance of psychological support, so that the collaboration of these two essential figures is not always optimal.

59 In these cases one has to physically entrap, chase, force the patient to take drugs and accept a forced admission, with policemen, sometimes firemen (to break down doors), nurses.

Some cases repeat traumatic experiences of forced hospitalization because these points are not well understood and applied.

60 Admission to a protective environment, that can absorb the incessant arousal, to protect the patient and his living environment, is another important support in this phase of the crisis. One should not believe that it is an easy task attempting to manage a manic phase at home, even with an adequate pharmacological treatment and family support staff.

61 In addition, social and psychiatric stigma themselves become the cause of deviant behavior; if one has been classified as "crazy" (a classic psychiatric saying goes: '*once psychotic, always psychotic*") well, then one can afford it, to do strange things, the role allows it. Society can use stigma as a means to manipulate the subject and control his behavior.

62 A lot of tact and humanity and affection are needed in the care of these patients; it is necessary to know how to build a good psychological relationship that lasts over time, based on trust and professionalism but also human esteem. It is so important in such moments to understand their fragility, sensitivity, inclinations, their hopes and fears, even unspoken ones, their dreams and even delusions. In such fragile conditions, even a wrong word or voice intonation can be sufficient to disturb or hurt. Therapists should know how to accompany, comfort, the patient, and to create and maintain a climate of positive transference that is indispensable for the administration of drug therapy and for its continuity.

63 However, there is also the *risk of over valuating psychotherapy*, of believing that psychotherapy alone can cope with and resolve a critical phase in its ability to manage the bipolar patient by means of talk sessions alone. In the acute phase in particular, it is almost impossible to initiate and maintain regular psychological sessions, and the patient does not benefit from interpretative methods aimed at elaborating the dynamics at play; the behaviour, both externally as internally, is dominated by "*acting out*", that is, by impulsive enactment, not elaboration and integration.

Chapter 7

Disorders with a predominantly identity crisis component

Identity, the central theme of this chapter, represents the *coherent sense of self that integrates our memories, emotions, perceptions, and behavior into a unified experience of* "who we are," *the body-mind complex, the* "me."

In healthy psychological functioning, identity provides continuity across time and different contexts, allowing us to maintain a stable sense of self despite life's changes and challenges. *However, when this integrative capacity is compromised*—particularly after *awakening—we can experience identity crises of varying types and degrees of severity*, ranging from mild identity confusion to severe fragmentation of consciousness. These conditions represent a *spectrum of disorders of the sense of self*, manifesting as a loss of coherence in what was previously a stable self-representation.[1]

Interest in the development of the ego and the study of ego-defense *mechanisms* is central to all schools of psychotherapy, which therefore recognize this as an important element in health and pathology.[2]

The degree and manner in which identity is deconstructed, and the different pictures that arise from this, will now be the subject of the next three chapters. In all these clinical conditions, *the identity crisis is in the foreground* of the energetic alterations we have examined so far.

Identity crisis disorders represent the *cognitive and identity aspect* of PC, whereas *SK describes mainly the energetic-affective aspect.*[3]

In this chapter, we will examine the field as a whole, including identity, defenses, and trauma.

The Derealization-depersonalization (DD) syndrome will be taken as an example of how the process of losing oneself, losing the self we knew, can be the prototype for all dissociative forms.

We will then devote a separate chapter to control disorders, where defenses are in the foreground to prevent this dissolution of the ego.

DOI: 10.4324/9781003676461-7

Finally, the chapter on psychosis will examine the most severe, unfortunate, and deteriorated cases in psychiatry, of those who have been lost and not found.[4]

7.1 The ego and defense mechanisms

Sigmund Freud (1856–1939) based his theory of personality and identity development on five stages of "psychosexual" development, which follow one another in childhood and adolescence.[5] He introduced the concept of defense mechanisms as unconscious strategies of the ego to protect itself from anxiety arising from conflicts of the ego and inner and outer world. He initially identified Removal as the primary mechanism, but in the course of his work elaborated other mechanisms (such as Projection, Negation, Rationalization, Sublimation, and Reactive Formation).

Later, these theories on identity development were *enriched and modified* by other important contributions from the Freudian tradition and ego psychology.[6]

We are particularly interested in the studies on the defense mechanisms of the ego, developed by *Anna Freud) and M. Klein*, who analyzed Splitting and Dissociation more closely.

Anna Freud organized and extended her father's work, identifying ten main defense mechanisms[7]; she emphasized that defense mechanisms are not necessarily pathological, but can serve adaptive functions in personality formation.

M. Klein described how defense mechanisms operate already in the first months of life.[8] She theorized that the child passing from fusion with the mother to the autonomous adult position passes through an initial *schizo-paranoid position*, (characterized by the defense mechanisms of Splitting, and Projective Identification (a complex mechanism in which parts of the self are pushed into the object, which serves to control the object, communicate, get rid of unacceptable parts); to this position the adult self can regress in defense.[9] *The depressive position*, on the other hand, is characterized by the gradual integration of "good" and "bad" objects, and by the development of the capacity for reparation, tolerance of ambivalence.

Numerous other researchers contributed in the following years to psychological theories on identity and defense mechanisms in relation to psychopathology.

They distinguished different defenses at work in different pathologies (different defenses in neurosis, psychosis, borderline), and saw, for example, the correlation between mature defenses and better physical and mental health, and immature defenses and greater psychopathology.[10]

Modern understanding of defense mechanisms integrates psychoanalytic, empirical and neurobiological perspectives[11] for understanding normal and pathological psychological functioning.

The importance of the ego's defense mechanisms is such that *therapies focusing on defense mechanisms* have been proposed; for example, interventions aimed at strengthening mature defenses, or techniques for modifying primitive defenses.

Indeed, defense mechanisms provide crucial information about the level of organization of the personality and help in treatment planning: different therapeutic approaches are indicated for different defense levels.

An assessment of ego defenses also helps in prognosis: the maturity of defenses predicts therapeutic outcomes and general functioning. Evolution towards more mature defenses is an indicator of therapeutic progress.

7.1.1 Dissociation and Splitting

The two main defense mechanisms involved in PC, where identity crisis is the central point, i.e., "losing oneself" (wholly or in part), are *Dissociation and Splitting;* these processes *give rise to dissociative disorders and psychosis.*[12]

These mechanisms show a dual aspect: on the one hand they underlie the ego's *de-structuring* processes, on the other, they *also serve as defense mechanisms* for the ego—to defend itself against this same process, and to maintain homeostasis, i.e., its own dynamic equilibrium.

1. The term *dissociation* refers to a form of disconnection of the individual consciousness from certain habitually integrated psychic functions, or a more comprehensive disconnection from one's own identity.

In dissociation from specific functions, the normal coordination and integration of the fundamental psychic functions (thought, affect, will) is lost: there is a separation or fragmentation between different functions of the ego, such as memory, emotionality, unconscious complexes, and a distancing, a dissociation of the consciousness from them. This condition of partial dissociation occurs during non-serious PC, in which the split, the loss of ego cohesion is only partial. It is like *being partially lost, or having lost parts, having lost pieces.*

The disconnection only concerns certain functions, which are thus misaligned, altered,[13] and there is a *distancing from functional parts of the ego.*

When, on the other hand, the dissociation is more overall, there are cases in which it may present itself in a *milder* form, as in DD, where there is only a sense of estrangement with oneself, but the ego remains as a point of reference, it is not lost altogether; *or it may manifest itself with a deeper distancing* of the ego from one's overall psychic life, a loss even total, as in psychosis.

Dissociation is thus a psychological process involving a temporary or prolonged disconnection between one's sense of identity and one's thoughts, feelings, memories, bodily perceptions, or even of oneself.[14]

For ego psychology, it represents a defense mechanism that allows the mind to separate itself from experiences that are too difficult to process as an integrated unit.

Dissociation creates *horizontal separations,* between self and parts of self, or between self and whole self.

2. *Splitting*, on the other hand, is a psychoanalytic term, that indicates the defensive mechanism by *which the ego divides representations of itself and others into opposite poles* (*all good/all bad*), keeping them separate and alternating, typical of borderline disorders and stages of childhood development.[15] The ego does not detach itself from reality or itself (as in dissociation), but creates internal and opposite compartments incapable of mixing.[16]

Splitting raises vertical walls, dividing the *ego complex into different parts,* attitudes or representations within itself; it mainly concerns the internal organization of the parts that the ego cannot integrate.

These processes arise in the ego and are enacted by the ego, to divide, defend, and split. The effect is the *reverse of the integration process*, *of the process that maintains the ego's cohesion.*[17]

7.1.2 Trauma and the split complexes

1 *In recent decades, psychoanalysis has rediscovered the importance of trauma*, examining with a new perspective childhood physical and sexual abuse and Post-Traumatic Stress Disorder (PTSD) in war veterans. Modern psychology has highlighted the importance of early childhood attachment and the lasting effects of relational attachment trauma on brain development and trauma symptoms.

Some traumatic experiences are so intense that they are universal, such as serious accidents and war situations. Life itself can be too much for many of us to bear, and it could be said that almost all children are, to some extent, traumatized.

A trauma is a situation, outward or inward, on a physical, psychic, or spiritual level, perceived as *too intense subjectively*, perceived as a danger beyond its objectivity, as a threat to identity integrity; a situation in any case unwelcome, and rejected by the ego, for which *the psychic system defends itself,* usually *with defense mechanisms such as dissociation, escape and control.*

The conditioned and conditioning mechanism could be summarized in a typical sequence:

- Encounter *with a traumatizing situation* (physical accident, psychic identity breakdown).
- Perception *of danger* to one's psychophysical integrity, due to the *interpretation of* this situation as dangerous: a *belief*.[18]
- Finally *intense defensive activation* (physical, psychic, neurophysiological reactions).

This may take different forms and be maintained over time, and include different degrees of avoidance, control, nagation, dissociation, and projection.[19]

Over time, some authors (e.g., Jung) have given less and less importance to external traumas in determining the formation of split complexes, revaluing instead fantasies and inner conflicts.[20]

On the other hand, the *most traumatic inner experience* is probably that of a PC, with its destabilization of identity, together with the great energy flow associated with the *awakening of Kundalini*; this activation can lead to a near-death experience (NDE); and, as we have seen, PC can be fostered or precipitated by external traumatic events.[21]

PC may well be considered the internal traumatic factor *par excellence*.[22]

2 According to *Donald Kalshed*, an American Jungian analyst, *trauma contains a spark of the transcendent, the transpersonal*.[23]

This author proposed an interesting theory on psychological trauma using Michelangelo's fresco of the *Creation of Man* in the Sistine Chapel to illustrate the concept. In the fresco, a small space, a separation, remains between the hand of God and that of man, through which life, the spirit, passes.

Kalshed calls this space "intermediate space," *a* "synapse" that allows or denies communication; it is the space where the divine creative energy, the life force, passes through.[24]

Dissociation, as we have seen, is both a fact and a defense: psychosis for Kahlshed would correspond to insufficient protection, to an invasion of the unconscious; a situation analogous to a high-voltage current which, arriving at the home network, would not find an adequate transformer.

As we have seen, the ego, in order to defend itself from this excess, traumatizing it from within, develops a dissociation, a protection which then persists, generating a dysfunction, a specific block: for Kahlshed, dissociation can be seen as a *damage to the capacity to feel*, a defense against the invasion of the unconscious, protecting the ego from an internal trauma.

The function of the Soul for Jung is to act as a bridge between the ego and the unconscious, between man and God, to reconnect, to cross this in-between space, to make the axis between the ego and the Self pulsate, to regulate its amplitude. When the ego-self axis during the child's psychological development does not develop adequately, the foundations are laid for dissociation. *The soul* is thus the function that reconnects the two worlds; it is a creature belonging to two worlds, representing the sacred vitality and divine spark of the personality, and is often represented by the divine child. *The soul thus links trauma and transcendence.*

The patient, in order to rediscover the soul, must cross this space within the therapeutic relationship. Therapy supports this reconnection: *it performs a cure from within, it supports self-care in the affective energy* system, recovering the possibility of the energy to flow through the system; this is perceived, for example, by the appearance of emotions in the patient's body, or dreams of rebirth in the transference.

3 Complex formation

When trauma strikes, the first response is not defensive but disintegrative, dissociative, passive. Like a vase that falls and breaks, the consciousness shatters under the impact, due to the inability to absorb and integrate the traumatic experience into the whole.

The first response is therefore an immediate passive absorption, a state of *internal shock*, where the ego withdraws into the nucellus, eventually leaving the periphery to itself. The direct effect is *an energetic contraction,* a lowering of the energy available to hold the whole together: in response to the danger the system paralyzes, protects itself, regresses, towards *more primitive forms of functioning, in which Splitting can more easily be activated.*[25]

On the other hand, in that situation of danger dissociation also becomes an active survival strategy of the ego, which tries to salvage what can be saved by using *fragmentation* itself. What is left of the ego—this "residual ego"—reorganizes itself, and actively contributes to Splitting as a defensive mode; the ego projects into the split fragment all that it cannot tolerate—pain, fear, anger, despair—in order to psychologically distance itself from it.[26]

Jung proposed the theory of complexes to justify the interference of this splitting with the ego's consciousness, favoring the development of neurosis and psychosis. In the Jungian view, *Splitting lies* "upstream" *of the formation of autonomous split complexes* in the unconscious.

According to this theory, when an experience is too conflictual to be integrated by the ego, the latter may use a basic defensive mechanism: the ego separates internally (splitting) thus generating a split complex.[27]

The ego "expels" by placing in the split-off complex whatever it cannot or does not want to integrate.[28]

Through Splitting, the individual is able to maintain the illusion of control over his or her own inner experience by projecting the shadow onto the split complex.[29]

The response to trauma is a *schizoid state of the ego.*

The complex becomes unconscious because the ego's consciousness moves away from it, withdraws its energetic investment in it, distances itself by dissociating from it and loses its relationship with it; the complex thus recedes into the semi-darkness of the subconscious or becomes completely unconscious.[30]

On the other hand, as we have seen, the ego also distances itself actively, defensively from the complex, thanks to a further separation between the ego and its contents, further dissociating itself from it.[31]

7.1.3 Neurosis

The unconscious complex behaves as a *dissociated part of the psyche.*[32] It behaves like a sub-personality, with a life of its own, a conglomerate of thoughts, emotions, and defense mechanisms, unconscious and sometimes partially conscious.

It most often remains silent, absorbing energy from normal life, giving indirect signs of itself rarely, for instance in dreams. In fact, in trauma, part of the psychic energy remains sequestered and another part is needed to defend against it. The split complex recedes into the shadow of consciousness, and as we have seen, it can even become completely autonomous.

However, complexes *can sometimes emerge (in dreams, symptoms, behavior) and temporarily* take control of the psyche, or even *invade it*, as in psychosis.

The unconscious split parts sometimes return (the return of the repressed), can *influence the ego equilibrium*, and typically produce strong *emotional oscillations* (e.g., of borderline disorder); when a complex is activated, it can "steal" psychic energy, influence dreams, memories, or actions, showing that the split has already produced separate psychic material.[33] This can happen when the complex is "constellated (i.e. activated)," for example, by conscious or unconscious association with those contents and fears, or even just with those physiological reactions (typical of a KS) that characterized the trauma (PC).

In these cases, the same alarm reaction can be reactivated, with intense activation of the intrapsychic defense mechanisms of avoidance and control, which ends up interfering with the conscious functioning of the personality.[34]

In this re-emergence of the complexes into consciousness we might also see *an attempt to regain contact, to reunite* what had been divided, to enrich the personality, defrauded of a part of its riches; but this attempt is *ego-dystonic,* inimical to egoic power and control, and generates anxiety and further dissociative defense reactions.

This dissociative defense is sometimes "remedy worse than the disease".[35]

7.1.4 Ego cohesion

In dissociation, in its most diverse degrees, several factors interact: *the strength of the trauma*, the activated *defences* (more or less archaic and activated more or less intensely), the *individual resources and the help* received.

However, there is probably also a predisposing factor, *internal cohesion, the tightness of the ego*. Indeed, it seems that the ego responds very differently to traumas, external but especially internal ones, and to awakening in particular, on the basis of its constitutional disposition to split. However, the ego's loss of internal cohesion may depend on the *interconnection* of multiple *factors:*

- *On the one hand*, as we have seen, there is a *spiritual factor*; the strength of the ego, (that is, the identification of consciousness with the me), depends on the degree of "sleep" of consciousness. In our "ordinary state", consciousness, as a sleeping beauty (i.e. unaware of itself,) is identified totally with the individual ego, the "me". In awakening, this "me", the individual ego, loses strength and cohesion, due to the withdrawal of identity and energy into the Self.
- *On the other hand,* the strength of the "individual ego", the "me", depends on a *psychological factor*, on the evolutionary level of the personality, on how much at the psychic level integration of the Self has occurred; it depends on the psychological constitution, on how the "ego" has built itself up over time, what phase it is going through, the validity of its defense mechanisms, etc. In awakening, the tightness of the ego depends on the level reached in the pre-crisis phase.
- *Finally*, one cannot exclude a *biological factor*, which could have a constitutional inbfluence, differing from case to case. Some authors have even hypothesized the presence of some *toxin*, preventing the healthy and valid cohesion of the ego in the face of internal and external changes, in the awakening itself.

As for the factors that condition the ego's cohesive force, we recall the work of Pierre Janet, who studied dissociation in particular in obsessive compulsive disorder.

This author described dissociation as a consequence of an "abaissement du niveau mental", i.e., a lowering of the psychic tension that maintains the cohesion of the contents of consciousness, favoring the formation of autonomous psychic automatisms. For Janet, therefore, dissociation and splitting are due to a *lowering of the cohesive force (or of the relationship between the drive for unity and the drive for division) that can favor splitting and can lead to mental disorders.*[36]

In schizophrenia, according to Eugen Bleuler, one is faced with a state of "*extreme dissociation*" whose cause ultimately remains unknown. He used the term *Spaltung* to indicate *the* "fracture," "splitting," *or* "segmentation" of the fundamental psychic processes (thought, affect, will), which become separate and unable to co-ordinate.

Jung was working at the time in the Burgholzli's psychiatric hospital in Zurich, in close contact with its medical director, dr. Bleuler.[37] Jung published his work on verbal association experiments that identified the unconscious split complexes,[38] suggesting their influence in the dissociation and psychogenesis of mental illness; through splitting and interference they would contribute to the weakening of ego cohesion.

Let us recall how from the transpersonal point of view we are interested not only in the ego's difficulties and its legitimate need to maintain homeostasis, with its defense mechanisms, but also in what emerges from its transformation, its death rebirth.

We might hypothesize that *the cohesion of the* "I" *depends on the degree to which the consciousness is rediscovered in the Self*; ego cohesion would thus be that cohesive factor allowing the integration of the Self in the me.

When consciousness remembers itself, recognizes itself, here it can act as a container, an alchemical vessel for the process of deconstruction and restructuring of the individual ego.

7.2 Personality disorders

Identity and personality are two terms that often overlap.

Personality is the (more or less stable) set of traits, patterns, motivational and emotional styles that describe "how" we are and how we behave. It is a set of *distinctive traits*, patterns of thought, perception, affective and behavioral modes, relatively stable over time, that characterize a person.[39]

Identity, on the other hand, is the subjective sense of continuity, unity, and recognition of self in time and space; it is the answer to the question "who am I?"

Personality is "what we look like" (traits, mannerisms, styles), identity is "who we feel we are" (integration, feeling of oneness).[40]

Personality is also observable by others, identity is experienced from within.

Personality theories propose various *personality structures*, indicating the internal organization of traits in a normal person.[41]

Personality disorders are *psychological conditions of the personality that deviate significantly from the* "norm" *in a given social culture*, a kind of *stable deformation of the personality*, which negatively influences the person's everyday life in a way that is dysfunctional.[42]

Personality *disorders* for official psychiatry are *mental disorders*, psychiatric conditions characterized by *rigid and pervasive patterns of thought, perception, emotion and behavior* that *deviate markedly from cultural expectations* and *cause discomfort or significant impairment of personal, social, and occupational functioning.*

A personality disorder is diagnosed as a mental illness when its traits are persistent, inflexible, and maladaptive, and lead to significant problems in the life of the person concerned. They are, however, *generally ego-syntonic.*

They emerge in adolescence or early adulthood, and tend to be stable over time.

Here are some of the best-known personality disorders, as classified by the DSM-5, which distinguishes them into three groups (or *clusters*)[43]:

A *Paranoid, Schizoid, Schizotypal*, characterized by strange, eccentric behavior, social isolation.

B *Antisocial, Borderline, Histrionic, Narcissistic*, characterized by dramatic, emotional, unpredictable behavior.

C *Avoidant, Dependent, Obsessive-Compulsive* (or *OCPD*), characterized by anxious or fearful behavior.[44]

Borderline personality disorder,[45] conversion disorder, and obsessive-compulsive disorder frequently present dissociative symptoms of depersonalization and derealization.[46]

7.3 Depersonalization and derealization[47]

Depersonalization-derealization disorder (henceforth "*DD*") is one of the *dissociative disorders*, i.e. a group of illnesses that have in common the alteration of subjective identity experience.

These syndromes often occur following a trauma or acute stress (abuse, violence, accidents, natural disasters), but can also occur without any triggering action.

Derealization-depersonalization disorder is characterized by a *loss of personal identity together with a loss of comprehensibility, coherence of the world.*

The two are inextricably linked, and to varying degrees these two components are always co-present.

For the DSM, a diagnosis of DD can be made based solely on these symptoms:

> *The subject must have a persistent or recurrent experience of feeling detached, or of feeling like an outside observer of his or her own mental processes or body (e.g., feeling as if in a dream).*

Although this disorder involves an alteration of the subjective experience of reality, it *is not a form of psychosis*. In fact, patients still retain the ability to distinguish between their internal experiences and the objective reality of the external world, and the difference between reality and fantasy (technically, *the Reality Test is* said to *remain* "intact").

DD is a very *frequent* symptom, affecting *when transient, up to 40 per cent or more of the general population*, most life-threatening experiences, acute intoxication by psychoactive substances (marijuana, hashish, hallucinogens, ketamine, ecstasy, etc.), sensory deprivation, or prolonged sleep deprivation.

From an epidemiological-statistical point of view, depersonalization/derealization *as a symptom* even ranks third among the most common psychological symptoms, just after anxiety and depression.

As a disease in its own right, it even affects more than 2 per cent of the general population (which in medical statistics is a huge number, corresponding to millions of people).

Depersonalization and derealization are transdiagnostic symptoms, manifesting in anxiety disorders, mood disorders, or trauma-related and psychotic disorders; they are common to all psychiatric conditions and represent the identity crisis present to varying degrees in these.; we also encounter find them during the activation phase in bipolar disorder, borderline personality disorder and dissociative psychosis.

7.3.1 Symptomatology

Dissociation simultaneously involves the perception of the self and of the external environment, leading to a fragmentation of conscious experience; this condition may evolve towards more severe complications, such as the more severe dissociative forms, *psychosis*, or towards the neurotic defensive organizations,forms such as *OCD*.[48]

Identity crisis: one's identity is perceived as altered: it may happen that one no longer finds oneself, no longer recognizes oneself when looking in the mirror. This process may evolve towards a true identity crisis in which the patient no longer knows who he is, what his body, thoughts, and emotions are, resulting in estrangement from external reality that appears fake, dreamlike, cartoonish.

Example:
"I had a sense of derealization, and a deep detachment from everything, so that if something was happening around me or towards me I wasn't sure what was happening to me."

"I almost seem as if I don't exist, I feel as if I don't understand, I can't understand; and if I do understand, after a few moments I forget, I repeat things so many times to my wife, to my daughters, I almost feel as if I am incapable of understanding. I can't make a speech, I can't do anything, I can't follow, I feel belittled, as if I no longer count for anything, luckily my wife is there and she has taken over the reins."

Distinguished lady who has been coming to me for years. Doctor: "How do you do, madam?"; *Patient* "Eh!, how do you do...? is a big word. You see: I don't even know if I exist!"

Very frequent is the *feeling of not being able to exercise one's will,* of not being able to control one's mind or one's actions. Patients often feel like robots, depersonalized, with a progressive loss of a sense of control over their inner experience.

Example:
"I get panic attacks with a feeling of strong derealization, with the fear of not being able to return to actual reality, as if one feels one's brain is shutting down. Associated with this is the fear of losing one's mind, of going mad, of no longer being able to control one's mind: and of not being able to do anything about it if it happens!"

Sensory alterations include numbness, tunnel vision, perception of blurred or distorted objects, changes in the quality of hearing, and even booming or distorted sounds. In some cases, there are "out-of-body" experiences (OBE), sometimes accompanied by hypnagogic images or a perception of separation between oneself and one's physical body.

Example:
"What is happening to me?" I asked myself; and I said to myself, "I am going out of the body." Then I thought: "I am afraid, I am not used to it, where do I go?" And I could not open my eyes. It took me a few seconds, then everything went blank."

"You seem to see in a distorted way, almost imperceptible. Sometimes it's as if I'm touching things with my eyes, and at other times as if they're distant and I see everything blurry."

"Sight. ... is too unreal ... that's what bothers me the most; sight and hearing. Hearing ... is like I hear everything distant ... I seem to hear sometimes louder and closer and sometimes more distant, almost distorted. Sometimes I hear other people's voices booming. As if one is drunk or 'high.'"[49]

Perceptual alterations are an important part of a *distortion of reality*, taking the form of a form of internal hallucination involving all sensory systems.

Experiences of detached self-observation are frequently observed, described as feelings of seeing oneself from above or perceiving as if the body, legs or arms are distorted, enlarged, or shrunken.[50]

Patients report *changes in reference to their bodily, psychological, and social self*, with a significant impairment of their relationship with their body.

In DD one often feels estranged *from reality, which is transformed,* or is not recognized, a feeling of being an "alien" in the world, a feeling of being estranged from the people one cares about. One perceives reality as if one were living in a dream or a film, with a painful awareness of a sense of detachment from reality, and a great fear of being—or about to become—"crazy."

The surrounding environment is perceived as unfamiliar, foreign, and unrecognizable: one does not recognize one's home, the people, as if living in a parallel dimension, in a film; the world is often described as fake, not real, dreamlike, a cartoon.

Perceptual alterations can give the sensation that the floor moves independently of one's movements, or that smells and sounds are altered, distant, or muffled.

Example:

"I was looking at the pavement, and it seemed to me that it was moving under my feet, and not that it was my feet walking on it. Then when I arrived at my destination, the feeling started to get stronger than before and I felt like I was going crazy: I can smell things, I can see things, but everything is estranged. What is the world? How did I see it before? I don't remember anymore."

Frequent *impairment of memory and sense of time,* with the perception that memories no longer belong to themselves or are blurred and emotionally meaningless.

Example:
"I don't forget ... but sometimes I don't remember, and although I concentrate sometimes I don't remember ... what I did yesterday I don't remember completely ... and that scares me. I remember that before having this DD ... I remembered memories perfectly... Now I don't remember anything and I don't feel anything, I don't remember, or if I do remember it's all blurred, dark, unreal: because it's as if that memory or period was not 'me', present in reality..."

A moderate presence of energetic sensations often accompanies these dissociative phenomena; these are of less importance than those perceived in the KS.[51]

When the energetic component is relevant in a picture of DD complicated by reactions as in ODD, we must take into acount the perceptual distortion that arises from egoic alarm, and put it into perspective. In any case, moderate symptoms of this series are often present, such as feelings of bodily vibration, dizziness, and/or a sense of imbalance that accentuate the sense of disconnection from the body and reality.

7.3.2 Reactions

The fundamental symptom is the loss of identity and the fear this "*residual ego*" may lose what little identity it has left; to fade away even more, and that this condition, this terrible feeling may reoccur.

This condition can be described metaphorically as a state in which *one is* "half-dead, and half-alive; however, it is the half-alive part that is on the alert, that worries about not ending up as badly."

DD is almost never pure, but from the very beginning the identity symptoms, of the first series, are almost always accompanied by the reactive symptoms, the third cluster of symptoms.

These egoic reactions are not yet organized though in a stable defensive system, as in OCD, (although DD symptoms are often present in OCD).

Two main forms of reaction are observed:

7.3.2.1 Refusal

The patient generally turns to the psychotherapist because of obsessive thoughts about the possible evolution of DD, to relieve anxiety about not being in control, rather than to come to terms with the new situation.

In neurotic forms such as OCD and PD, the ego- dystonic reactions, of avoidance, or escape, are in the foreground.

Underneath the reactive symptoms, however, one can easily recognize the identity crisis syndrome of demotivation, confusion, uncertainty, fear. The reactive component, although not produced by the process itself, nevertheless sets in very rapidly contaminating the symptomatology. Thus, a fear of fear often sets in, a true paranoia: even in the absence of symptoms, one lives in a state of alarm at the possibility that they may sooner or later manifest themselves.

Examples:

"I have episodes of derealization but the problem is the phases in which it becomes an obsession ..."

"For example, I had a very bad time at work, I started getting panic attacks more and more often, and I had to put myself on leave for fear of them coming, a real obsession."

"One day in April while driving I had a bad episode of derealization .... From that moment on I felt strange every day ... it was a perpetual feeling/obsession of feeling strange, as if there was something wrong, as if you were going crazy ..."

"I was terrified of it all: I thought I was losing my mind; I felt completely detached and even dull, and at the same time it was so easy for me to be overstimulated. Everything was too much for me."

7.3.2.2 Acceptance

At other times, or over time, the subject may come to tolerate these intrusive, repetitive, negative thoughts, showing how the reactive component is not as important as in other reactive syndromes. He or she may even end up enduring these symptoms patiently, no longer paying too much attention to them; sometimes they go away on their own.

This attitude towards symptoms is very important: the difference in the way one deals with things, or changes one's reactions to what is happening, directly influences prognosis and treatment. Let us look at some clinical examples:

Examples:

"I have decided to surrender to DD and let them take their course without trying to oppose them and chase them away; I don't feel like it anymore, the more I try to make sense of it, the worse I am ... Does this seem strange to me? Peace, sooner or later I'll get over it ..."

> "We 'derealized' people are aware of the illusory reality of matter. I think we are healthier."
> "DD has made me realize slowly that there is much more than a material world ... a kind of pre-perception of a multidimensional universe ...
> In the last few years that it has been present it is no longer so heavy ... I accept it, and the obsessive thinking has practically vanished ... Sometimes I think about it, and almost smile, about the gift she left me ... empathy, emotionality, sensitivity, and so many friends ..."

These reactions are so different from those who reject DD; this different attitude depends essentially on the degree of identification, on how much the consciousness is still identified with the character, with his mind and his world.

7.3.3 Etiopathogenesis of DD

From the perspective of mainstream psychiatry and psychology, the fact that the ego can no longer recognize itself or external reality, which appear changed, is considered a *pathology*. Even patients habitually experience this as undesirable, *ego-dystonic*, still being partly identified with what they would not like to collapse.

However, from the TP point of view, the painful process of loss is at the same time realizing a *healing*—a reunion with the self: *a difficult path through which one must pass for change; that ending is actually the beginning* of a journey back to a unified, undivided vision of reality and oneself as consciousness—a return home.

Thus, this crisis of identity, this "vanishing" of consistency and credibility in the ego and in external reality, this *dissociation from identification*, can be welcomed by those who have a certain degree of spiritual evolution as an intermediate phase that is possible to endure, as we have seen in some of the clinical examples reported.

From the TP point of view, this picture therefore expresses the *emergence of a perception of reality observed from the point of view of a different consciousness, from a transpersonal point of view.*

This new perception imposes itself as a new awareness, as inevitable, inexplicable, irreversible: in short, tremendous. Now the consciousness "sees" that what was true until yesterday was not true at all: it wakes up, rather like when one realizes, in a dream, that one is dreaming.

7.3.4 Evolution of DD

DD is not a psychosis, but it can develop further and proceed towards greater dissociation and splitting, as in psychosis.

In DD the splitting is less intense and complete, and an internal observer always remains to witness the process.

This splitting corresponds to an incomplete awakening, in which there is not really a complete losing and not even a complete finding; the process is almost always accompanied by unstructured ego-dystonic reactions.

The reason for this incompleteness in the process may lie in an insufficient intensity and depth of the awakening, and in the unpreparedness of the ego to accept the dis-identification, which then interprets the symptoms of the process in an ego-referred manner.

In these cases, due to the ego-dystonic nature of the process, it will tend to transform, and the symptoms of the third series will soon emerge, and may tend to organize themselves; in fact, DD is often found in comorbidity with neurotic pictures, as in the control syndromes (OCPD and OCD).

Notes

1 In general, psychological schools recognize that *a* "healthy" *development of* identity enables the individual to integrate past, present, and future, maintain coherence between different self-images, and show adaptive capacities in the face of crises. It is the outcome of secure attachment, developmental crisis resolution (Erikson), and integrated object relations. A healthy identity includes flexibility, self-esteem, and the capacity for self-narrative.

On the contrary, a "sick" identity shows a lack of self-integration, a fragmented, insecure identity, oscillating between opposite poles ("good me/bad me"), characterized by an existential emptiness. In borderline personality disorders, for instance, one observes a prevalence of splitting mechanisms and identity instability; in psychosis, one observes a severe disorganization of the sense of self, loss of identity boundaries, and an inability to distinguish between internal experience and reality.

2 In psychoanalysis, for example, the work of A. Freud, Freud's daughter, and those of M. Klein, the work on the formation of split complexes in Jung, and many others later paved the way. In the cognitive-behavioral schools, too, much emphasis is placed on healthy and pathological defenses.

3 In both cases (Identity crisis or enerrgetic alteration) we find the basic symptom of *fear, panic.*

4 This chapter will speak of "those who live at the crossroads of the winds and are burnt alive," of "those who go and do not return, and who have lost their souls and their wings," as a song by F. De Gregori, "Santa Lucia," so beautifully puts it.

5 *Ego development* stages: *Oral stage* (0–1 years): Pleasure focused on the mouth; suckling and sucking respond to drive needs. *Anal stage* (1–3 years): Focused on sphincter control and control-autonomy issues. *Phallic*

stage (3–6 years): Gender difference and the Oedipus/Electra complex emerge. *Latency stage* (6–puberty): "repressed" urges and the child develops sociality, skills and values. *Genital stage* (puberty onwards): Sexuality turns towards the other; complete maturation of identity.

6 *Freud's followers and the post-Freudian psychoanalytic schools develop these studies. Erikson*, for example, replaces the drive perspective with a sequence of eight psychosocial stages extending from childhood to old age, each characterized by a central conflict. He places great emphasis on adolescence (identity crisis), coining the term "ego-identity." The *object relations school* (Klein, Fairbairn, Winnicott) argues that identity is constructed through the early internalization of "object figures" (objects of love, care, frustration). The *school of self-psychology*, on the other hand (Kohut) favors the idea that identity formation depends on the empathic integration of experiences of the self (mirror experiences, idealization, otherness). Finally, contemporary psychoanalysis (Kernberg) believes that identity formation is related to the ego's modes of defense, particularly in the "borderline spectrum" between neurotic and psychotic organization. *For other psychological schools*, identity formation (e.g. Piaget, Kohlberg) is seen as the result of cognitive and moral stages: the child gradually develops the ability to reflect on himself, on others, and to internalize rules and values through social interaction. In the attachment model (Bowlby, Ainsworth), healthy identity originates from secure attachments in the early years; the establishment of insecure patterns may predispose to identity disorders in adult life.

7 Anna Freud (1895–1982), see *The Ego and the Mechanisms of Defense* (1936), and *The Psychoanalytic Treatment of Children* (1947).

8 E.g., Splitting (division of the object (breast/mother) into "all good" *and* "all bad," which constitutes the mechanism of Splitting, a fundamental mechanism for managing infantile ambivalence, and for protection from persecutory anxiety); or *Projection and Introjection* (expulsion of "bad" parts of the Self onto the external object, incorporation of "good" objects to strengthen the Self). M. Klein: "The Psychoanalysis of Children" (1932), "Notes on Some Schizoid Mechanisms" (1946), "Envy and Gratitude" (1957).

9 *The schizo-paranoid position* (Klein, 1946) is an early mental organization in which the ego, still poorly integrated, copes with primitive anxieties by splitting, projection, introjection, and projective identification: the world and the self are divided into all-good/all-bad and intolerable contents are kept at a distance. Schizoid functioning represents, according to the Kleinian and post-Kleinian tradition, a particular, defensive structuring of the self, which seeks isolation, retraction, and closure in order not to be overwhelmed by persecutory anxieties.

10 These include *H. Hartmann* (1894–1970), who studied ego psychology and autonomic functions, and neutralization, i.e., the process by which drive energy is "neutralized" and made available for ego functions. *O. Kernberg*, who identified a constellation of primitive defenses characteristic of the borderline organization (splitting as central defense, primitive idealization, devaluation, projective identification, denial, omnipotence and omnipotent control). He proposed a hierarchy of personality organizations: Neurotic (where defense mechanisms are mature—removal, sublimation); Borderline: (where defense mechanisms are primitive but reality testing is maintained); and Psychotic (with loss of reality testing). *G. Vaillant* developed a four-level classification of defense mechanisms based on longitudinal studies: Level I—Psychotic defenses (Psychotic denial, Delusional projection, Distortion); Level II—Immature Defenses (Schizoid Fantasy, Projection, Hypochondria, Acting out, Passive

Aggressiveness); Level III—Neurotic Defenses (Intellectualization, Removal, Displacement, Reactive Formation, Dissociation); and Level IV—Mature Defenses (Sublimation, Suppression, Altruism, Humor, Anticipation). In the study of identity and defense mechanisms, *rating scales* have been developed, such as the Defense Style Questionnaire (DSQ) (Michael Bond), or the Defense Mechanism Rating Scale (DMRS) (J. Christopher Perry).

11 Neurobiology of defense mechanisms: the neural correlates of defense (prefrontal cortex, limbic system) have been studied, and neuroimaging studies on defense processes have been carried out.

12 Dissociative disorders and psychosis are described in the fifth edition of the Diagnostic and Statistical Manual of Mental Disorders (DSM-5) and the tenth edition of the International Statistical Classification of Diseases and Related Health Problems (ICD-10) as two categorically distinct diagnostic categories.

However, several studies indicate high levels of co-occurrence between these diagnostic groups, which could be explained by overlapping symptoms. From https://pmc.ncbi.nlm.nih.gov/articles/PMC5216848/

13 Example of before and after a not too severe CP: "and everything seemed fine, between me, my words, and my soul..." De Gregori's song, "La nevicata del '56."

14 *There are ordinary dissociations and pathological* ones, depending on the intensity of the dissociative process.

A *normal dissociation* would be, for instance, absorption during reading or automatic driving, daydreaming, mild meditative states; a *pathological dissociation*, on the other hand, would be, for instance, dissociative amnesia (the patient not remembering traumatic events), the feeling of observing oneself from the outside as in depersonalization, or the perception of the world as unreal or distant, as in derealization, or when it is deeper still, as in dissociative identity disorder (temporary loss of personal identity). In schizophrenia, pathological dissociation presents itself as a disconnection between the self and external reality, with loss of ego boundaries, experiences of external influence, and hallucinations as voices dissociated from one's own will.

15 For example, a borderline patient may see the therapist or partner as "totally good" at one stage ("idealization"), but after a sudden disappointment, experience the same person as "totally bad" ("devaluation"), suddenly alternating between these two views without being able to integrate them.

16 *There are different levels of dissociation*, ranging from primary dissociation (an apparently normal personality, PAN, and an emotional personality, PE), secondary dissociation (one PAN and several PEs), to tertiary dissociation, which corresponds to dissociative identity disorder, where multiple apparently separate "selves" coexist (Onno Van der Hart).

17 *These mechanisms are not simply successive—they mutually reinforce each other*. Vertical fragmentation creates more content to keep at a distance, increasing the need for horizontal dissociation. In turn, horizontal distancing prevents the integration of fragments, maintaining and aggravating vertical fragmentation. It is a vicious circle where each attempt by the ego to protect itself through distance ends up increasing fragmentation, and each new fragmentation requires more distancing. The ego finds itself trapped in a dynamic in which the survival strategy itself becomes a source of further destructuring.

18 We wish to emphasize that *what consciously or unconsciously keeps the* associated *reaction active, and alive*, is believing that that experience or those associated conditions were indeed (and, above all, still are) a danger: a *believed interpretation, a belief*.

The definition of trauma includes the control reaction, the individual reaction, and not only the causal factor.

Trauma is what a person carries within him or her because of how he or she reacted and continues to react. The traumatic event remains so insofar as it remains dissociated and unconscious; it tends to re-emerge and give signs and symptoms of itself, but does not dissolve because of the persistent *resistance* to reliving it and allowing oneself to be transformed by it.

19 A *traumatized* "survivor" may appear almost normal on the surface but hide deep-seated emotions; they may present states of emotional hypo- or hyper-activation (from emotional numbness to hypervigilance) and numerous post-traumatic symptoms such as flashbacks, anxiety, sudden reactions, and self-injurious behavior (Onno van der Hart).

20 Today it is recognized that a significant part of traumatic consequences concerns the *internal mental dimension, memory, representation of self and the world*, and not only the physical reaction to external events. The trauma theory of complexes would explain dissociation as a defensive reaction of the ego. An external trauma could also act by activating and/or sustaining a PC, in which the identity and energy of the system become unbalanced. Among the authors who have explored the subject in depth are Bessel van der Kolk ("The Body Accuses the Blow"); Cathy Caruth ("Unclaimed Experience"), Onno van der Hart ("Ghosts in the Self"), and others, such as Giovanni Liotti, Benedetto Farina, Michele Giannantonio, etc.

21 *Also many childhood traumas* can find an explanation in an *awakening* that occurred during childhood or adolescence, resulting in *an early activation of Kundalini,* when the vehicle is not mature enough and ready to channel it. This activation, which occurs in a condition of early physical and psychic maturation, can be excessive and unmetabolizable, an overload in the subtle system that gives rise to a defensive reaction of interference in the channels and *Chakras*. Hormonal activation in adolescence, on the other hand, implies in itself a strong energetic activation, which in turn fuels awakening, since these two elements, as already mentioned, are intimately linked.

22 We could say that every ego-dystonic situation includes an interpretation, a judgement of unpleasantness for the ego, for the very fact that egoic is questioned; for the ego every internal threat is an experience of encountering death.

23 Kalshed Donald: *The Inner World of Trauma: Archetypal Defenses of the Personal Spirit* (Routledge, 1996); *Trauma and the Soul: A Psycho-Spiritual Approach to Human Development and its Interruption* (Routledge, 2013).

24 Winnicott used the term "transitional space."

25 As we shall see, Janet argued that the cause of this disassociation of psychic functions was "*abaissement du niveau* mental"—that is, a lowering of the "*mental*" level (we would say: consciousness level), a reduction in the energy available to maintain the cohesion of the self.

26 See Caruth's *theory of the double wound*, which emphasizes, drawing inspiration from Freud, how trauma is composed of two wounds: the first is the traumatic event itself, the second is the return of this experience in the form of delayed, obsessive, and non-voluntary symptoms. Trauma, thus, is not simply belonging to the past, but persistently manifests itself in the present.

27 A *complex* for Jung is an autonomous psychic set of ideas, emotions, and memories linked to a thematic core; for example, the "mother complex." The split complex is composed of contents, interpretations, emotions, unwelcome

physiological reactions, generated by the trauma, and placed in it by the compartmentalization, the projection of the ego. The complex therefore contains the memory of this disturbing experience, the "disturbing" material, segregated in a separate compartment: a dangerous psychic content, from which to distance oneself.

28 In the gospel (Mark 9:43-47), Jesus says that "If your hand is an occasion of scandal to you, cut it off: it is better for you to enter into life one-handed, than with both hands to go into hell, into the unquenchable fire..." This passage seems to indicate how splitting one part can save the rest.

29 *Splitting plays a key role in the phenomenon of projective identification*, a term introduced by Melanie Klein and further developed by W. R. Bion. Projective identification is the process whereby the subject not only projects the unwanted part of him/herself into an external object (into another or into a part of him/herself experienced as "non-self"; when acting within the same mind (i.e. between psychic subsystems of self) we speak of "intrapsychic projective identification"), but also identifies with the projected content and remains bound by it in some way, in an attempt to manipulate the split part or control it so that it acts in ways that are in line with these projections. This dynamic amplifies the distance between the healthy core and the foreign content, making the latter less integrable. From www.lilianstrobl.com/splitting-a-psychoanalytic-exploration-of-defense-and-the-fragmentation-of-the-self/

30 See C. G. Jung, *Psychic Energetics*. The very concept of the unconscious indicates the loss of contact with the ego complex. Alan Watts compared the ego-consciousness to a ship's radar, which scans the environment to detect the world, and possible dangers to the ship's survival. Beyond its beam there is perceived nothingness, not objectlessness.

31 *It is one thing not to see* because the object is lost in the distance, because night is coming, *and quite another* to close one's eyes because one does *not want to see* the object;

32 The ego defensively develops a dissociation, an inhibition, which can express itself not only at a physiological level, but also somatically, with an inhibitory regulation, even a more or less prolonged interruption of pathways and connections at a neurological level.

33 Caruth: *Trauma is what* "speaks through the wound" *rather than through the rationality of discourse.*

34 This better explains that vicious circle, that neurotic preventive defense, the alarm of the possibility to become alarmed, the fear of fear "He who has scalded himself with hot water, is also afraid of lukewarm water."

35 Dissociation is initially activated as a defense mechanism, to defend the frightened ego; however, if this process intensifies, it in turn generates conditions of intrapsychic conflict and estrangement from oneself, which in turn can be a cause of worry for the ego, reverberating in the circuit of fear, alarm, defense.

36 For Jung, too, psychosis stems from this cohesive energetic weakening of the ego.

37 Bleuler was among the first to have proposed a psychological explanation for psychosis, diverging in this from the prevailing contemporary biological theories of psychosis of Kraepelinian origin. In 1903, Bleuler appointed Jung as the director of research on the Word Association Test at the Burghölzli. The experiments were conducted under Jung's direction but as part of the broader research programme at the Burghölzli led by Bleuler. Bleuler and Jung also co-published an article entitled "Komplexe und Krankheitsursachen bei

Dementia praecox" (Complexes and aetiology in dementia praecox). The concept of "complexes" that Jung developed through associative studies was fully embraced by Bleuler, who used it in his theory of schizophrenia.

38 1904–1907: "Studies in Word Association" – originally published in the *Journal für Psychologie und Neurologie* as a series of separate articles. 1906: *Diagnostische Assoziationsstudien: Beiträge zur experimentellen Psychopathologie* (*Diagnostic Studies in Associations: Contributions to Experimental Psychopathology*) – Volume I, Leipzig: Johann Ambrosius Barth. 1906: Specifically, Jung published "Psychoanalyse und Assoziationsexperiment" (Psychoanalysis and Association Experiment) as a chapter in the volume *Diagnostische Assoziationsstudien* Vol. I. 1910: "The Association Method" – lectures delivered at Clark University in 1909 and published in the American Journal of Psychology in 1910.

39 Examples of personality traits include extroversion, conscientiousness, openness to experience, friendliness, and equanimity.

40 In psychopathology, identity disorders do not always imply a severe personality disorder, while many pathological personality traits can coexist with a relatively intact perception of identity. A personality may be highly structured and yet the person's identity may be fragile or blurred (as in dissociative or relational syndromes).

41 One only has to think of the study of *psychological types* in psychology, for instance in C. G. *Jung*'s analytical psychology, or to *astrology*, which classifies psychological types in great detail. *In astrology*, one recognizes, for example, the typical functioning of signs based on signs and ascendants (12x12, 144 types just by examining sign and ascendant alone), and the typical configurations of certain syndromes, such as that of control or avoidance (e.g., with regard to control, the importance of planets such as Pluto and Mars, their relationship to Mercury or the Moon or Sun, the position of planets in Scorpio or the Eighth House, etc.).

42 Perhaps it can be said that each personality, each person, corresponds to a specific way of functioning: it is already a deformation of the archetypal man; each horoscope is therefore a description of a *personal personality disorder, the person*.

43 In the latest classifications, a "dimensional" approach is adopted, whereby not only the traditional "all-or-nothing" categorization (present/absent) is assessed, but also the severity gradients and combinations of specific traits, such as impaired personality functioning (identity, self-direction, empathy, intimacy) and the presence of pathological traits (e.g. negative emotionality, detachment, disinhibition).

44 In total, the DSM-5 defines ten personality disorders: here is the list with the main characteristics:

Paranoid: distrust and suspiciousness of others; *Schizoid:* detachment from social relationships, limited emotional expression;

Schizotypical: acute distress in intimate relationships, cognitive distortions, eccentricity;

Antisocial: contempt and violation of others' rights, impulsivity, deception;

Borderline: instability in relationships, self-image and affects, impulsivity;

Isthrionic: excessive emotionality, attention-seeking; *Narcissistic*: grandiosity, need for admiration, lack of empathy;

Exciting: social inhibition, feelings of inadequacy, hypersensitivity to judgement;

Dependent: excessive need to be cared for, submissiveness, fear of separation;

Obsessive-compulsive: perfectionism, order, control, rigidity.

45 In particular, much has been said about the *borderline personality;* the concept, now obsolete, once referred to a "borderline state" *between neurosis and psychosis*. Borderline personality disorder (DBP) is now specified by the DSM criteria, and corresponds to a pervasive pattern of emotional instability, chaotic interpersonal relationships, impulsivity, fear of abandonment, and self-harm. *Kernberg* studied this condition in depth, observing how a borderline personality structure is characterized by primitive defenses (splitting, idealization/devaluation), diffuse identity, and a preserved reality test.

46 See "Dissociative symptoms and dissociative disorders comorbidity in obsessive compulsive disorder: Symptom screening, diagnostic tools and reflections on treatment" (Hasan Belli, 2014).

47 In 1935, the German psychiatrist *Wilhelm Mayer-Gross* coined the term "derealization" to describe feelings of unreality relating to the external world. Psychology has approached these psychic states with some trepidation, perhaps because of their deceptive proximity to serious psychopathological phenomena. According to Nicola Ghezzani (*Life Is a Dream*, F. Angeli ed.), depersonalization and derealization disorder is on its way to becoming one of the most widespread disorders in the contemporary world, plagued by anxiety in human relationships, drug and psychotropic drug abuse, and increasingly isolated and virtual lives. Until 2015, it was thought that these were two different disorders, but today it is assumed that they are two sides of the same coin.

48 In fact, we will shortly see how dissociation can be complicated by an internal split in which one part of the personality maintains an apparently normal functioning while another is in a state of profound destabilization. This mechanism of fragmentation represents an extreme defensive attempt to preserve at least a portion of the functional identity, while the "insane" part contains and absorbs the traumatic load or the experience of loss of control.

49 This disturbing alteration of reality can also occur in a dream: "I was looking at faces, and I saw the eyes transform, and I had a feeling of danger, of gloom, of unreality, and I wanted to run away, but a greater force told me to stay, to go and see... then I found myself sucked into another reality, into a liminal state, fearing the worst, and this woke me up from this nightmare."

50 The patient may also report experiences similar to *OBEs (*Out of Body Experiences); such experiences involve the sensation that one's body, parts of it, or one's thoughts are "detached" from one's self; this sensation gives rise to a process of estrangement as if one's thoughts and body were being observed from outside.

51 Here too, as in the SK, one can observe waves of internal energy, tremors, sudden sensations of heat or cold, and ascending energy movements along the spinal column.

When energy sensations become important, the DD syndrome is joined by the symptoms of SK; this would not allow these conditions to be classified either as purely identity disorders or as purely energy disorders; it would then be a matter of considering them as an attenuated form of schizoaffective syndrome.

Chapter 8

Control disorders

These disorders are part of the neurotic syndromes related to control defences.

On the one hand we will have the drive of the awakening process, in identity and energy; on the other hand, we will have the unwillingness of the residual ego to accept this process of death rebirth, this transformation. In disorders of control, we will therefore have a *civil war* that can be prolonged for life, a *chronic neurosis*.

We will examine this particular psychiatric pathology in depth, since the defensive core that sustains it is transdiagnostic to many other psychiatric syndromes.

OCD has been called "the black sheep of psychiatry" due to poor cooperation of patients with therapy, its limited response to pharmacological treatment, and its tendency to become chronic.

This syndrome in fact excellently represents how the third set of symptoms of a psychiatric crisis (PC) (the reactive ones, related to ego resistance) can greatly complicate the awakening process, interfering with it and making it chronic, thus making these syndromes so difficult to treat.

For prognostic and therapeutic reasons, it is important to distinguish situations where ego defenses are less intense and the ego complex is less dissociated—i.e., ego-syntonic conditions (as in OCPD)—from the more severe, dissociated, and exaggerated forms (as in OCD), where the syndrome is ego-dystonic.

For this reason, we will describe the symptomatology of the two syndromes, highlighting the differences as well as the similarities, and provide clinical examples.

Both OCD and OCPD are relatively frequent conditions, and account for a significant proportion of psychiatric disorders in the general population.

For MS psychiatry, the two disorders do not appear to be related. However, when looking at psychogenesis from of these two conditions, we see how they both revolve around the neurotic defensive mechanism

DOI: 10.4324/9781003676461-8

of control. From this perspective, the two conditions are significantly correlated, and actually lie on a *continuum,* representing distinct points in a process that differs in terms of degree of dissociation, intensity, and negative impact on daily life.

Comorbidity between OCD and OCPD is frequent, but many people present with only one of the two disorders; furthermore, OCPD can often complicate and turn into OCD.

8.1 Obsessive-compulsive personality disorder (OCPD)

OCPD is a personality disorder characterized by an *excessive preoccupation with order, perfectionism, and control* at the expense of flexibility, openness, and efficiency.

It is one of the most common personality disorders.

The problem of a *hypertrophy of control,* both individual and social, is *omnipresent in our world.*[1] In OCPD, these traits are deeply rooted in the personality structure, *contribute to personal identity* to a large extent, and are therefore defended by the ego as its own. These defensive traits become the *default* mode through which the individual manages the internal and external world.

The person with OCPD tends to perceive their obsessive needs and desires as an integral part of themselves, often showing little awareness of the discomfort they may cause themselves and others. With this in mind, these patients may be more inclined to try to change their environment rather than questioning their own patterns of thought and behavior.

Within this syndrome (unlike OCD, who could be considered his sick older brother) these psychological actions are structured in an *egosyntonic* manner, *and are not very disabling.* On the contrary, they can *also* be *positively exploited* in a society where control is valued, if not part of the system.[2]

OCPD is present in a large percentage of the population, and present in almost every psychiatric disorder.[3] It is more common among males than females (a ratio of two to one), and occurs more often in people who have suffered trauma or abuse during childhood.

It is so widespread and so unrecognized as a psychological problem that there is always a risk of underestimating it.[4]

8.1.1 Symptomatology

In general, people with OCPD tend to *seek control and order in every aspect of their lives, including in interpersonal relationships.*

Hence the need for others to *act exactly according to the subject's dispositions, to the point of a manic control over people,* which makes family and friendship relationships difficult and burdensome.

This can create difficulties due to a tendency to be rigid and inflexible in expectations, with difficulty in accepting the differences and opinions of others; or a tendency to be overly critical and judgmental, both of others and of oneself, and to have high and unreasonable standards for oneself and others.

Excessive preoccupation *with organizing, doing, achieving, tidying up (trying to make sure that* "everything is in order"*). Time is never enough, and they are often late.*

Constant preoccupation with cleanliness, control of spaces and environments.

This also results in *excessive pedantry and adherence to social conventions, rigidity, and obstinacy.*

Excessive tendency to try to understand, to find *reasons*, *explanations*, which one does not find or does not consider satisfactory and decisive.

Often the excessive attempt to understand psychic dynamics in psychotherapy stems from this need to control with knowledge, in order to be better prepared to control with rationalization.

Over-rationalization of feelings, which leads to experiencing affects in a limited way.

In OCPD there is a tendency to exert strong control over emotions, as affectivity and emotions are considered a loss of control by the ego. There is a tendency to suppress emotions or to express them only indirectly, such as through ritualistic or compulsive behavior.[5]

The most frequent emotions are *anxiety*, *anger*, *frustration*, and *envy*; there may also be *difficulty in expressing* anger and frustration, and adoption of *passive-aggressive* behavior, which manifests itself in indirect hostility and sabotaging behaviors.[6] They therefore have *difficulty empathizing*, that is, understanding and appreciating the ideas, feelings, and behavior of others that do not coincide with their own value system, and they have difficulty trusting and establishing *relationships of intimacy and emotional closeness* with people.

Unexplained anxiety in situations that differ from the subject's routine, to the point of showing rigidity and difficulty in adapting to changes.

Many patients who seek psychotherapeutic help experience a constant state of anxiety, and a fear of feeling it, so they are "afraid of fear," and would like to eliminate it with psychotherapy.

They attribute their uneasiness to external situations (such as "when I am at work," "when I am traveling"), and so *associate such conditions with the defense mechanism* of avoidance to control this state of theirs; at other times, they use *self-medication* methods (such as cannabis, music, psychotropic drugs) as habitual sedatives.

Excessive preoccupation with details, rules, lists, order, and organization, to the detriment of the general purpose of the activity. Their lifestyle is driven by a sense of duty, excessive responsibility, due to egocentrism, which combined with *perfectionism, scrupulousness*, however, interferes with getting a job done quickly. This is why they struggle to meet deadlines.[7] A certain *inflexibility on ethical and/or moral positions* (not justified by political or religious affiliation) is observed.

A variant of the above involves an *excessive dedication to work and* productivity (not justified by economic necessity), resulting in *a devaluation of leisure activities and interpersonal relationships*; these people never relax and enjoy themselves.

Control leads to *reluctance to delegate tasks or work in groups.*

Feeling of *self-pity or excessive blaming* in case of minor or even trivial mistakes. The same can be said for *excessive fear of criticism*, even if constructive, *pessimism. Tendency to doubt*, which may lead to *excessive indecision and caution.*

A tendency to accumulate, in a lesser form than in OCD stemming from not "letting go" of life and things, such as the inability to throw away old or useless objects, even when devoid of emotional or economic value (hoarders). *Thrifty lifestyle* (money is seen not as a source of pleasure but as protection, to be accumulated in case of future misfortunes or problems).

It is difficult for these people to seek psychological help.

In fact, these people generally have *little insight*: their way of functioning is for them a blind spot, they do not see themselves; and even when they do see such rigidity, they justify it, being ego-syntonic (i.e.: ego-favorable) they see it as part of themselves: *that is how I am,* they say.

However, the same excessive preoccupation with control, perfection and order can make it difficult for them to admit that they *have problems or need help* from others: it is difficult for them to admit that they are imperfect, or sick, and they fear being judged or criticized by others or rejected when they reveal their weaknesses or limitations.

Thus, they may be reluctant to accept the fact that they have a problem or need psychological or psychiatric help.

8.1.2 Etiopathogenesis

For mainstream psychiatry, the genetic predisposition to obsessive personality traits is considered a relevant factor, as is the learning of perfectionistic behavioral patterns through identification with similar parental figures.

According to ego psychology, the psychogenesis of this syndrome is due to *the development of rigid personality traits in response to childhood experiences of excessive control, parental perfectionism and criticism.* From the perspective of ego psychology, "OCD can be viewed as a defense mechanism through which a person attempts to manage their emotional conflicts and maintain a sense of control over their life." Obsessive-compulsive behavior in the OCPD would thus serve to reduce anxiety and uncertainty in the ego, acting as defensive strategies to maintain a psychological, ego-syntonic, albeit rigid and limiting, balance.

In a TP perspective, on the other hand, this personality structure arises and organizes itself in childhood or adolescence as a reactive response to a weak awakening, mainly involving identity. Thus, the person finds its equilibrium in an adaptation of the personality, which bends, deforms itself in the sense of preventive control and stiffening.

8.1.3 Clinical example

A professional with OCPD spends hours reviewing and re-reading documents, even when not strictly necessary, in fear of making the smallest mistake.

This exasperated meticulousness, although it may lead to an apparent accuracy in work, often results in delays in delivery, significant difficulty in prioritizing tasks and a chronic sense of dissatisfaction with the work done, as it is perceived as never quite perfect.

Relationships with colleagues can be strained due to her inflexibility, tendency to impose her own high standards and difficulty in delegating tasks, fearing that they will not be carried out with her own precision.

On an affective level, there is difficulty expressing and managing one's emotions, particularly anger, which is perceived as a threat to one's control, and which leads to rigid and unspontaneous relationships.

Such an individual would adhere scrupulously to lists and schedules, and experience discomfort and anxiety when faced with the unexpected or change.

Her home reflects this need for order and control, with every object in its place and a marked intolerance for disorder, even the slightest. She does not primarily complain about his traits; on the contrary, she often considers them a strength, a guarantee of efficiency and reliability.

Rather, suffering emerges from the consequences of this rigidity in interpersonal relationships, work performance and general well-being.

8.2 Obsessive-compulsive disorder (OCD)

Obsessive-Compulsive Disorder (OCD), once classified among anxiety disorders, is now recognized as an autonomous nosographic entity, characterized by the coexistence of obsessions and compulsions that profoundly impair quality of life.

OCD manifests itself with *two pivotal symptoms*: *obsessions and compulsions*.

1. *Obsessions* are intrusive, recurrent, and unwanted thoughts, images, or impulses that generate intense anxiety.

2. *Compulsions* are repetitive behaviors (such as washing hands, checking), or mental acts (such as counting, repeating words) enacted to neutralize or prevent the anxiety associated with the obsessions.

The obsessive perceives his or her thoughts as *internal enemies*, experiencing a condition of psychic *siege*[8] in which *he or she desperately tries to* "tame" *or appease* them.

The unease does not derive so much from the presence of the thought as from the *absolute belief in its veracity and the need to defend oneself against it*, thus configuring a dynamic of internal blackmail.

> **Example:**
> "If I resist compulsions, the anxiety becomes unbearable, as if I were about to die; if I perform them, I lose hours stuck in endless rituals.
> It is like being locked in a mental cage, a nightmare with no way out."

A hallmark of OCD is the *awareness*, present in most cases, *of the irrationality of one's fears and behavior*. The subject recognizes the excessiveness of compulsions but still feels compelled to carry them out.[9]

What differentiates OCD from OCDP, besides the severity of the disorders, is the constant presence of a state of *dissociation* of a part of the personality.

The most common forms are "checkers," "cleaners," and *accumulators*. Let us take a closer look.

8.2.1 Prevalence, onset, course, and prognosis of OCD

The lifetime prevalence of OCD is between 2 and 3 per cent of the general population.

The *onset* of *OCD* occurs predominantly in childhood, adolescence, or early adulthood; the onset is typically early, often before the age of 25, with a higher incidence in males between the ages of 6 and 15 and in females between the ages of 20 and 29, the latter being likely related to emotional-hormonal factors.

The prognosis of OCD is negatively influenced by the presence of *comorbidity with anxiety, mood, autism spectrum, or tic disorders.* An unfavorable prognostic factor is also the *delay* in starting treatment, which on average occurs seven years after onset. Further negative elements are poor compliance, a particularly early onset, and the presence of stressful life events.

The clinical literature shows a *significant correlation between the severity of OCD and the presence of dissociative* symptoms, and that patients who do not respond to treatment have elevated dissociative symptoms. This confirms the central role of splitting in the genesis and maintenance of the disorder.[10]

OCD significantly impairs quality of life, leading to difficulties in interpersonal relationships, work or school functioning, and carrying out daily activities.

Not infrequently, the pathology *also influences (infects) close family members* (spouses, parents, children), who may be involved in avoidant rituals and justify or support the compulsions, thus contributing to the maintenance of the disorder.

The course of OCD is predominantly chronic, with significant individual variability. Both episodic forms, characterized by remissions and relapses, and forms with a continuous course are observed. Symptomatology may fluctuate over time, but the chronic course is predominant. In some cases, symptoms may persist subclinically between episodes.

8.2.2 Clinical examples

In these clinical examples, the different traits of defensive organization, such as obsessions and compulsions, are present to varying degrees in the different example. One can clearly see how the impact on the OCD's life is quite different than in the case of the OCPD.

Examples

35-year-old woman with contamination obsessions. Following the birth of her first child, she developed an obsessive fear that the baby would be contaminated with pathogenic germs. This led her to wash the bottles for over two hours each time, following a strict ritual that included the use of three different detergents in a precise sequence. If interrupted during this ritual, she had to start again from the beginning. Although she recognized the irrationality of her behavior and the fact that she was compromising her relationship with the child (she could not devote enough time to him), she felt unable to interrupt these rituals.

Patient with pathological doubt obsessions and control compulsions. Constantly plagued by persistent doubts about past actions, such as forgetting to turn off the gas, shut the door, or having made important mistakes at work. These doubts generate anxiety and worry, leading the patient to engage in repeated control compulsions. He or she might check the gas is shut off dozens of times before being able to leave home, meticulously check his or her work tasks, even the simplest ones, or continually seek reassurance from family members about his or her own adequacy. These compulsions, while providing temporary relief from anxiety, consume an enormous amount of time and energy, significantly interfering with his life. Patients with pure obsessions are often assailed by unacceptable thoughts, such as profanity, intrusive sexual thoughts or violent fantasies. While not engaging in overt motor compulsions, the patient may react internally through compulsive mental acts, such as repeating prayers, seeking mental reassurance, or avoiding situations that could trigger such thoughts. This generates a constant state of anxiety and a strong sense of guilt or disgust.

8.2.3 Symptomatology

Constant state of anxiety: Obsessive patients often seek psychological or psychiatric help for an underlying state of anxiety that often lasts for years and has no plausible cause.

They often abuse anti-anxiety drugs, or use cannabis continuously as self-care. They often experience panic attacks," or rather, "dreaded panic attacks": at the mere thought they panic.

Intrusive thoughts of a violent, sexual or blasphemous nature: Obsessions involve disturbing impulses or images that the person fears they might act out. People have the thought that they might do or have done something unacceptable, or unseemly, or dangerous, such as blaspheming or having homosexual relations, and they consider this idea coming as real, and then they become anxious, and engage in an inner dialogue of reassurance to prove otherwise.

A classic example is that of a parent who is obsessed with the thought of harming their child, even though they have no intention of doing so.

Contamination: Excessive fear of being contaminated by germs, harmful substances, or bodily fluids, leading to exhausting cleaning rituals.

> For example, the exhausting compulsion to disinfect, and to avoid dirty substances or places, syringes, blood, detergents etc., avoid hospitals, buses, gardens.

If they think they have come into contact, they enact rituals of washing, of hands, of objects, with disinfection, to reassure themselves about the idea of contagion. The alarm can be extremely high if the person convinces themself that they are infected.

> **Example:**
> "I spend hours in the bathroom, to be sure I have cleaned myself well. I have doubts of contamination on the towel; even if I have it changed, I then have doubts that the person who changed it had infected hands. I wash my hands many times in a day, for a long time, and my skin has cracked."

A person might wash their hands to the point of causing skin lesions, or avoid public places completely for fear of contamination.

A variant is having to *keep everything clean,* as well as tidy, an obsession with cleanliness, of the body, of the environment.

Fear of losing control, reassuring compulsions: Persistent fear of having caused damage or accidents through negligence, leading to repetitive checking rituals.

In this case, patients enact repeated and prolonged checks to avert possible misfortunes, enacting control rituals. The control is aimed at reassurance with respect to constant doubt.

Patients may check the front door, the car, or if the gas has been turned off, or the lights off, or if the door has been locked, and even return home several times to check. They might check whether they have filled out a form correctly or counted money correctly, or whether they have carefully studied the page before the examination.

> **Example:**
> "If I absolutely have to check, it's because if I don't, all hell breaks loose inside."

Order and symmetry: The need to arrange objects in a perfectly symmetrical manner or according to strict rules. This disorder may concern objects, such as pencils, the position of shoes: there are patients who do not tolerate seeing things out of place, everything must be aligned, symmetrical, ordered in shape, color, or size, otherwise they do not feel right with themselves, in harmony with the world. *Everything* has to be "right."

Example:
"I get anxious if my slippers are not placed properly and parallel to the foot of the bed, I can't sleep."

A person might spend hours arranging books in a bookcase in a precise order, feeling intense discomfort if someone moves them even slightly.

Pathological doubt: Among the recurring thoughts is the thought of doubt—pathological doubt—about oneself, one's sexuality and performance, one's partner or honesty, having done something wrong and not remembering it.

Examples:
"My thoughts tell me that I am a loose woman, but I am not!"

"I have this disorder of always wondering whether I am gay or not."

Obsessive repetition: The patient mentally repeats mental actions such as praying, repeating words, counting.

Delay, slowing down: Often people with OCD do not respond immediately when you talk to them; in the dialogue they perhaps slow down, or leave moments of silence, during which it is as if they are thinking about it, whether and what to respond; walking by your side they stop and talk, they control their own and others' movement. The relationship is never direct and spontaneous, but always calculated and blocked.

Example:
"I am 15 years old. It takes me so long to do anything. It's tiring, really."

Obsessives *always* arrive *late*, for rituals, accumulate constant delays, until the final avoidance as a solution. The opposite symptom, however, namely *the obligation to always be on time,* also expresses the same control problem.[11]

Accumulation and hoarding: These patients do not throw anything away, they keep useless objects (even of little value), because they hope they will be useful sooner or later, which leads to an accumulation of things to the point of occupying all the space, the whole house, to the point of making it difficult even to move around inside.

Examples:
The accumulation in the house of empty cans, bottles, rubbish, bottle caps, magazines, empty food containers, etc., such as to make the house even uninhabitable due to the occupation of space, the stench, etc..

Collecting CDs, books, stamps, files on the PC, etc.

Excessive superstition: Superstitious thoughts, e.g., that doing or not doing certain gestures, saying certain words, seeing or not seeing certain objects, may have catastrophic consequences; thus, they may enact superstitious, or propitiatory, preventive rituals so that the feared events do not occur.

Example:
I remember the case of a patient of mine who, if he happened to come across a hearse in the street, he had to return home immediately, on pain of the imagined death of his father.

A famous tennis player always had to perform a certain ritual before hitting a shot, at the risk of failure.

8.2.4 Etiopathogenesis of OCD

8.2.4.1 Ego psychology

The classical Freudian psychodynamic model interprets obsessions and compulsions as manifestations *of unconscious psychic conflicts, often linked to unacceptable aggressive or sexual impulses that are controlled through defense mechanisms.*

In the less severe obsessive-compulsive disorder (OCD), defense mechanisms that are defined as "neurotic" or relatively mature generally predominate. Among the most frequent and characteristic defenses are *reactive formation,*[12] *isolation of affect,*[13] *and retroactive undoing.*[14] In more severe forms of OCD, especially when there are comorbidities or a more disorganized ego structuring, more primitive and disabling defense mechanisms prevail, such as *denial*,[15] *repression*,[16] *splitting*,[17] and *schizoid projection*.[18] This gradation reflects a progression from the prevalence of relatively adaptive defenses in less severe forms, towards rigid and primitive defenses in more severe forms of OCD.[19] According to this perspective, the internal conflict between unacceptable impulses and rigid superego generates distress that is managed through compulsive rituals.

In contrast, *the behavioral model,* developed in the 1960s and 1970s, views OCD as the result of classical operant conditioning: *anxiety is associated with certain stimuli and compulsions are reinforced through the temporary reduction of the anxiety they produce.* This model provided the basis for the development of exposure and response prevention therapies, which remain among the most effective interventions for OCD.

8.2.4.2 Transpersonal psychology

In the transpersonal perspective, OCD is not simply a neurobiological or behavioral malfunction, but rather represents the *manifestation of a profound evolutionary crisis of consciousness, which seeks to go beyond the limits of the personal ego.*

The anamnesis of many OCD patients usually reveals a *premorbid* personality characterized by obsessive-compulsive traits (OCPD): a personality based on control, subject to cyclical flare-ups that overlap and reinforce the basic configuration.

In the TP perspective, the *traumatic experience is determined as a consequence of the opening of the PC,* often as early as childhood or adolescence, *primarily due to the destabilization of identity,* almost always associated in this first experience by a strong energetic activation, the awakening of the *Kundalini.*

The trauma derives from the disproportion between the intensity of the destabilization, which can be variable, or even more so from the ego's difficulty in accepting the transformation process, preferring instead to hinder it and thus favoring the chronicization of the disorder.

The ego's main defense is to try to restore at least part of the old identity. And this, as we have mentioned, happens mainly through the mechanism of *splitting*: the ego separates and isolates the part of itself experienced as disturbing, thus creating a split complex. In practice, the consciousness splits and compartmentalizes the "disturbing factor"—that is, that evolutionary impulse that pushes beyond the old set-up—relegating it to an unconscious split complex. We have also seen that the result of all this is the development of a *schizoid condition of the ego*, which feels threatened by that which it has itself excluded; the severity of the OCD is directly related to the degree of splitting.

Moreover, *any attempt at reunification* is blocked: walls are put up (the so-called *vertical split*) between the ego and the split complex, which is kept away from consciousness, rendered unconscious (through a *horizontal split*, i.e., a real psychological distancing from the undesirable contents). These defense mechanisms are activated by the ego to avoid being overwhelmed, and *remain in operation continuously and rigidly, consuming a lot of psychic energy and generating anxiety, depression and favoring the chronicization of the disorder.*

Once rendered unconscious and autonomous, *the complex functions as an* autonomous *sub-personality*, acting independently of the conscious will, and expressing itself through obsessive thoughts and compulsions experienced as extraneous and intrusive (*ego-dystonic*) with respect to the subject's conscious control.

The ego's uncompromizing defence has a fundamental function: it maintains internal separation. This, though, has a prize for the ego: he remains locked in a schizoid logic, where division and confrontation (*the two*) rather than integration and the meeting of the parts (*the three*) predominate.

In this sense, OCD can be seen as a "spiritual disease": internal separation never gives way to encounter and synthesis, to the logic of union, to love, and so the psychic landscape turns into an eternal conflict, fueled by fear, when in fact there would be the possibility, if only the ego would allow it, to transform the crisis into a process of sacrifice, integration, and harmony.

In this condition, *an inversion of the parts* takes place: it is not the awakened consciousness that drives the process, but the part of the ego that resists change, wanting to remain in power.

It is metaphorically a *psychic* "coup d'état," in which the old regime remains dominant and exiles the new part, experienced as threatening. Thus, a clear division is created in the individual between a "white self" (apparently healthy, which identifies with control and the accepted part of oneself), and a "black self," which represents all that has been demonized and rejected, creating the conditions for the dissociated and controlling life typical of OCD.

The schizoid ego, therefore, is not only a victim of the situation: it is itself the *tyrant*, the persecutor, the one who orchestrates this separation, applying the principle of "divide and rule" to maintain control.

When it dissociates and tries to defend itself, *the ego represents itself as a victim* with respect to the return of those parts of itself that it had excluded; on the one hand, it had expelled and isolated these internal instances in an authoritarian way, on the other hand, when they re-emerge and demand to be recognized, the ego behaves as if it is being attacked, reinforcing its position as the "good part."

In OCD, this translates into a *central deception*: the ego convinces itself that it is in the right, while the unconscious and disturbing part is demonized, manipulated, and kept at a distance, because to accept it would mean abandoning habitual defenses and facing an experience subjectively felt as catastrophic, as if every barrier were to fall and one were to sink into psychosis.

In this dynamic, the ego remains trapped in an *emotional state dominated by paranoid anxiety and a feeling of impending threat.* Every attempt to integrate what has been excluded is read as a danger and becomes the cue to further stiffen the defenses against itself: thus, *the defense put up by the ego not only does not solve the problem, but turns itself into the source of suffering*, as if the psyche had an internal enemy, as if it were turning against itself (think, as an analogy, *of an autoimmune disease*).

The ego, in its desire to preserve itself, promotes fragmentation instead of integration, obsessive control instead of trust, dissociation instead of expansion of consciousness. This creates a *vicious circle with no exit*, where defense itself ends up complicating the inner evolutionary crisis, worsening and chronicling a process that, if supported and understood, could have evolved naturally.

In fact, *the symptoms are typically ego-dystonic*: negative obsessive thoughts—often related to death, catastrophe or harm—creep into the mind with compulsive force, accompanied by emotions perceived as extraneous or uncontrollable, making the subject feel constantly under attack from their inner as well as outer world. These thoughts and compulsions are experienced as alien intrusions that possess the mind and take away personal control.

8.2.4.3 TP reinterpretation of symptoms

One of the most common symptoms of OCD is *depression*. It is more properly a deep dissatisfaction, a gloomy sadness, the perception of always being wrong or at fault: it is therefore not a mood disorder in the technical sense, but a form of chronic anguish and demotivation, a subjective death experience. The constant internal attack prohibits all spontaneity and trust in life, generating helplessness and despair, without any hope of real change. The experience of the obsessive patient often remains an internal world marked by conflict, deception, and darkness, with a relentless war against an unconscious enemy. It is therefore not primary depression, but a condition of psychological hell.

Anxiety, for its part, is a clear manifestation of the conflict with the unconscious. This conflict is perceived internally, almost physically (actually in the subtle body) as an obstruction in the flow of energy, and is then projected onto external situations, and then interpreted as the cause of the tension.[20]

The fear of contamination—from microbes or "dirty" thoughts—must be read symbolically: the perceived threat actually comes from the disturbing unconscious material, while the germs or external situations are merely supports for the projection. The feared external contagion, the dangerous contact, is in fact about the rejection of internal contact with the disturbing complexes.

In the initial stages, *confusion* is experienced as the most distressing symptom; the rejection of confusion fuels the compulsive repetition to clarify, to understand; this fruitless activity, while attempting to restore order and clarity only reinforces the paralysis and dependence on doubt. Good and evil become confused, one enters a cloud of not-knowing, in which the mind seems incapable of thinking and understanding. If only this confusion were accepted, it could turn into mystical openness; in OCD, however, it is declared unworthy and threatening, and therefore actively rejected.

Similarly, one can *read hypochondriac obsessions and thoughts of death in a TP view*: the obsessive repeats medical examinations incessantly to reassure himself, but the fear remains, because the real object of the threat remains the experience of psychological death, that is, the encounter with his own split complex, the tyrannical "shadow" of the ego.

In this syndrome, anxiety is self-feeding: the mind fears an internal disaster, they had experienced in the past on occasion of the first PC, imagined in the present as a situation from which one absolutely must flee. But the danger is not real: it is evoked by the defensive mind, and each attempt to defend itself increases the fear itself.

Thus, the repetition of rituals only serves to further feed this vicious circle: compulsions are an attempt to placate an enemy that the ego has generated but does not really want to encounter.

In the end, the knot remains the same: *the OCD sufferer desires liberation but unconsciously defends the very structure that holds him trapped*. The real healing process only begins when the patient accepts *responsibility* for himself, overcomes the projection of the disorder as "other than himself" and begins to see the pain as an internal part to be integrated, not controlled.

From the transpersonal point of view, the return of repressed material can be interpreted as a *self-healing attempt* of the psyche, a constant call for the integration of dissociated contents, which, however, are rejected, and thus return more and more insistently.

8.3 Differential diagnosis between OCPD and OCD

OCPD shares some characteristics with *Obsessive-Compulsive Disorder (OCD)*, such as anxiety and obsessions, although these two clinical entities actually remain distinct.

We see some differences between the two syndromes (see Table 8.1).

In OCD, the obsessions and compulsions are more circumscribed and specific, whereas in OCPD, concerns are often about order, control, and perfection.[21]

In OCD, obsessions cause anxiety and compulsions serve to reduce it, creating a vicious cycle of negative reinforcement. In OCPD, on the other

Table 8.1 Differential Diagnosis between OCPD and OCD

Characteristic	*OCPP*	*OCD*
Nature of symptoms	Pervasive pattern of perfectionism, rigidity and control	Obsessions (intrusive thoughts) and compulsions (repetitive behavior)
Awareness of illness	*Ego-syntonic* (perceived as appropriate and desirable)	*Ego-dystonic* (perceived as irrational and problematic)
Function of behavior	Expression of values and principles the person considers correct	Reducing anxiety generated by obsessions
Onset	Gradual, typically develops in adolescence or early adulthood	Often acute, may occur at any age
Course	Stable and persistent over time	Fluctuating, with possible periods of remission
Emotional impact	Distress mainly related to interpersonal difficulties	High subjective suffering
Control	Excessive need for control over the environment and others	Feeling of loss of control over one's own thoughts

hand, obsessive behaviors are an integral part of the person's personality and identity, and are not perceived as problematic.

It is important to note that OCD and OCPD can occur in *comorbidity*, further complicating both diagnosis and treatment. In these cases, a thorough clinical assessment that considers both dimensions is essential for effective therapeutic intervention.

There is some overlap between OCD and *other personality disorders*, but OCD is distinct from these disorders in its main features and consequences on behavior.[22] There is a high comorbidity between OCD with psychotic manifestations and Schizotypal Personality Disorder, anche with BP as mentioned.

OCD also borders on psychosis due to the poor insight of many patients. Although awareness of the irrationality of symptoms (insight) has historically been considered distinctive of OCD ("folie lucide"), clinical observation and the DSM-5 recognize a *continuum of insight*, down to cases where it is absent, bringing OCD phenomenologically closer to psychosis; indeed, *insight varies in OCD along a continuum.*

Thus, *between obsessive-compulsive disorder (OCD), psychosis and borderline personality organization, there are complex overlaps. Otto Kernberg* offers a crucial interpretative model with his *borderline personality organization* (*BPO*), seen as an intermediate area between neurosis and psychosis.[23]

8.4 OCD and *Chakras*

OCD is the expression of a separative ego identification, which is reflected in the various energy levels represented by the *Chakras*.

We are all subject to an "impure" *vision*, as karma veils clear consciousness. This impurity, or stain,[24] is distributed differently in the different *Chakras*, but usually affects one or more of them differently.

By identifying more precisely the *Chakras* affected by this obscuration, we can get an idea of the kind of obsessive energies and thoughts and the specific resistances we will encounter in therapeutic work.

All obsessive thoughts revolve around egoic identification, creating a *revolving door* syndrome (i.e. repetition) to confirm and express consciousness from that point of view (egocentrism).

Consciousness is identified with the *person*, i.e. with the *separate body-mind*: this is the *first of all obsessive, repetitive thoughts,* the assertion (believed) to *be the* "me."

The individual obsessions all derive from this first belief, functioning in a dissociative sense from the true nature of being, and reconfirming the separation, thus reinforcing the pivot of the *ego-centered* carousel.[25]

For example, sexuality indicates separation from unity, and the desire to return to it; anger indicates separation at the level of ego affirmation and the desire to remove the obstacle.

From each *Chakra* originates specific psychological and emotional dynamics that in the OCD we see distorted and exasperated in each *Chakra*; symptoms express a form of interference, attachment, or dysfunctional control of the separate ego.[26]

8.4.1 Analysis of the main Chakras

- *First Chakra*: Associated with *survival* and identification with the physical body. In OCD, it manifests as material attachment and fear of loss. Obsessive thoughts revolve around the *loss* of psychological integrity, psychological or social destabilization, uncertainty about health or money, of that which gives security.
- *Second Chakra*: Connected *to sexuality, creativity, and pleasure.*
- Here we observe dynamics of pleasure control, as in pornography or perversion; attachment to this energy can express in relationships, where control and power can lead to pathological jealousy, stalking, relational and manipulative seduction. Pathological jealousy, for example, is also about not letting go of sexual pleasure.
- *Third Chakra*: This is where the energy of *self-assertion, the emotion of anger,* is expressed.

The egocentric aspect of control is expressed as competition and aggression.

Pathological anger (outbursts of rage, inability to express self-assertion) arises from blockages at this level, and thoughts revolve around self-value, thinking oneself worthy and capable.

- *Fourth Chakra*: This is where *affective energy, love and emotional relationships* are expressed.

Control over affections generates toxic attachments, jealousy, and relational suffering, incapacity to love.

Limerence is an obsessive disorder centered on not being able to overcome separation in a relationship; prolonged mourning, the inability to let go of a person, even an animal, if exaggerated can become an obsession, with compensatory compulsions based on affective blackmail and toxic attachments.

- *Fifth Chakra*: Related to *communication, distinguishing reasoning*, and therefore *doubt* that becomes pathological.

Obsessive thinking manifests itself as sterile rationalization and mental control, pathological doubt, an obsession focused on reasoning, wanting to understand, finding differences and details and divergences.

- *Sixth Chakra*: This *Chakra* is the gateway to the integration of opposites (Sun–Moon) and the *overcoming of duality*. The *Moon* is the mirror of light, of the Sun, they are one; it is where consciousness is mirrored in form.

In OCD, we see the consequences of attachment and dissociation: difficulty in letting go of images and fantasies, and the tendency to believe in them as external, real objects.

It is ultimately a matter of *not letting go of the formal dimension of reality*. The tendency to imagine, to produce images, might be an individual characteristic, but the not letting go of them, the believing in them, as in hallucinations, wanting to control them, stems instead from the ego reference, the resistance to extinguish the separation.

As always, the problem is spiritual but presents itself as psychological.

In a room of mirrors, one could travel for miles,[27] under the illusion of arriving somewhere.

- The sixth *Chakra* (*Sun*) is the core of the individual vision. Going beyond form is the final frontier, and this happens only reaching the seventh *Chakra*: thoughts and images are the frontier where one crosses the separation of oneself from Self (God).

Let us remember that *just as symptoms are specific pathways of expression of resistance*, differentiated according to the *Chakras* most involved, *so they are also pathways of access and return to unity*, through self-recognition: each specific energy is an area of psychological work and differentiated alchemical transformation, an opportunity for the awakening of consciousness in each *Chakra*.

In this sense, the suffering resulting from obsessive thoughts can be transformative, indicating a way to overcome egoic identification.

8.5 Therapy

As already mentioned, OCD responds poorly to any kind of therapy.

Between the onset of obsessive-compulsive symptoms and recourse to specialist help there is usually a very long time lapse (7–15 years); usually these patients have poor *compliance*, and are not as responsive to therapy. During this long time they face obstacles and suffering in all important areas of functioning. Sometimes patients try more than one route in their long journey through suffering, various types of therapies.

The therapeutic approach of mainstream psychiatry and psychology is mainly based on Cognitive Behavioral Therapy (CBT, especially with Response Prevention (EPR)), and *Pharmacotherapy,* with Selective Serotonin Reuptake Inhibitors (SSRIs). The combination of the two approaches seems to offer the best results.

OCD's therapy is generally outpatient, and hospitalization is not recommended, except when a high suicidal risk is detected, or when physical conditions are poor due to rituals, or when patients are aggressive. During an in-patient stay, however, it is possible to apply higher doses of medication or propose a higher frequency of psychotherapy sessions.

8.5.1 Psychotherapy

8.5.1.1 Cognitive therapy in OCD

Cognitive therapy in OCD focuses on identifying and modifying the dysfunctional beliefs that underlie the obsessions, such as excessive responsibility, overestimation of threat, and intolerance of uncertainty. *EPR* consists of gradually exposing the patient to the situations or thoughts that trigger the obsessions, while preventing the compulsions from taking place. The aim is to break the association between obsession and compulsion, allowing the patient to experience anxiety without neutralizing it through ritual and gradually learning that anxiety decreases even without the compulsion.

For example, a patient with contamination obsessions might be gradually exposed to touching objects perceived as dirty, being instructed not to wash their hands immediately afterwards.

Compliance with behavioral therapy is often poor, and a significant proportion of patients discontinue treatment prematurely. Dropping out may be due to various factors, such as low motivation, unclear expectations of the therapy, criticism of the therapist, and lower initial severity of symptoms. Furthermore, patients with predominantly obsessive symptoms and little compulsive component tend to respond less effectively to EPR.

In the treatment of OCPD, the primary focus is on *long-term psychotherapy*, often of a psychodynamic or cognitive-behavioral orientation, aimed at modifying rigid and inflexible personality traits. The goal is to help the patient develop a greater awareness of his or her own patterns of thought and behavior, tolerate ambiguity and imperfection, improve their interpersonal skills, and develop greater flexibility in handling situations.

In OCPD, given the ego-syntonic traits, motivation to change may be lower than in OCD. Therapeutic work requires patience and a focus on understanding the origins of these traits and their long-term negative consequences. The goal is not the elimination of obsessive-compulsive traits per se, which in a mild form can also be adaptive, but *their modulation and integration* into a more flexible and functional personality.

8.5.1.2 Psychoanalysis

Freud distinguished between a "terminable" *analysis*, which leads to recovery, and an "interminable" *analysis* in which the patient continues to suffer despite the treatment, which is therefore prolonged.[28] This essay marks a phase of critical realism in Freudian theory: Freud had often obsessive patients in therapy, and he himself admits that psychoanalysis is not omnipotent.

In his reflection, he attributes this prolonged "duration" to the *patient's difficulty in overcoming unconscious resistance. He identifies three factors* that can make an analysis interminable: the force of the *drives* (when *the Id* is too strong and the drive energy is so intense that it resists any analytical elaboration), the rigidity of the *superego* (which is too severe), and above all the *compulsion to repeat.* Freud thus observes a *disposition to* "persevere" which he nevertheless attributes to a force the patient suffers, a disease for which the patient is not responsible: he is a victim, he tends to relive the same pathological patterns even though he recognizes them rationally.

8.5.1.3 TP psychotherapy

It is appropriate to integrate cognitive-behavioral and psychodynamic aspects with a TP approach, in order to have a more complete understanding and to favor more significant therapeutic results for the OCD and the OCPD.

In this perspective, as mentioned, obsessions and compulsions may represent distorted attempts to respond to deep spiritual needs or to address fundamental existential issues that CBT therapy does not provide an answer to.

Thus, in a TP therapy that simply seeks to bring the spiritual dimension back into therapy, one can *explore the existential meaning of symptoms* and help the person understand their obsessions and compulsions not only as symptoms to be eliminated, but as expressions of deeper issues related to meaning, identity, morality and transcendence. *Mindfulness* and *meditation practices* can be *incorporated*, i.e. techniques derived from millennia-old spiritual traditions that foster non-judgmental awareness of obsessive thoughts and the ability to distance oneself from them without reacting compulsively. *Spiritual experiences* can be *recognized and valued*, distinguishing between healthy expressions of spirituality and pathological manifestations that can feed OCD. During psychotherapy, *spiritual metaphors and narratives* can be *used* to offer new perspectives on inner conflicts and possibilities for transformation. It should be recognized that the meanings attributed to symptoms may vary considerably according to the patient's cultural and spiritual background, rather than imposing a foreign medical model.

However, in a deeper TP approach, the critical factor for therapy is the *presence of a non-dual state of consciousness in the therapist and the therapeutic field*, within which only the fundamental split between the ego and the self can be healed.

The treatment of OCD should not be limited to the suppression of symptoms, but should favor the reintegration of the split contents and the recognition of the underlying evolutionary impulse; one will have to help the patient tolerate the transformation by accompanying the process of individuation in a safe and gradual manner.

One should recognize the negative transference always present in the OCD as an element to which one should give due dignity, instead of seeking a dualistic, ameliorative, symptomatological solution; one should recognize the individuative potential of the ego's resistance in order to transcend that duality.

On closer inspection, *the repetition compulsion of which Freud spoke does not seem so innocent*: the ego itself, which undergoes the compulsion, coercively repeats the dynamic of interposing itself. The first compulsion remains its own survival instinct: its tendency to remain separate, to oppose its merging with the whole.

This dynamic depends on the contamination with the shadow, on the internalization of the principle of separation, which is the first thing to be dealt with, so that the consciousness can disidentify itself: this is, in fact, the true source of suffering.

It is said that "if you have never seen the devil,[29] look at your self." And it is also said that *to persevere is diabolical.*

This persevering in opposition to the principle of love, of reunification, is an issue of spiritual choice (certainly not religious or confessional); it is the foundation of the control system, which finally extinguishes the sacred fire.

It must therefore be recognized that the ego in this view is an active impediment in the transformative process. Any therapy that truly aims at integration (be it psychodynamic or transpersonal) must necessarily confront the ego's long history of attachment to its own defensive system and resistance, and analyze the *negative transference.*

In fact, many of these therapies merely support the patient in constant, stagnant suffering, or are interrupted by the patient himself when he approaches real change. *Change, in fact, is perceived as the main enemy by the OCD*: complaining about chronic suffering always goes hand in hand with strategies that keep it unchanged.

The patient wants to heal in order to stop suffering, but at the same time he does not want to give up the defenses that keep him attached to that suffering, as this would open the door to the process of inner death and rebirth.

From the transpersonal point of view, *the return of the repressed material* can be interpreted as an *attempt at self-healing* of the psyche, a constant call for the integration of dissociated contents, which, however, are rejected, and thus return more and more insistently.

8.5.2 Pharmacotherapy

Pharmacological therapies are based on *high-dose SSRIs*, or *clomipramine* (a tricyclic)*; neuroleptics*, *benzodiazepines* are also used.

Psychotropic drugs administration could be prolonged, even lifelong. Usually high drug dosages are used (e.g., double or triple the dosage of antidepressants used for uncomplicated depression).

Patients often leave treatment without consulting the psychiatrist.

8.5.3 Intervention with family members.

It is important in OCD therapy to involve the family, to help them not to cooperate with the patient's pathology. In short strategic therapies (Dr. Nardone) this point is essential: it is recommended to stop cooperating with the rituals the patients ask them to perform. The family is often unclear as to what kind of problem there is, does not accept it, and is afraid of this disorder, also because of the violent reactions that these patients display towards others and themselves; in these patients, as we shall see, the suicide risk is high.

8.6 The problem of suicide in OCD

In my experience, patients with OCD are among those at highest risk of suicide, followed by bipolars in a driven manic phase, and often delusional, and deliriant psychoses. This risk is also present in other self-destructive psychiatric conditions such as anorexia and drug addiction, but we must consider that an obsessive component is always present in them.

According to the DSM-5, *suicidal thoughts are present in 50% of individuals with OCD, and about 25% of patients attempt suicide*. Thus it can happen that they commit that murder, called suicide (which has the aggravating circumstance that the victim cannot defend himself), when they fail to integrate the dissociated oppositional part, which can then take over.

The dissociated destructive complex is not a *victim*, but rather a *persecutor*; its logic could be expressed as follows: "rather than die I will kill myself." The opposition will not give in and is willing to *break the bank* in order not to give way.

Catastrophic thoughts originate from the split ego-complex, from the "destructive me," which fears to vanish into thin air, to be eliminated, and for this it may rather menace to eliminate itself; the ego-consciousness often has little insight into *who is speaking inside the head, who is speaking into the microphone*: consciousness is totally identified, and believes that those thoughts are its own, and in these cases the risk is greater.

A less serious variant of suicidal thoughts are *violent thoughts of self-damage*, against the psychic "me", or benefactors, or towards life itself, or even towards one's own belongings, which we often find in the OCD.[30]

Self-devaluation and self-harm in young people today is on the rise due to the increase in identity crises and collective dissociation, but it works with a similar mechanism to that of OCD. Here, too, the negative thought is considered alien to oneself, and yet neurotically one consents to it thanks to dissociation: the patient does not take responsibility for recognizing, accepting, and integrating the anguish.

A frequent form of physical harm is *to compulsively cut oneself*: obsessive thoughts of guilt and the compulsion to self-damage can generate a ritual that provides a form of relief, while at the same time punishing the supposed perpetrator with pain.

As we said, even in *eating disorders or drug addictions* the will to self-damage or elimination is often transparent, even when it does not lead to direct suicide.

Again, in *paranoid psychoses* one only finds thoughts of being harmed or of harming oneself or one's family members, which arise from a hounded, besieged ego that resists and projects the threat of being eliminated out of itself.

People do not always take action, but if the dissociation is strong, they may commit reckless and unconscious actions, such as suicide.

The subjective perception in OCD can have a *positive component*, if properly understood: it is a drive to psychologically step out of one's own path, to come out of egocentrism, and to recognize our higher nature; after all, we can recognize in this call a healing purpose. But in OCD this call for death of the limitation of ego identification and transfromation is very easily misunderstood, and interpreted literally, as a destructive drive, stemming from the logic of dissociation: the separated ego is a prisoner[31] of separation, it is identified with that anti-love logic of death. And the ego is a master of deception, and can take things literally, believe these thoughts, and take action, with tragic results.

The overcoming of the self-destructive position lies in the *shift in consciousness from* "I" *to* "Self," in the shift *from* "my will be done" *to* "*His will be done*," which will also allow the integration of the split complex into this new, broader awareness. Then suffering and dying do not only happen *to you* (the person, the character with whom you still identify), but above all they happen *within you* (i.e., self-awareness).[32]

When disidentification is possible, healing and hope begin: the way out of this destructive loop is to meet the psychological sensation of death, to be with the sensation, to welcome it: not to deny it and repress it, nor to express it or enact it.

Thus, dying to oneself (not physically!) is the way to awakening, as Jesus says "He who loses his life will save it"; the Master is certainly not here recommending mass suicide.[33]

The obsessive on the contrary often is dangerously unaware of this destructive identification, and may fatally "literally" believe the voice in his head telling him that he must die, or that he must kill himself.

Notes

1 Our society is evolving towards a society based on control, increasingly refined, internalized, and pervasive. Today, the more physical and outward forms of behavioral guidance and control, such as brute force (a *hard control)*, are increasingly giving way to psychic control; self-control (a *soft control)*, is managed from within, by the *super-ego,* an internalized autopilot fueled by education and society's mental conditioning (e.g., through films and the media).

2 In the normal individuals we encounter everyday, pathological traits of the OCPD can be traced, but they are considered normal because they are common.

3 Some sources estimate it to be on average around 4.4 per cent, i.e. *one in 20 individuals*; this figure rises to *10 per cent in people who present for a psychiatric examination*. My opinion is that it is even more widespread. However, an accurate estimate is difficult due to the fact that many people with this disorder do not seek professional help. Furthermore, the diagnosis of OCPD can be complex due to the similarity of symptoms with those of OCD and Avoidant Personality Disorder.

4 I believe that almost every patient who comes to psychotherapy suffers to varying degrees from a control problem; in other words, *they do not suffer*

because of the way things go, inside or outside of them, but because *they do not agree with the way things go, and would like to control them.*

5 This control over one's life and emotions may lead to repressing or hiding one's emotions, and may go so far as to avoid situations altogether that could trigger negative emotions, such as conflict or criticism.

6 Passive-aggressive is a term used in psychology to describe a pattern of behavior in which a person indirectly expresses hostility, anger, or resistance instead of manifesting it directly and openly. This attitude manifests itself through actions or omissions that hinder, irritate, or frustrate others, while maintaining an appearance of conformity or neutrality. Passive-aggressive behavior can cause problems in personal, work, and social relationships, as it makes authentic communication and conflict resolution difficult. It can be a source of frustration for both the perpetrator and the sufferer, fueling vicious cycles of misunderstanding and resentment. Examples of passive-aggressive behavior are intentionally procrastinating on tasks requested by others, "accidentally" forgetting important commitments or responsibilities, showing sarcasm, irony, or ambiguous responses, giving the "silent treatment" (ignoring or not answering), showing obstinacy or deliberate inefficiency.

7 A sense of duty ("I must always be one hundred per cent"; "I must always give my best") does not necessarily benefit performance. On the contrary, such patients have difficulty prioritizing their tasks and often find themselves stuck, feeling that time is never enough and effort never enough, and as a consequence they struggle to meet deadlines.

8 "Obsessive" comes from the Latin word "obsessio," meaning "siege." This term, in turn, derives from the verb "obsidēre," composed of "ob" (in front) and "sedēre" (to sit), thus literally "to stand in front of" *or* "to besiege." In medieval Latin, "obsessio" also came to mean *demonic possession.*

9 This is a crucial element in differentiating OCD from psychotic conditions.

10 The prevalence of psychotic symptoms (particularly delusions) in OCD patients is about 20.5 per cent, often associated with increased severity, early onset, and impaired functioning. In addition, patients who did not respond to treatment were found to have elevated dissociative symptoms.

11 With regard to a specific movement disorder, *tics*, not infrequently present in obsessives, are probably discharges of energy through the subtle system, *Kundalini* energy, acrtivating motor structures (at the level of the motor cortex), as a short circuit with respect to an impeded psychic processing of them. Tics, like mannerisms, are reminiscent of the movements and mudras of Indian dances. The tics-mudras correspond to the movements of energy and consciousness that accompany awakening, and which are present in certain phases of OCD.

12 In reactive formation the unacceptable impulse or thought is transformed into its opposite; this often results in hypermoral behavior or obsessive rituals that serve to manage forbidden or distressing impulses.

13 In the isolation of affect, there is a split between the obsessive thought and the corresponding feeling, whereby the subject thinks recurrently about distressing content without fully experiencing the emotion.

In other words, the person may think or talk about traumatic events, desires, or impulses without experiencing (or showing) the emotions that would normally be associated with those contents. This is a form of dissociation. *Clinical examples*: A person who recounts a severe bereavement or trauma without showing any emotion, as if they were talking about something extraneous; a patient who describes aggressive or transgressive thoughts without feeling guilt or anxiety, as if they were abstract ideas.

14 In retroactive cancellation, the subject tries to mentally "erase" unwanted acts or thoughts through rituals or symbolic actions. For example, after doing or thinking something that is deemed "forbidden" or guilty, the person enacts an opposite or reparative action, as if he or she could thus retroactively eliminate the effect or reality of the previous act. In obsessive-compulsive disorders, retroactive undoing is often manifested in rituals (e.g., washing hands, counting, repeating gestures) that serve to "neutralize" unwanted thoughts or actions.

15 Denial: defensive refusal to acknowledge distressing impulses, emotions or realities.

16 Repression: exclusion of psychic contents from awareness.

17 Splitting: rigid separation between "good self" and "bad self," or between "pure" and "contaminated" thoughts.

18 Schizoid projection: attribution of unacceptable contents to external objects, often with experiences of internal alienation.

19 See recent research and psychoanalytic literature (Anna Freud, Melanie Klein, Otto Kernberg).

20 During transitional, seasonal, or life periods there is a worsening of symptoms due to increased energy that exacerbates defensive tension.

21 In particular, OCPD shares with a specific variant of OCD the tendency to engage in perfectionistic behavior mainly related to order and symmetry. In both cases, there may be excessive attention to details and rules.

22 The differential diagnosis also arises with subjects with *narcissistic personalities* based on the sense of self-criticism that is present in OCD, absent in the former, with *antisocial personalities*, who are prodigal towards themselves in contrast to those with OCD, and with schizoid personalities, where the social distance is not due to discomfort but to an inability to be intimate and a fear of others' aggressiveness. Compared to *Narcissistic Personality Disorder (NPD)*, it shares with it an excessive preoccupation with success and performance, an excessive focus on appearance, the importance of self-image, and a sense of superiority over others. However, unlike NPD, OCPD does not seek the attention of others and does not try to draw attention to itself). *Compared to Schizoid Personality Disorder (SPD), it* shares social isolation and emotional indifference. However, in OCPD, social isolation may be the result of excessive preoccupation with control and order, whereas in DPS, social isolation is the result of an inability to feel empathy and a disinterest in social relationships). OCPD and Avoidant Personality Disorder (APD) have some features in common, but are also distinguishable by some key differences. These two syndromes are united by a tendency to avoidance in order to better control external or internal conditions: people with OCPD may avoid situations that could cause anxiety or stress.

23 BPO is characterized by ego weakness, aggression, massive use of *splitting* as the main defense, chaotic thinking, and projective identifications. While maintaining the reality check (unlike psychosis), the borderline structure helps to understand cases of OCD with poor insight or psychotic manifestations, interpreting them as a shift towards more primitive defenses along a continuum of severity.

Dissociation (fragmentation of identity/consciousness, often linked to trauma) is present both in narcissism (linked to BPO, to protect a grandiose self by splitting vulnerable parts) and, in more radical forms and with a breakdown of the reality check, in psychosis.

In OCD with psychotic traits, it may manifest in the rigid attempt to control intrusive thoughts. *Splitting* (dichotomous good/bad division), central in BPO and narcissism to manage conflicts while avoiding ambivalence, differs from psychotic disintegration. Kernberg emphasizes how these mechanisms, although pathological, are attempts to preserve a coherence of identity under conditions of vulnerability.

24 In the Catholic tradition, the "*stain*" is sin, (original and in general); it is a matter of purifying with the fire (*Piur*) of the Holy Spirit (*Prana*) this first dark matter (the Mother, matrix, obscured *Shakti*: the Addolorata, the guilty conscience) and bringing it to be without stain (Immaculate); only then can it give way to the ascent (Assumption)

25 The sense of separation, the hindrance is usually thought to be caused by an external factor, due to unconsciousness and the resulting projection. Thus, we habitually see people engaged in solving external difficulties without succeeding: just as one cannot lift oneself up by the hair, so it is not the ego, the origin of the obstacle, that can remove it, except by eliminating its own resistance. The subject goes towards the other with the intention of healing the separation, of reuniting with love; however, he confuses attachment with love.

26 That is an ego contaminated with the principle of separation, with the shadow; as we may find in pathological jealousy, where love is so selfish as to be destructive.

27 From the song "Brainwashed" by George Harrison, opening track of his album "Brainwashed," released posthumously in 2002.

28 "Terminal and Interminable Analysis" from 1937, one of the last of Freud's life.

29 From the Greek "*dia ballein*," meaning that which separates.

30 In the Divine Comedy, the sin of violence is of three types: violence against oneself, against one's possessions, and against God.

31 *Captivus* in Latin means prisoner (e.g., in captivity).

32 "In this room there is only one exit / and it is the one invisible only to you."

33 For if "I and my father are One," who can ever die but ignorance, the illusion of being separate, a false belief? Only deception, the hiding of truth, can die, and all this leads to self-discovery: it is God playing hide-and-seek with Himself.

Chapter 9

Psychosis and dissociation

As we have now made clear, awakening proceeds by overwhelming all that is not yet allienated, ready, willing, and when the process becomes extreme, the situation can become very difficult.

Three possibilities may occur in the context of deeper awakenings, each with its own variations:

- *The first* one refers to what we will examine in *this chapter*: *psychoses and schizophrenic syndromes*.

  In these cases, the ego is quite unprepared to recognize and integrate awakening, is overwhelmed, fragments and becomes dysfunctional; the process does not recede, the result is a shipwreck. In psychosis, the identity impairment is deeper than in dissociative forms such as DD, and we find a fragmentation of the personality, a collapse of the ego: its boundaries may vanish, leaving a world dominated by chaos and terror to emerge.

  We can consider them severe forms of dissociation, *dissociative psychoses*, from the point of view of MS psychiatry, (keeping in mind that for the DSM, the dissociative forms constitute a separate category from psychoses), then we will consider the TP interpretation.
- *A second possibility*, which we will see in the next chapter, is that the PC encounters a more favorable and receptive ground, and could give birth, through a psychotic difficult labor, to a better outcome, resulting in what is known as a Spiritual Emergency (SE). Various diagnostic and prognostic indicators allow us to identify these cases and to intervene appropriately.
- *Finally, there is the possibility*, in the best cases, that the PC will resolve without excessive suffering and with a clear, positive outcome. These are referred to as "excellent" or complete awakenings. They are rarer, and reported in the history of all religious traditions. They can be found around us even today, if recognized. They bear witness to the possibility of the self_realization of consciousness, of its rebirth in peace and light.

DOI: 10.4324/9781003676461-9

9.1 Dissociative psychoses

The term "psychosis" was introduced in the 19th century with the meaning of mental illness or insanity, and currently denotes psychiatric disorders that involve a detachment from one's surroundings and severe difficulties in initiating activities and experiencing authentic feelings towards other people.

The DSM-5 (Diagnostic and Statistical Manual of Mental Disorders, fifth edition) classifies the main forms of psychosis into the category: "schizophrenia spectrum and other psychotic disorders"; schizophrenia and related disorders are part of this category.

These disorders *share some fundamental characteristics, such as psychotic symptoms* (delusions, hallucinations, disorganization of thought).

They are classified according to the severity of symptoms and functional impairment, described along a gradient: some diagnoses are at the extremes of severity (such as pure schizophrenia), while others are at the other extreme, as milder, briefer forms (brief psychotic disorder, schizophreniform disorder). Some forms include mood symptoms or are associated with organic causes or substance abuse.[1]

We wish to emphasize here that these syndromes represent conditions of identity crisis. They are marked by profound destructuring of the organizing instance—the ego—influencing various levels (thought, perception, mood). We will now examine these aspects in depth, focusing on the syndrome in which they are most prominent: schizophrenia (see Table 9.1).

9.2 Schizophrenia

The DSM-5 *does not separate* "psychosis" *from* "schizophrenia": *schizophrenia is one of the main psychoses,* characterized by the duration of symptoms, the simultaneous presence of several positive and negative symptoms, and the severe impairment of the person's global functioning.

Schizophrenia is considered the *prototype of psychotic disorders*, which is why we dedicate an entire chapter to this disorder; when speaking of psychoses, we will refer to it in particular.

Schizophrenia is considered *a severe mental disorder, characterized by the persistence of altered cognitive and perceptual functions, behavior and affectivity, with a course of more than six months, and with a strong maladjustment of the person.*

In 1893, *Emil Kraepelin* used the term *schizophrenia* to make a distinction (known as the Kraepelinian dichotomy), between the two psychoses: *dementia praecox*[2] and *manic depression* (now called bipolar disorder).[3]

Table 9.1 Classification of Psychosis in DSM-5

Disorder	*Main features*	*Duration Symptoms*	*Functioning*	*Cardinal Symptoms*	*Clinical Example*
Delusional disorder	Persistent non-bizarre delusions without other prominent psychotic symptoms	≥1 month	Slightly impaired	Delusions	Believes neighbor wants to poison him, lives normally
Brief psychotic disorder	Sudden psychosis with delusions, hallucinations or disorganization, complete resolution	1 day – 1 month	Returns to normal	Delusions/ hallucinations, disorganization	After intense bereavement, delusional episode lasting a few weeks
Schizophreniform disorder	Typical schizophrenic symptoms but lasting <6 months	1-6 months	Often impaired	Delusions, hallucinations, negative	Isolation, neglect, delusions for 3 months then remission
Schizophrenia	Typical psychotic symptoms (delusions, hallucinations, disorganization, negative symptoms), global impairment	≥6 months	Severe impairment	Delusions, hallucinations, negative symptoms	Delusions of persecution, social withdrawal, incoherent speech
Schizoaffective disorder	Major affective episodes together with psychotic symptoms; psychosis even beyond mood phase	Varies	Often impaired	Psychosis + mood disorder	Expressions of mania + delusions of grandeur
Substance/ drug-induced psychotic disorder	Substance/drug-related psychosis (onset during/ shortly after use or withdrawal)	During use/ shortly after	Varies	Delusions/ hallucinations	Auditory hallucinations 1h after taking LSD
Psychotic disorder due to medical condition	Psychotic symptoms due to known medical condition	During or after medical event	Varies	Delusions/ hallucinations	Delusions and hallucinations in a patient with a brain tumor

The word schizophrenia translates as "splitting of the mind" and is modern Latin from *schizein* (from ancient Greek: schizo, σχίζειν, lett. "to divide") and *phrēn* (φρήν, lett. "mind"), thus "divided mind." Its use was intended to describe the separation of functions between personality, thought, memory, and perception.[4]

It is therefore a dissociation within the mind, between the ego complex, psychic life, thoughts; the term indicates the "separation of mental functions," a dissociation of them.

9.2.1 Diagnosis

In DSM-IV schizophrenia was subdivided into different subtypes: *paranoid, disorganized, catatonic, undifferentiated, residual.*[5] Today, in DSM-5 (2013), it is categorized within the group of psychotic disorders, which has eliminated the division of schizophrenia into several subcategories, and introduced a *dimensional assessment of symptom severity.*[6]

The elimination of these subtypes was due to their low stability over time, limited clinical reliability, and lack of prognostic significance.[7]

In order to make a diagnosis of schizophrenia, *significant symptoms* must be present *most of the time, for at least six months.*

These symptoms may include: *positive symptoms* such as delusions, hallucinations, disorganization of speech, disorganized or catatonic behavior; and *negative symptoms* such as limited affective openness and reduced cognitive functions.

9.2.2 Symptomatology

Overt symptomatology is generally preceded by certain specific *signs known as prodromes.* Some time before the overt disorder, prodromal symptoms appear that should already raise suspicion of a dissociative psychosis; They represent abnormalities that will later evolve into the overt picture of dissociative psychosis, but, at this stage, emerge insidiously, with less prominence and intensity.

Gradually, *changes in lifestyle and the way of reacting* then manifest, such as loss of interest, reduced performance in studies or at work, emotional withdrawal in relationships[8] strange behavior, physical complaints ("my brain is burning"), episodes of unjustified anger or aggression, poor hygiene and appearance, insomnia.[9]

Reasoning is impaired: the person may have difficulty in logical thinking, with disorganized thoughts or logical leaps, difficulty in concentration and organization, manifest irrationality or strange beliefs, have bizarre, irrational, or delusional thoughts or beliefs.

The patient exhibits *changes in mood* (e.g., mood fluctuations, including irritability or apathy; may exhibit reduced affection or inappropriate emotional expression), difficulties in coping with stress.

Often at this stage the patient and family members psychologize the symptoms, seeking an external stressor as the - one that would be relatively insignificant for most people, and on closer evaluation prove to be clearly disproportionate both in intensity and duration.[10]

9.2.2.1 Positive symptoms: Delusions and hallucinations

Delusions: *a delusion is defined as a clearly false belief that the person continues to hold even if proven wrong.*

The most common delusional ideas in schizophrenia from a TP perspective can be understood as expressions of an identity crisis; in other words, they are related to the collapse of the ego reference, and what remains of the ego attempts either to attribute the experience to an external cause and/or to defend itself against it through flight or aggression.

Although the reference to the old ego as it was previously known has more or less definitively vanished, the consciousness retains a certain tendency, without true identification, to interpret what emerges during the CP in ego-referential terms. However, there is usually no longer a complete conviction that things depend on one's ego. *What prevails, is the loss of ego-boundaries*, and the fragmentation of the world formerly unified by the ego and in the ego. Consciousness has shifted to a position without clear boundaries, and yet a tendency towards ego reconstitution remains, although this ego is clearly incapacitated and confused.

One finds oneself like a small boat in the middle of the sea, or like an "idea" in a storm, without being too clear about what is happening and to whom. The ego lives and interprets reality in a delusional manner in a failed attempt to maintain the old ego-centric vision, although by now the new condition is that of having lost this ego reference.

One can observe delusions of

- *Persecution* ("they are after me," "I am being followed by the mafia," "they have tapped my mobile phone").
- *Reference*, of self-reference of what is happening ("a passer-by was whistling in the street to let everyone know that my wife is cheating on me"; "during the crisis, I was the awareness operator, and my brother was Bin Laden").

- *Influence and control* ("they put a microchip in my brain, with which they condition my thoughts and behavior")
- *Delusional ideas of greatness* ("I am the most famous singer in the world"), of *ruin* ("I don't even have the money to pay the bus fare"); and along the same lines, *delusions of nihilism or denial* ("the world does not exist"), *or of guilt* ("ten years ago I stole a book from a classmate and for this I shall be damned forever").
- *Hypochondriac delusions* ("even though the doctors assure me otherwise, I am sure that I have pancreatic cancer and that I will soon die").
- *Mystical delusions* have to do with the inflation of the ego (e.g., "I have received from God the task of saving humanity").
- Loss of ego boundaries is at the root of symptoms such as the *delusional belief in thought theft* ("the neighbors with a magnet pick up my thoughts"), *thought transmission* ("what I think is divulged through the radio"), and *thought reading* ("I feel naked: everyone knows perfectly well what is going on in my head"), typical of schizophrenic forms.

Hallucinations: consist of *an altered way of perceiving things, which can affect all five sense organs.*

The most common hallucinations involve the five senses:

- ***Voices*** that the person, but not others, hears and whose content is sometimes reassuring, more often offensive or threatening.

  Voices may also give orders, such as running away, hurting or harming oneself, which the person sometimes, fortunately rarely, obeys.
- Other forms of hallucinations consist of ***seeing*** *objects or people* (e.g., an image of the Madonna or the devil) that others do not see.
- *Sensing* ***smells*** (e.g., an intense perfume of roses).
- *Sensing* ***tastes*** (e.g., of rotten food) that no one else feels.
- *Perceiving a* ***physical sensation*** (e.g., being touched or stung) without anyone else being near.[11]

9.2.2.2 Negative symptoms

Negative symptoms are less prominent but no less severe and disabling manifestations.

In the identity crisis, in which identity vanished, the *motivation* to perform tasks or have interests related to it also vanishes.

Not understanding the reason for this, the patient (and his environment) react negatively to this process, judging it to be an obvious pathology.

The person becomes *apathetic* (inability to participate or take an interest, either affectively or intellectually), *abulic* (marked loss of volition, rendering the person unable to carry out even very simple tasks or projects), *anhedonic* (inability to take pleasure in anything), *demotivated* (not interested in being with others, does not take care of one's own hygiene), and often presents a *social withdrawal* (ending up living locked in one's own world, without feeling the desire to leave it).

The presence of negative symptoms is often a source of stress for the person and makes it difficult to lead a normal life and do a job.

9.2.2.3 Cognitive symptoms

The person suffering from schizophrenia *is unable to link his thoughts together in a logical way* resulting in strange speech that is incomprehensible to the listener; *sometimes he or she freezes while speaking* without being able to give an explanation as to why. He is clearly disconnected (dissociation).

He also has *difficulty concentrating* (e.g., maintaining attention on specific tasks or following a conversation), *remembering* (especially difficulties with short-term memory, i.e. remembering recent information or performing everyday tasks), *understanding what he is told* and using it to make decisions.

He therefore manifests *a reduction in executive skills* (planning, organization, and abstract reasoning), *slow thinking, reduced cognitive flexibility* (i.e. the ability to change one's way of thinking or adapt to new situations), and *difficulties in social comprehension* (i.e. the ability to understand the mental states of others).[12]

Again, *from a TP perspective,* these symptoms are typical of someone who has taken a plunge into the unconscious, who has lost himself in Nothingness, who is in the amorphous, homogeneous state of the Self, and can no longer find *him-self* or any sense of direction.

9.2.3 Epidemiology, Incidence, Evolution, Prognosis

Worldwide, schizophrenia *is the most common psychotic disorder*: approximately 1 per cent of the population suffers from it (other estimates indicate a global prevalence of between 0.3 and 0.7 per cent), with no significant differences between men and women. However, onset generally occurs between 15 and 25 years in males and between 25 and 35 years in females.[13] The frequency of schizophrenia varies worldwide and in different conditions, even by as much as fivefold. It is rare for a person to become ill with schizophrenia once they have passed the age of 50.

The development is often worsened by the fact that the person does not think he or she is ill, so he or she refuses treatment or discontinues it as soon as possible, thus increasing the number of relapses and hospitalizations.

Its evolution is generally towards *chronicity*: if left untreated, in most cases, schizophrenia follows a *recurrent course*, with alternating periods of intense symptoms and periods of amelioration or remission.

As the episodes recur, the intensity of the "positive" symptoms (delusions and hallucinations) diminishes, while the "negative" ones (apathy, emotional detachment, social withdrawal) gradually become more pronounced.

The disorder may manifest gradually or suddenly. More rarely the disorder consists of a single episode that may either gradually resolve or become chronic.

The *prognosis* depends on the type of schizophrenic form: in the past, they were classified in detail, whereas today, as we have seen, the old classifications are outdated. However, attention must be paid to a number of *prognostic indicators to assess the severity of the picture.*[14]

Schizophrenia *has a heavy impact* on the lives of those affected and their families impairing the ability to function in daily life, maintain relationships, pursue life goals, and social integration.[15]

People with schizophrenia may have *comorbidities,* including *major depression and anxiety disorders.* There are also frequent cases of *substance abuse* (found in almost 50 per cent of patients), or cases with *dual diagnosis*, or *social problems,* such as unemployment and poverty.

The most serious *complication* of the disorder is *suicide* (about 5–15 per cent of cases), sometimes as a consequence of overlapping depression, sometimes in obedience to *voices* inciting the person to kill themself.[16]

9.2.4 Differential diagnosis

- Schizophrenia is to be distinguished *from dissociative forms of shorter duration*, which when productive of delusional symptoms are called *acute delusional bouffée*, precisely to indicate the temporary nature of the ongoing major symptomatology.
- *Autism spectrum disorders*[17] must be differentiated as they can have psychotic-like symptoms and in some cases can be diagnosed in comorbidity.
- Depression or *bipolar disorder with psychotic features*, differing from schizophrenia in that the symptoms (delusions or hallucinations) occur only during a depressive or manic episode; these are forms in which the dissociative component is mixed with energetic symptoms typical of the bipolar series, forms defined as *schizoaffective* due to the propensity of psychotic symptoms to show exacerbations and aggravation according to recurrent energetic cycles, the dissociative symptomatology though remaining in the foreground.
- *Schizotypical personality disorder*, which has subthreshold symptoms that may resemble schizophrenia,

- *Obsessive compulsive disorder and body dysmorphism*, in which obsessions can take on delusional characteristics.
- There are also *medical conditions* that cause psychosis: for example, *strokes, brain tumors, some forms of epilepsy, AIDS, syphilis.*
- *Other biological causes* that can disrupt the cohesion of individual consciousness are the consumption of *psychoactive substances*: alcohol, marijuana, cocaine, hallucinogenic substances, NMDA receptor antagonists, such as ketamine.

At present, there are no *specific diagnostic tests* for schizophrenia, but various tools can assist with diagnosis and prognosis, even though no test is definitive; these rest on the *overall clinical evaluation.*[18]

9.2.5 A clinical example

A patient reports the persistent presence of voices communicating to him contents of a religious and grandiose nature: he is told that God can transform himself into anyone, including his interlocutor, and that he himself is destined for a journey to Rome with a figure identified as Divine Providence. The voices attribute divine qualities and supernatural powers to him, claiming that it is possible to transform into other people or animals.

The patient describes a system of supernatural beings (Gods, Saints, Mortals, Copies) and reports experiences of visions in which he sees himself as part of the Holy Family, and endowed with symbolic objects (cloak with inscriptions from the past, present and future).

He also relates episodes of dialogue with the devil, visions of the soul traveling between paradise and Nothingness, and the belief that he is a "script" of Nothingness itself, endowed with special powers and destined to disappear by divine will.

In spite of these experiences, the patient perceives himself as lucid and not confused, and regrets and resents being considered insane, even though he manifests anxiety and fear at the possibility of disappearing as a script, claiming that his destiny has been cancelled by God.

Auditory hallucinations (voices with religious and imperative content), delusions of grandeur and religiousness (identification with divine entities, belief in supernatural powers), magical and symbolic thinking (transformations, magical objects, travel between worlds), disorganization of thought (construction of complex and incoherent systems), alteration of identity and self-perception, and episodes of anxiety and fear linked to delusional beliefs are present in this case. Formal awareness is preserved, at least partially (he claims to be lucid, but disputes the diagnosis of schizophrenia made by psychiatrists). The patient believes himself to be a "script" of a director, of God himself, who creates with thought-forms. He affirms that he realizes he is a character generated by consciousness, a thought-form: one who had been erased from the face of the earth, from roles and from life; one who from being only a "script", a creature, becomes a creator, self-conscious.

A few observations can be proposed here. From the TP point of view, the *spiritual biography*, is rather confused. From his affirmations one comes to know that, first at age 4 then at seven, he had transcendent experiences, visions; and that from there he began a personal and beyond-form communication with the transcendent.

The patient also claims to have experienced, at the time when this process had begun, "sensations in the head" presumably due to the movements of the powerful and transcendent energy of the *Kundalini*, that was activated and had moved upwards in him; this he interpreted as intentional phenomena personally referred to him.[19]

He was lost (at the level of his *identity*), but not completely; and found again, (at the level of the Self), but only partially.

9.3 Etiopathogenesis of psychoses (dissociative syndromes)

MS Psychiatry: modern interpretations of biological psychiatry insist on finding biological *neuro-structural alterations* in psychoses.[20] Recent studies suggest that psychoses share a *common biological substrate* (such as alterations in the brain connectome or delays in frontal myelination), regardless of the specific diagnosis.[21]

Cognitive-behavioral perspectives: Cognitive theories emphasize the role of *distortions in information processing*, such as hyperactivity of the dopaminergic system in amplifying irrelevant signals (the "aberrant salience" hypothesis).

Interventions such as CBT for psychosis aim at *modifying dysfunctional beliefs* related to delusions.

Psychodynamic theories derived from the work of Freud and Jung propose that psychosis represents a regression to early developmental stages: psychosis would be due to *unresolved unconscious conflicts and identity fragmentation:* early traumas (e.g., abandonment) can activate primitive defenses such as *splitting* and *projective identification*, compromising the formation of a cohesive self. For example, *Henri Ey* and *Werner Janzarik* interpret psychoses as regressions to archaic states of consciousness, where unconscious dynamics (e.g., conflicts between split parts of the personality) generate symptoms such as delusions or hallucinations.[22] Delusions could represent attempts to make sense of chaotic experiences, where unconscious contents (e.g., repressed aggression) are expressed in symbolic form.[23]

Undoubtedly, *Jung* is the author who first dealt systematically with the psychological aspect of psychotic disorders.[24] *In particular, Jung* argued that *delusions and hallucinations contain a psychological-existential core that can be interpreted.* Jung believed that delusions are "archetypal" psychoses, i.e. spontaneous manifestations of universal images and themes that the ego-consciousness cannot integrate.[25]

Jung believed that two important features of schizophrenia were evident from Janet's concept of "abaissement": the fragmentation of psychic functioning into a multiplicity of *active and independent complexes* and, correlatively, a *physiological and non-systematic disintegration of psychic elements.*

Carl Gustav Jung contributed significantly to the study of psychosis by developing the concept of "emotionally charged complexes"; he studied delusions as manifestations of the collective unconscious. In psychosis, as a consequence of the identity crisis, *the ego would lose the ability to* "filter" *the archetypal contents. Psychoses would thus be existential crises linked to the breakdown of the balance between individual consciousness and the mystery that is behind of the term* "collective unconscious".[26] Delusions and hallucinations would reflect the irruption of archetypal images (e.g., mythological figures, symbols of death/rebirth) that the patient does not recognize as parts of himself.

It remains a mystery for ego psychology, *however,* what is the reason for this irruption of unconscious contents into consciousness, and for the disintegration of the complexes among themselves.

Theories that propose an interfering organic element (a toxin, a genetic alteration) do not, after all, provide exhaustive answers; they *refer to a further mystery: to the relationship between psyche and matter*, to something that precedes the symbol. Jung proposed the term ***psychoid*** for this mysterious place on the border between physical reality and psyche; by this term he referred to the *physical, as well as psychic, character of the unconscious.* Archetypes in fact operate as organizing principles that transcend the distinction between mind and matter, between individual and collective, between microcosm and macrocosm.

According to Jung, *the psychoid is the unitary basis of the archetypes*, which are not just psychic structures, but universal patterns that act at both the psychological and physical levels, connecting the individual to the cosmos *(unus mundus)*.[27]

TP Interpretation: transpersonal psychology, influenced by Jung and Wilber, interprets psychosis as *a failed attempt to transcend the ego, where the collapse of identity boundaries in the encounter with transcendent dimensions generates chaos instead of growth.*

For Wilber, hallucinations and delusions could reflect the irruption of archetypal contents (e.g., mythological figures, death/rebirth symbols) not integrated by consciousness.

In this view, the dissociation of mental processes would be rooted in the incompleteness and deviation of the process of disintegration and reconstitution of identity during the PC.

In the case of psychosis, it is a process of identity crisis that involves both a dissociation between consciousness and its contents, but also the connection between the very functions of consciousness. In these cases, therefore, there would be a dissociation involving different levels of the functioning of the system previously believed to be stable, a complete and mad disorientation of it, its disappearance as an aggregating center.

9.4 Therapy

In the treatment of schizophrenia, modern psychiatry often begins with *pharmacological interventions*.[28] The introduction of effective so-called antipsychotic medications—especially second-generation antipsychotics—has significantly improved patient outcomes: reducing the severity of symptoms, lowering relapse risk, improving family and social functioning, and helping individuals regain the ability to study or work.[29]

Drug therapy is usually planned over three main phases: the *acute phase* (symptom control), the *consolidation phase* (stabilizing progress), and the *maintenance phase* (relapse prevention). Multidisciplinary collaboration among psychiatrists, psychologists, and social workers, alongside family support, is considered essential for long-term stability and reintegration.

In the acute phase of dissociative crisis, it is very difficult to propose any psychotherapeutic "work," the patient being distraught and lost while his mental faculties are disconnected. When it then becomes possible to interact with him, in a more stable framework, one still encounters enormous difficulties in any kind of psychotherapy. Psychotherapy is offered as a supportive practice for the ego.[30]

Although therapy will be discussed at length in the last chapter, we want to say here some specific issues that we must confront in schizophrenic patients.

In parallel, *different psychotherapeutic approaches* aim to address cognitive, emotional, and relational dimensions of psychosis. *Cognitive–Behavioral Therapy* (*CBT*) remains the most widely recommended adjunct to pharmacology,[31] as it can help reduce both positive symptoms (such as delusions and hallucinations) and negative symptoms (such as apathy and social withdrawal), while building social skills and self-awareness.[32]

Metacognitive and *phenomenological* therapies focus on restructuring dysfunctional relational patterns and deepening self-understanding. *Family psychoeducation* and *systemic-relational*[33] or *multi-family therapy*[34] help improve communication, reduce relapse rates, and foster a more supportive environment.

Psychoanalytic[35] and *Jungian approaches*, while generally unsuitable in the acute phase, can be valuable in more stable phases, especially when exploring symbolic meaning and personal narratives, always with a cautious, gradual pace. *Jungian psychotherapy* of schizophrenic psychosis, although not a rigidly codified technique, adopts a series of specific methods and strategies born out of the clinical experience of Jung and his students. Thus, first of all it is important to *protect the patient from* "archetypal pressure" (images, mythical motifs, universal symbols) by showing how these images have a universal meaning, here translated into a personal key; an attempt is made to *attribute meaning and universalization to the experiences,* to help the patient recognize and integrate the delirium or hallucination in a comprehensible language, for example, by linking it to mythical, universal, artistic, or symbolic narratives. Jung attaches great importance on the personal, affective, and empathic relationship between therapist and patient; the countertransference is not neutral, but a therapeutic tool for "sharing the world" and emotional acceptance. Space is also given to *expressive techniques*, *art-therapy*, *dramatization of archetypal themes*, trying to help the patient recognize his own symbols and reintegrate them into consciousness. Psychotherapy usually requires a very long time and advancing step by step, in these cases, with a certain gradualness is fundamental, never forcing the interpretation and respecting the patient's rhythms and defenses.[36]

9.4.1 The transpersonal turn

Beyond these well-established methods, some clinicians advocate for a *Transpersonal* perspective—one that does not replace conventional therapies but enriches them by addressing an often-overlooked dimension: the *spiritual* aspect of human experience, the search for existential meaning, and the exploration of non-ordinary states of consciousness that sometimes emerge in psychotic episodes.[37]

In acute psychosis, the patient often struggles with confusion, lack of insight, and an inability to cooperate with any structured therapeutic process. What he is lacking is a founding, stable organizing point in psychic life, and awareness of this dissolution.

At this stage, the most important contribution a transpersonal therapist can offer is *containment*, *empathic presence*, and an ability to "*hold the field*" without forcing insight or interpretation.

The transpersonal vision rather than simply "rebuilding the ego" to its pre-crisis state, aims to *support the patient in re-decovering a deeper center of identity—the Self-aware Self, or pure consciousness—which has remained intact throughout the psychotic storm.* This deeper Self can become the new axis around/in which the sense of self reorients and stabilizes. The crisis is thus not seen solely as a breakdown to be repaired, but as a possible gateway for transformation, if navigated with great care.

9.4.2 TP approach to psychoses

This therapeutic approach begins with a *radical shift in perspective,* a *simple yet profound premise: at the core of every person lies, and always has, an intact Self*—a pure, unbroken awareness untouched by the psychotic process. Rather than aiming solely at "restoring" the pre-crisis condition, therapy could be directed at helping the patient establish a direct, living relationship with this deeper dimension of themselves, allowing it to become a new center of orientation.

For the therapist, this means cultivating a rooted, impersonal presence—a stable, non-reactive state of consciousness that acts as a field of resonance in which the patient can feel safe and free from judgement. More than explaining or interpreting, the therapist offers a non-verbal attunement, embodying calm awareness so that the patient may have an immediate, lived experience of being met without pressure to change stands as a witnessing presence rather than casting themself as a savior figure, refraining from "fixing" the person, and instead supporting the recognition that something within them has never been damaged.

The patient can thus be helped to perceive, to experience, to direct himself towards that space beyond the mind that is untouched by the psychotic crisis. This may be for him the new point of reference.

This may reduce the anguish of fragmentation for the patient, when he realizes that what is happening in the dissociative crisis is not only happening *to him- or herself-the* "person" but is also taking place "within" *self-consciousness.*

In acute phases, the therapist's role becomes even more one of a steadying presence—a fixed diffused-point in the storm—without forcing interaction or understanding. The symbolic and archetypal load is reduced to protect the patient from unnecessary cognitive or emotional stimulation; instead, the therapist focuses on helping the mind find micro-points of stability, such as familiar sounds, steady eye contact, or the rhythm of shared breathing. Simple, grounded phrases like "I'm here with you" or "This moment is okay as it is" could help sustain a connection with something constant and safe.

When the patient is in a stable or sub-acute phase, various gentle tools can be introduced. Sensory or perceptual anchors—noticing the contact of the feet on the floor, the support of the chair, or the rhythm of natural breathing—can help connect experience to the present moment without overloading it with symbolic meaning. The language used is that of direct experience, with simple, open-ended questions like "What is here right now?" that draw attention to the immediacy of the present rather than to past stories or imagined futures. There may be brief moments of non-identification, helped by the therapists' pauses and transmission of his consciousness state, in which the patient experiences themselves as the observer of even their most disturbing thoughts or sensations. Creative expression—through drawing, movement, or sound—can be encouraged not for analysis, but as a way for the body-mind to self-regulate naturally. Small shared activities, such as having tea together, walking side by side, or observing an object in the room, can work as quiet rituals linking the patient's inner world to the shared external reality.

The ultimate aim of this approach is to build a durable bridge between a functional ego and the Self-aware Self. In this configuration, the ego is neither the dominant ruler nor entirely dissolved; it becomes a flexible and adaptive interface. The Self—steady, whole, and unfragmented—remains the reference point, even amid turbulence in the ego. With this inner anchor, the person can engage with the world effectively, while remaining rooted in a deep space of integrity and presence.

In the transpersonal–Self-aware framework, the therapist's *state of consciousness* is not just a background condition; it becomes an *active therapeutic ingredient*. By holding a non-dual field, the therapist models a state in which the patient can gradually stabilize, sometimes even before they can cognitively grasp what is happening. The patient may sense, perhaps for the first time during the crisis, that there is a "place" inside untouched by fragmentation—and that this place can be inhabited. Over time, this can act as a *cohesive agent* for dissociated parts of the personality. As the patient grows accustomed to residing in this deeper awareness—often in synchrony with the therapist—they may start to observe the processes of deconstruction and reconstruction of the ego without being overwhelmed by them. Functions once managed by the old, fragmented ego can be taken up by this new organizing principle: the Self-aware Self, which is no longer ego-centered yet remains fully capable of engaging with life.

This is not a quick or protocol-driven process; it requires patience, humility, and the therapist's willingness to step beyond an exclusively clinical mindset into a shared field of conscious presence. But in those crises with transformative potential—the so-called *spiritual emergencies*—this can make the difference between a chronic downward spiral and a gradual re-emergence into a more integrated, expanded way of being.

We are well aware that psychotic schizophrenic breakdown often does not allow for easy solutions, and often entails a lot of suffering; nevertheless, this approach offers some hope to the patient's soul, since it addresses the mystery itself, and embraces the patient's madness.

Notes

1 Schizotypal personality disorder has certain features in common with the psychotic spectrum (reduced emotional expression, magical thoughts, unusual perceptual experiences, ideas of reference) but does not have true delusions or persistent hallucinations and does not result in a net loss of contact with reality; rather, it represents a a personality disorder at risk of evolving into (in a minority) into full-blown schizophrenia. This is why the DSM-5 places it among the psychotic spectrum personality disorders in the notes, recognizing a continuity but also a clear distinction from frankly psychotic disorders.

Social impairment is due to oddities of thought, eccentric behavior, and discomfort in close relationships, but true psychosis is not usually manifested.

2 When it became evident that the disorder was not degenerative dementia, it was renamed schizophrenia by Eugen Bleuler in 1908.

3 *Premature dementia* was the term used in 1891 by Arnold Pick to classify a case of a psychotic disorder. In 1893, *Emil Kraepelin* introduced a distinction in the classification of mental disorders between *dementia praecox* and mood *disorders* (which included unipolar depression and bipolar). Kraepelin believed that dementia praecox was primarily a disease of the brain and in particular a form that is distinct from others, such as Alzheimer's disease, which generally occur at a later age. Kraepelin distinguished psychoses into a few main types: *Hebephrenia*: characterized by disorganized behavior, inappropriate affectivity, and early onset, often associated with progressive deterioration; *Catatonia*: dominated by psychomotor symptoms such as stupor, muscle rigidity, or uncontrolled agitation; and *Dementia paranoides*: focused on delusions of persecution and grandiosity.

Eugen Bleuler (1857–1939) redefined dementia praecox as schizophrenia, emphasizing the "splitting" (from the Greek *schizein*, "to divide") of psychic functions. He introduced the concepts of *primary symptoms* (dissociative association, autism, ambivalence) and *secondary symptoms* (delusions, hallucinations), expanding the diagnostic boundaries. Bleuler retained the Kraepelinian subtypes, while adding *simple* schizophrenia, characterized by an insidious decline without overt psychotic symptoms.

4 The dissociation of the ordinary egoic consciousness and the transfer to a space of homogeneous, amorphous consciousness, in the Self, explain well this difficulty of orientation, of fixation of the ordinary mind, experienced in an ego-dystonic manner due to the non-recognition of the new identity condition.

5 *Paranoid* schizophrenia was mainly characterized by delusions and hallucinations, often with a distorted perception of reality; *disorganized schizophrenia*, by severely disorganized speech and behavior and inappropriate emotions; *catatonic* schizophrenia by abnormal motor behavior, which may include complete immobility or excessive motility; *undifferentiated* schizophrenia did not fall into any of the above categories; *residual* schizophrenia described cases in

which schizophrenic symptoms were attenuated, but the person still had some residual symptoms.

6 *Dimensional assessment* in psychiatry is an approach that measures the intensity and severity of different symptom dimensions. The DSM-5 introduced a specific scale, the *Clinician-Rated Dimensions of Psychosis Symptom Severity* (C-RDPSS), to assess a number of key symptom dimensions, such as delusions, hallucinations, thought disorganization (informal language), abnormal motor behavior (including catatonia), negative symptoms (e.g., reduced emotional expression or motivation), cognitive deficits, the degree of depression, and any manic symptoms. Each dimension is assessed on a *severity scale* from 0 (not present) to 4 (severe), so as to obtain a detailed profile of the patient's clinical state instead of a simple diagnostic label. It does not replace the diagnosis, but enriches it by making it more useful, dynamic, and person-centered.

7 In the ICD-10 (*International Classification of Diseases*, not just psychiatric therefore), the second major classification tradition, the traditional categories have been retained instead: *Paranoid* Schizophrenia (predominant delusions and hallucinations), *Hebephrenic* Schizophrenia (behavioral and affective disorganization), *Catatonic* Schizophrenia (psychomotor impairments), and *Residual* Schizophrenia (persistent negative symptoms).

Psychotic spectrum disorders also include: *Schizoaffective disorder* (combination of psychotic symptoms and mood disorders, e.g., major depression or mania), *Brief psychotic disorder* (episodes lasting less than a month, often triggered by acute stress), *Delusional disorder* (non-bizarre delusions, e.g., pathological jealousy, without other *psychotic symptoms*), *Substance-induced psychosis* (drug- or drug-related hallucinations or delusions, without other *psychotic symptoms*), *Organic psychoses* (caused by medical conditions, e.g., brain tumors, epilepsy use), and *Pathological jealousy* (without other psychotic symptoms).

8 The patient isolates himself, withdrawing from others, or manifests difficulties in social relationships,

9 The patient presents variations in sleep patterns, such as insomnia or excessive daytime sleepiness

10 Many of these symptoms are non-specific and can occur under different conditions.

11 As we shall see, *these alterations in sensations can be explained as altered activities in the Chakras*, interpreted in an ego-referenced manner. For example, for voices and sounds it is a hyperactivation of the sixth *Chakra*.

12 *Cognitive symptoms* may vary in intensity and severity from person to person and may also vary over time. Psycho-educational and rehabilitation interventions can be helpful in managing the cognitive symptoms of schizophrenia and improving daily and social skills.

13 "In this country, two out of every single person are schizophrenic."

14 German psychiatrist Kurt Schneider, shortly after Kraepelin helped to differentiate it from other psychoses, distinguished its characteristics into: *first-rank* symptoms, which included hallucinations (e.g., auditory, such as voices commenting or arguing), and thought disturbances, delusions (such as thought transmission or subtraction, delusional illusions); and *second-rank symptoms*, which included confusion, perceptual alterations, feelings of emotional emptiness, mood alterations, and other symptoms. This distinction has been dropped over time as characterizing schizophrenia. However, the attempt to distinguish indicators of a tendency towards dissociation or chronicity remains valid. One

type of classification in the past distinguished catatonic schizophrenias (in which motor symptoms, paralysis, or hyperactivity were in the foreground), productive (positive symptoms in the foreground), hebephrenic (undifferentiated), and others.

15 "...The mind is terrible, you know..."

16 This is also why the average life expectancy of people with the condition ranges from 12 to 15 years less than the general population.

17 *Autism* is a complex and variable neurodevelopmental disorder, now classified as "*autism spectrum disorder*" (ASD). It mainly involves verbal and non-verbal communication, social interaction, and manifests repetitive behavior and narrow interests. Peculiar difficulties in perception, thinking, and relating to others are present from early childhood, and the spectrum is very broad and variable in severity and manifestations. In DSM-IV it was divided into five subtypes, but in DSM-5 a single term is used that encompasses all previous diagnoses, emphasizing continuity and different levels of severity rather than separate categories. The levels of support needed (Mild, Moderate, Severe) are specified. The incidence is increasing, worldwide it is 0.5–2 per cent, in the US it is as high as 3.2 per cent (1 in 31 8-year-old children receive this diagnosis). The causes are multifactorial, strongly genetic (damage to the genome), but also an environmental component. There are no specific therapies, only support for the patient and family.

18 In addition to the aforementioned scale, here are some tools that can be used as part of the assessment process: structured interviews, such as the *Structured Clinical Interview for DSM* (SCID), to guide the diagnostic assessment; questionnaires and rating scales, such as the PANSS (*Positive and Negative Syndrome*), to assess the severity of schizophrenia symptoms; *laboratory tests and brain imaging*, useful for ruling out other medical conditions and assessing possible brain abnormalities. And finally, *neuropsychological evaluation*, useful to better understand the impact of schizophrenia on the patient's cognitive abilities. At present, the diagnosis of schizophrenia remains mainly based on in-depth clinical evaluation.

19 I met this patient when I was a young novice psychiatrist; I was sent to his home to hospitalize him, as he was showing signs of insanity and did not accept to be treated. At the time, his speech, which I transcribed, seemed to me merely delusional, pathological, meaningless. Today, beyond the veil of those words, I would see in those experiences his attempt to communicate to me his experience of death and resurrection, and how he was amazed by it, and sought meaning in it. Many years later I met this patient by chance, in the street: he had put on weight, because of the medication, and he had a relaxed, perhaps resigned face; he lived in a residential facility run by the Mental Health Service. His gaze was aware, and at the same time lost, kind, and loving; and he remembered me with affection for the way I had listened to him and understood him at the time.

20 We refer to the first chapter for biological theories on mental disorders.

21 This perspective takes us back to the old theories of *unitary psychosis* (already mentioned in Kraepelin's time); it downgrades rigid nosographic entities, proposing a continuum between schizophrenia, bipolar disorders, and other conditions.

22 *A proposed hypothesis* is that the collapse of intersubjectivity first, and then of subjectivity, would give rise to a form of pathological reorganization of a disembodied and fragmented self and, at the same time, to a compensatory mode

of object relations of an adhesive-imitative type, replacing the organization of an attachment system. See "Structural characteristics and a etiopathogenetic mechanisms of psychotic functioning: an integrated model between psychodynamics and interpersonal neurobiology," Caporale R. [1], Battisti V. [2], Ricci F. [3] at www.irppiscuolapsicoterapia.it/meccanismi-eziopatogenetici-del-funzionamento-psicotico-un-modello.
-integrated-between-psychodynamics-and-interpersonal-neurobiology/

23 M. Garrett, *Psychotherapy of Psychosis*, Raffaello Cortina ed. (2021).

24 "We can safely argue that in *dementia praecox* there is no symptom that can be defined as psychologically unmotivated and senseless ... What the patient says is by no means absurd but is full of meaning, so that those who know the key can understand it without undue difficulty."

25 "From the psychological point of view, psychosis is a mental state in which previously unconscious elements take the place of reality" (Jung, 1919)

26 Jung recognized the phenomenon of *Kundalini awakening* as a powerful archetypal symbol and as a possible psychic dynamic, especially in relation to the process of individuation and confrontation with one's deep unconscious. He also observed that certain experiences of spiritual awakening, such as the *Kundalini*, could be accompanied by psychological conditions of strong confusion or disorientation, which could sometimes be confused with or associated with psychotic episodes or schizophrenia-like conditions.

27 Jung introduced the *concept of the psychoid* in the 1940s *The Structure of the Unconscious* (1946), *Man and His Symbols* (1964, posthumous), see also correspondence with physicist Wolfgang Pauli in the 1950s, discussing the theory of synchronicity and the relationship between psyche and matter. Ego cohesion, i.e., the feeling of continuity, identity, integrity, depends on the way the ego manages to relate to (and integrate with) the deep, impersonal levels of the psyche, the field of (archetypal, psychoid) forces that give it structure, but also constantly challenge it: ego cohesion becomes a dynamic result of the balance between the conscious and psychoid poles. Jung argues that the archetype is a transcendent factor, which does not belong entirely to the soul (conscious psyche) nor to the body, but acts as a dynamic and invisible bridge between the two realities; the archetype "is never conscious in itself, but only in its manifestation, as an archetypal image," and in its root it is "psychoid-extrapsychic." Jung thus postulates a *psychoid base*, unconscious of itself, which gives birth to all those expressions named as archetypal; it is "something" inconceivable but at the same time actual, real in its own way, or surreal, i.e. hyper-real, or more than real.

28 "Neuroleptic" and "antipsychotic" are terms often used as synonyms, but in reality they have different origins and meanings: *the former* is a term introduced in the 1950s to indicate the first drugs such as chlorpromazine, capable of inducing a "neuroleptic state," i.e. a reduction in psychomotor activity, agitation, and emotional response, without any real hypnotic effects. The term is derived from the Greek ("grasping the nervous system"). The *term antipsychotic* is a more modern term, and indicates the broader class of drugs used to treat psychotic symptoms (hallucinations, delusions, disorganization), both in classical psychosis (schizophrenia) and in other conditions. Atypical antipsychotics (second-generation; e.g., clozapine, olanzapine, risperidone) have a more complex pharmacological profile than the first neuroleptics, and often do not induce the classic neuroleptic state.

29 The development and efficacy of antipsychotics *are tested* in the laboratory on cells and animals. *In vitro testing* (on cells): human or animal cell lines are used

to assess the drug's ability to bind to and modulate key neurotransmitter receptors (e.g., dopamine D2, serotonin 5HT2), studying receptor affinity, agonist/antagonist activity, and effects on intracellular signaling pathways. The complexity of the human mind and the verification of actual effects on neurotransmitters in vivo, however, remain largely indirect.

Prior to human testing, the drug is administered *to rodents or primates* to observe the behavioral effects related to psychosis (stereotypies, motor activation, avoidance tests). Finally, *in humans*, functional magnetic resonance and PET techniques offer important data, but *do not show precisely what happens to synaptic neurotransmitters in the living human brain*. The human response depends on genetic, epigenetic, and environmental factors and the extraordinary complexity of the neuronal network. Separate Phase I (safety in healthy volunteers), II, and III (efficacy and comparison in psychiatric patients) clinical trials are conducted in humans, in which the drug is administered to progressively larger population groups. See again Dold, M., Leucht, S. (2014) "Pharmacotherapy of schizophrenia: Recent advances and future prospects."

30 "Whether the case is at the onset or in an advanced stage, and regardless of any particular theoretical model, all therapeutic techniques used for psychosis have as their main objective the re-establishment of the reality plane, ... the restoration of that psychic instance known according to the psychodynamic conception by the name 'I'."

From *Psychosis: Integration of Symptomatology, Restructuring of the Ego, Reorganization of the Self*. Fulvio Marchese, Caterina La Cascia, Alessandro Bruno, Daniele La Barbera. Giovanni Fioriti eds (2015)

"The ego is thus the filter between the external and internal world, between the subjective and objective dimensions ... and all models of care, whether consciously or unconsciously, are ultimately grounded in fostering its empowerment."

31 The most effective treatment of schizophrenia appears to be that which combines drug therapy with psycho-education, cognitive behavioral therapy, and art therapy.

However, although cognitive behavioral therapy (CBT) for psychosis is recommended by major international guidelines, its actual efficacy in the treatment of schizophrenia and psychosis is still a matter of controversy. See "Efficacy of cognitive behavioral therapy in the treatment of psychosis: a meta-review," Alberto Barbieri, Federica Visco-Comandini, at www.rivistadipsichiatria.it/archivio/3249/articoli/32182/

32 See Aucello E., Pastore V., "Schizophrenia and cognitive-behavioral therapy: introduction to the subject and elements of effectiveness," at https://www.stateofmind.it/2015/12/schizofrenia-cbt-efficacia/

In particular, culturally adapted brief CBT (CaCBT), and cognitive behavioral therapy for negative symptoms (CBT-n) seem to be useful.

Other modern techniques have also shown promising results in this field: social skills training, cognitive rehabilitation, and mindfulness interventions or third-generation therapies complement the treatment framework. These include mindfulness, metacognitive therapy (MCT), compassionate mind training (CMT), and the method of levels (MOL).

33 TSR considers the family a "system" where all individuals influence each other. It works on communication, alliances, and non-functional family dynamics, trying to reduce the rigidity of interactions and the repetition of "games" that

can maintain psychotic symptoms. Generally, the involvement of the entire involvement of the entire family unit is generally necessary.

34 Multi-family group interventions: they involve several families at the same time in a protected environment, favoring shared experiences and solution-focused strategies. They lower feelings of isolation, create mutual support, and increase therapy adherence. Self-help groups also provide practical psychological support, thanks to the direct exchange between family members, sometimes mediated by professionals; they help to overcome feelings of guilt and social stigma related to the illness.

35 Freud himself considered "narcissistic psychoses" scarcely treatable with pure psychoanalysis.

A "sustained" and adapted psychodynamic approach may, however, be useful in stable/residual phases, to help patients make sense of the psychotic experience, working on relational aspects, ego-qualities, and symbolic processes. Some current authors suggest using psychoanalytic references very cautiously and creatively, paying close attention to the therapeutic alliance and the limits of the relationship (as proposed by Bollas, Jung, Fromm-Reichmann and others).

36 Collected Works, Vol. 3, 8, 14: Studies on psychosis, experimental psychoanalysis, the collective unconscious and the archetype.

37 In the field of TP therapy, as we have seen, there is a *current that proposes to broaden the focus of treatment by integrating the spiritual dimension, crises of meaning and the exploration of* "non-ordinary states of consciousness" *into psychotherapy,* recognizing that the spiritual dimension is also involved in the crisis as a fundamental factor. I believe that this type of contribution, with due caution, could be useful in supporting those crises that tend, as we shall see in the next chapter, to evolve positively, in those psychotic episodes that are experienced as spiritual crises or "transpersonal emergencies." These persons, *after the acute phase, often feel the need to elaborate the existential meaning of their psychotic experience.* However, the techniques proposed in this area can be unfruitful and sometimes even *counterproductive* in those psychotic crises where deconstruction takes a turn for the worse. I am referring here to the proposal of *meditation and mindfulness* techniques to help in controlling anxiety and dissociation, which these patients can scarcely use; or to *deep breathing techniques* (holotropic breathing, guided visualizations), to encourage self-reflection and the emergence of symbolic meanings, which in these patients are also too intrusive and difficult to manage. Even *dream work, art therapy, biographical support,* tools that are proposed to help the patient find mental calm, are often impractical, and interpretation is often not accepted or may generate further internal difficulties for the patient. In Psycho synthesis, work aimed at *the integration of the self is* proposed: *work is done on the cohesion of identity and on the relationship with a broader and more sacred dimension of life*; this could be applied with caution where it is recognized that the crisis evolves towards a spiritual emergency.

Chapter 10

Transpersonal psychiatry

10.1 Introduction

In scientific circles, spirituality is considered to be the result of ignorance, superstition, primitive, or childlike magical thinking. Mainstream psychiatry and psychology define these experiences, these non-ordinary states of consciousness (NOSC), as fantasies or pathologies.

Spiritual experience, for example, could be interpreted in this light as an *attempt to satisfy the desire to be cared for by a* "good mother," or as *a sign of a fragile ego*, unable to distinguish between internal images and external reality.

The psychiatric literature contains numerous articles and books discussing what the *appropriate clinical diagnosis* might be *for many of the great figures of spiritual history.*

For example, as Harner reports,[1] "St. Anthony has been called a schizophrenic, St. John of the Cross has been labeled a 'hereditary degenerate', St. Teresa of Ávila has been dismissed as a 'severe hysterical psychotic', and Muhammad's mystical experiences have been attributed to epilepsy.

Many other religious and spiritual figures, such as the Buddha, Jesus, Ramakrishna, and Sri Ramana Maharshi have been seen as suffering from psychosis due to their visionary experiences and beliefs. Even Buddhist meditation is described in psychopathological terms, and is referred to as 'artificial catatonia'.[2] Similarly, some anthropologists believe that shamans are schizophrenics, walking psychotics, epileptics or hysterics. Western psychology and psychiatry describe the rituals and spiritual life of ancient and native cultures in pathological terms.

However, the madness of our world, which risks self-extinction, is so much considered normal that it is not recognized as pathological by doctors and researchers."

DOI: 10.4324/9781003676461-10

In bio-medically oriented psychiatry, mystical images and experiences are considered the *result of biochemical alterations in the brain and seen as manifestations of serious mental illness*. Believing oneself to be a messiah or God, in this view, is certainly attributed to a biochemical disturbance. Psychiatrists[3] are called in to resolve the crisis and restore the patient to their previous state, though results are often partial and precarious.

Let us first clarify the distinguishing features of TP psychiatry compared to MS psychiatry and TP psychology.

10.2 TP psychiatry, characteristics

As we have seen, *MS psychiatry has ended up medicalizing states of transformation of consciousness as mere pathologies,* thus losing their deeper meaning. Following medicine, it has increasingly espoused a scientific conception based on objectivizing materialism, in the direction of a transhumanism that denies the soul and the spirit, and that risks distancing it from a true reintegrative and evolutionary cure.

It is psychiatry without hope, without future, *without soul.*

Patients with these non-ordinary states of consciousness are taken into public health care by doctors who usually operate with a *limited awareness of their own limits of vision and preparation,* disconnected from their own souls in the name of science.[4]

From these limits, *TP psychiatry* has emerged *as an evolution and not only as a reaction*, which *broadens and reorients the clinical approach*, basing it on a *different vision of the human being* and a different use of medical aids.

As previously noted, the *conception of a PC* also differs, as it is recognized to have an *intrinsic evolutionary potential.*

The intervention also differs, aiming not to suppress but to *contain and support* these delicate moments, using medications to regulate subtle energies in support of TP psychotherapy.

Perhaps the most radical element of this different approach, however, is the centrality attributed *to the TP psychiatrist's state of consciousness within the therapeutic relationship.*[5]

10.3 TP Psychiatry and TP psychology

Let us then consider in more depth the *similarities and differences* between psychiatry and TP psychology.

Both disciplines recognize NOSC as *evolutionary states of being* and observe their increasing frequency in the present context. They also share the view that the *suffering experienced in CPs stems primarily (though not exclusively) from the resistance and unpreparedness of the individual*—understood as consciousness and subtle body—to accept and integrate the ongoing transformational process. Finally, they share the *holistic view of man* as an inseparable unity of body and mind, individual and society, matter and spirit.

However, TP psychiatry proposes a *specialized medical intervention integrated with the TP psychological one*; *it* recognizes *the need for a medical intervention that is more evolved and conscious, a conscious psychiatry, that integrates the TP orientation into medical training.*

This is because the TP doctor has the possibility of using psychotropic drugs, and has *more experience with cases of psychosis or bipolar disorders*, managing the diagnosis, pharmacological treatment, and in-patient and out-patient containment of these acute cases.

Furthermore, medical training can be important where it is necessary to also monitor physical health and the risk of acute medical complications, such as heart failure.

The difference isn't just in the prescription of medicines: TP psychiatry is based on a model that integrates mind, body, medicine, and spirit, while maintaining the possibility of intervening on the organic/pharmacological side as well. TP psychology, on the other hand, deals exclusively with mental, emotional, creative, and spiritual processes without medical tools.

It is important, however, to *avoid falling into the error of devaluing (some go as far as total denial) MS psychiatry*; it still represents the only help available for people going through a psychotic crisis, for medication or for hospitalization.

We cannot *have a different psychiatry, however, if we do not have a different kind of psychiatrist working in a different organization.*

The diversity concerns the level of consciousness, the vision of man, of suffering, of treatment: different principles therefore from the current ones, a holistic vision of man, not flattened on the materialist paradigm only; a reintroduction of the centrality of consciousness and its evolution, of awakening, in the theory and practice of psychiatry; a different selection and training of doctors, to accompany and develop a real understanding of mental disorders. The role and training of psychiatry residents must be profoundly reconsidered.[6]

Ultimately, TP psychiatry aims to offer a broader and more integrated vision of suffering and care, which takes into account the complexity of human experience and the transformative potential inherent in crises.

It paves the way for a new psychiatry, a *psychiatry of the future*, for a *Conscious Psychiatry.*

This is not a utopia, but a call to rethink the psychiatric clinic as a place where science and spirituality come together to transform crises into evolutionary turning points, to approach them as an art—a sacred art.

10.4 Psychosis or spiritual emergency?

Let us start with the observation of Assagioli that "the incidence of disorders of spiritual origin is increasing rapidly today, in parallel with the growing number of people who, consciously or unconsciously, seek their way to a fuller life."7

After spiritual awakening, however, there is much difference between one PC and another in terms of symptomatology, evolution, and favorable or unfavorable prognosis.

PCs can be more or less severe, and up to now they have been considered in terms of their intensity within the two series (energetic and identity).[8]

As we saw for the energetic series (when we talked about the KS), also in the identity series we will have to know how to discern how deep it is, so as not to consider each CP of the identity series as a form of dissociative psychosis with a difficult prognosis.

Some of these crises do indeed evolve positively, passing through a symptomatology similar to that of dissociative psychoses, but with greater insight, with less alarm, with more acceptance of the loss of boundaries, of confusion, needing lower dosages of drugs and containment.

The concept of *spiritual emergency* (henceforth SE) was introduced to describe *those transformative crises that can be mistaken for mental disorders, but characterized by a favorable prognosis.* The lack of a conceptual view that is open to understand SE in Western culture can lead to their pathologization.

The term SE was coined by *Stanislav Grof and Christina Grof* in the 1970s and formalized in 1980, who defined them as:

> *Critical and experientially difficult stages of a profound psychological transformation involving the whole human being. They take the form of non-ordinary states of consciousness and involve intense emotions, visions, various out-of-the-ordinary sensory phenomena and numerous physical manifestations.*[9]

The term SE is derived from the verb to *emerge, to* manifest.

TP psychiatry sees in this type of crisis the potential for spiritual evolution; it sees in the difficulty and crisis an *emergence of a new consciousness*, as well as the sinking of the old, a "spiritual emergency" (in the sense of emergence of Spirit), and considers a PC an important and valuable experience on the path of evolution.[10]

In this view, SE should also not be treated with drugs, but rather supported in their evolution with TP psychotherapy, appropriate to the process underway, validating and supporting it.

SE at their onset are indistinguishable from other states of consciousness of the psychotic type; the latter, unfortunately, do not turn out to have a favorable evolution, while the first ones do; hence the importance of distinguishing the two through some indicators.[11]

In general terms, it can be said that in SEs we find symptoms of the first and second series, while manifestations related to the third series of symptoms are scarcely present (or are present for a short time): In SEs, in fact, the ego manages, albeit confusedly, to perceive the final positivity of the process; there is insight into what is happening. Spiritual symptoms such as expanded states of consciousness, spiritual symbols, transpersonal harmonic NOSC are often present. However, such crises may manifest with intense emotional symptoms, visions, perceptual alterations, unusual mental states, and physical symptoms (trembling, heat, feeling of energy rising up the spine, etc.).

On the basis of the more or less favorable prognosis, we can therefore position PCs of the dissociative -psychotic identity along a *spectrum*, with severe *psychotic PCs* at one extreme, and the more favourable cases, such as *SEs*, at the other, bearing in mind that all the intermediate conditions exist, on a *continuum* within a continuum that it is clinically important to recognise in order to assess prognosis and treatment appropriately.

Not all SE, in the various forms that we shall now examine, are so mild or easy to pass through; and perhaps not all dissociative psychoses have an unfavorable outcome, over time, if well treated initially and well accompanied later.

We may hypothesize that *the reasons* why syndromes unfold differently lie in the modality of the awakening, the preparation of those going through it, and the help they receive.

When the process of awakening takes place in an evolved, fairly purified *consciousness*, the crisis will tend to have a more benign course; it is within this group that SEs can be framed.

In those situations in which the awakening occurs in more unprepared persons, in whom the ego has never reached a higher, more integrated level of functioning, (or when it regresses for various reasons to the lower levels of functioning), suffering, personal disorientation, will be more intense and in the foreground; these are the situations that can be placed among *traditional psychiatric crises*.

These may then require pharmacological and/or restraining of the kind commonly used as we usually apply in psychiatry.

These situations tend to manifest more severe symptoms and have a more unfavorable evolution.

10.5 Symptomatology of spiritual emergencies

In the spectrum of severity of clinical conditions that appear during awakening, from the most painful conditions, dissociative psychoses, to a successful and resolved awakening, free of impediments. SEs can be seen as those conditions that occupy the middle range of the continuum.

If we were talking about little boats crossing the sea, going from the shore of the dead to the shore of the living, then dissociative psychoses could be represented by those boats that do not make it, that drown: they are best kept close to the shore from which they started, if possible.

Spiritual emergencies, on the other hand, can be represented by larger boats, perhaps even more consistent, that manage, if well guided, to approach the opposite shore. Those, on the other hand, who have crossed over completely, and are in the land of the living, who came to life, to the light, are spiritual masters, as we will see them in the following chapter: in this case we are dealing with "excellent awakenings," where the symptomatology of the labor has not prevented their journey or been too difficult, those that have gone beyond, beyond all and beyond the individual self.

In the SE, one finds symptoms of the identity crisis and also, to a certain extent, of the energy series; reactive symptoms, on the other hand, are scarcely present (if at all temporarily).

Identity symptoms are often connected to the activation of the upper Chakras.

The sixth *Chakra* allows one to *see* deeper, due to the opening of the third eye; one can have psychic experiences in this opening such as *extrasensory perception; spontaneous trance states, out-of-body experiences; memories of past lives; astral travel; direct awareness of auras and Chakras; contact with spirit guides through inner voices, dreams or visions; healing powers.*

We speak here of symptoms related not only to the sixth *Chakra*, but also to the *transition between sixth and seventh*, i.e. experiences of consciousness that transcend egoic identification. For example, mental confusion; difficulty concentrating; "strange" activity and/or feelings of bliss in the head, or sometimes pain, particularly in the crown area; mystical experiences.

For the coronal Chakra in particular, the symptomatology is generally *one of expansion of consciousness*, loss of boundaries, sense of infinity, heightened awareness; states of ecstasy, bliss, and intervals of extraordinary joy, love, peace, and compassion. Increased creativity: new interests in self-expression and spiritual communication through music, art, poetry, etc. Heightened understanding and sensitivity: insight into one's own essence; deeper understanding of spiritual truths; exquisite awareness of one's environment (including the "vibrations" of others). Enlightenment experiences: direct knowledge of a more expansive reality; transcendent awareness.

Symptoms related to *the sixth Chakra, the transition from the sixth to the seventh, and those peculiar to the seventh* fade into one another and are often coexistent, depending on the evolution of consciousness.

Energetic hyperactivation on the other hand manifests sensory phenomena dependent on the activation of *the upper Chakras in relation to the senses of sight and hearing* located here. Lights are seen, sounds or voices are heard; these are inner sounds, often described as the sound of a flute, a drum, a waterfall, birds singing, bees buzzing, but which can also sound like a roar, a hiss, a clang, or a ringing in the ears. Other more general energetic symptoms are the feeling of heat, or sometimes cold, sometimes one-sided, depending on which side channels are most active.

The symptoms of the energetic series are also more more closely associated with the upper *Chakras* than with the lower ones; however, more general energetic symptoms are also often present. These symptoms are often in the background, or appear mainly in the acute opening phase, then receding again once consciousness expands and is able to contain and absorb the energetic movement and imbalance.

10.6 Examples

We report some paradigmatic cases, also to indicate how SE can initially easily appear as dissociative psychotic crises. It will then be other factors, as we shall see, that will help us to distinguish these conditions, and to assess the prognosis:

Case 1: 24-year-old woman. She presents with poor self-care, social withdrawal, inappropriate laughter, and abnormal body movements (repetitive pelvic lifting, accelerated breathing, head swaying). She had been practicing *Kundalini* yoga for a year, describing the opening of the *Chakras* and a flow of energy from the base of the spine to the head. She expressed a desire to become a "sannyasin" (renunciate). Despite treatment with olanzapine during psychiatric hospitalization, she showed no improvement.

Case 2: 18-year-old boy. He manifests social withdrawal, suspiciousness, reduced speech, and academic decline. Spends hours watching yoga videos on YouTube. Initially reserved, he later reveals that he believes his *Kundalini* energy was awakening thanks to online yoga gurus. He reports sensations of heat in his abdomen, interpreted as a sign that the *Kundalini* had reached the third *Chakra*. He exhibits delusions of thought transmission, persecutory ideas, and grandiosity. He was treated with risperidone (2 mg).

Case 3: 44-year-old man. Presents a chronic delusional disorder (lasting 12 years) with well-structured delusions of grandiosity. He believes he has experienced enlightenment and possesses special powers (immortality, control of the weather) through *Kundalini* yoga practices. Shows disinhibition and disorganized behavior. He rejects conventional psychiatric drugs, convinced that they "steal beauty from him" and interfere with the benefits of yoga. After an attempt at treatment with olanzapine (which, according to him, caused a "sensation of energy leaving the body"), he is followed on an outpatient basis with family support.

10.7 Classification of spiritual emergencies according to Grof[12]

According to Grof, spiritual awakening experiences *can be recognized and grouped by certain characteristics that distinguish them*, for example, depending on whether visionary aspects prevail, or the sense of union, or the opening of telepathic or mediumistic faculties, etc.

According to Stanislav and Christina Grof, SE stem from the same undelying process, the awakening of consciousness, and can be of three types: *biographical* SE (linked to personal history), *perinatal* SE (linked to the trauma of birth), and *transpersonal* SE (which go beyond individual identity). Let us look at them individually:

1. *Peak experiences* (such as those described by *Maslow*).[13]
   These are episodes of "unitive consciousness" *(Peak Experiences)*, characterized by the dissolution of personal boundaries and a sense of unity with all things (a feeling of being one with others, with nature, with the whole universe, with God), accompanied by intense positive emotions, space-time transcendence, and a sense of the sacred that can lead to self-realization.
2. *Kundalini awakenings* (see Sannella), which can trigger ecstatic or dramatic experiences, release trauma, and lead to extrasensory perceptions, but can also be dangerous to the psychic and physical balance.[14]
3. *Spiritual Renewal crises,* characterized by a symptomatology *strongly* focused on the *strong tension and then transcendence (individuation) of light and darkness* (Perry).[15] These are transformative crises with dramatic sequences. Often one experiences a *return to the origins*, or to the center, or being dead and reborn; the *symbolism of the* "sacred wedding" often appears in this renewal; contact with the Self leading to a new awareness and integration.[16]
4. *Crisis with Psychic Opening.* In these cases, there is an awakening of extra-sensory perceptions, with the emergence of *paranormal gifts* such as remote vision, precognition, telepathy, synchronicity, which

can provide unconventional information but may also disorientating if excessive, which can, in advanced stages, can integrate with a mystical worldview.

The most extreme manifestations of this type of emergence are *Out of Body Experiences (OBEs)*. Here, consciousness appears to separate from the body, acquiring varying degrees of independence and freedom and gaining the ability to perceive the environment without the mediation of the senses. Those who experience these states of "disembodiment" are able to observe themselves from the ceiling, to witness events taking place in other parts of the building, to "travel" to distant places perceiving exactly what is happening there.[17]

These states are particularly frequent in *near-death experiences (NDEs)*, the authenticity of which has been confirmed by systematic clinical research.

5. A variant of psychic openness is *communication with spirit guides and channeling*. These experiences involve perceived contact with distinct entities offering guidance and information, or becoming a "channel" through which messages from external sources to the individual consciousness are transmitted. Such experiences may benefits personal growth but also carry risks of ego inflation.[18]
6. *In these encounters in other dimensions*, we may recall close encounters with *UFOs*.
7. *Shamanic crises*: these can begin with an involuntary dramatic episode with visions, often a journey into the underworld with trials of death and rebirth, which can lead to improved physical and psychic health if experienced fully, (but in the West there is often a lack of community support for these experiences).
8. *Emergence of memories of past lives*, with *regressions to birth and before*.
   One category of transpersonal phenomena that occur during spiritual crises deserves special mention because of the great therapeutic importance (e.g., resolution of phobias) and the key role they play in the religions of many cultures: *memories of past lives, or karmic experiences*. These are experiences related to emotionally charged events, with often very detailed representations of protagonists and circumstances occurring in historical periods and/or in countries different from the present. These experiences can be activated with regressive hypnosis.[19] An important characteristic of these experiences is the deep conviction of the experiencer that they are memories of a previous life.
   Sometimes they can cause discomfort or conflict with one's own belief system.[20]
9. *States of Possession*: characterized by the feeling that one's body and psyche are invaded by a hostile foreign entity or energy with personal characteristics.[21]

This sensation may be transient and intermittent, or persist for long periods of time. The entity is perceived as *malign*, hostile, disturbing: it is alien to the I, it is believed it comes from outside, as if not belonging to one's personality. If one can identify it, it is *disembodied*, a demonic presence, or the consciousness of an evil person trying to take over through witchcraft and black magic rituals. This condition can manifest itself in different forms and with varying degrees of intensity.

According to Grof, states of possession rightly belong to SEs: the underlying demonic archetype is in fact transpersonal by nature, and represents the counterpart of the divine, of which it constitutes the opposite polarity, or negative mirror image. It often constitutes a screen concealing access to the divine, like the terrifying figures guarding the gates of oriental times.[22]

10.8 Psychiatry and spiritual emergencies: Differential diagnosis

Given the prognostic importance of an adequate diagnosis, we will now set out the criteria for distinguishing these clinical syndromes.

SE should be distinguished from psychiatric crises in terms of symptomatology, prognosis, and treatment. Not all states usually diagnosed as psychotic correspond to crises of psycho-spiritual transformation or have the potential for healing. Just as mystical states should not be considered pathological, neither should psychotic states be romanticized.

Let us examine the factors indicating the difference between CPs that follow the path of psychiatric deterioration and those that instead manifest tendencies in an evolutionary, spiritual direction.[23] *The key distinction lies in the meaning attributed to the experiences and their impact on the subject's life and capacity for post-crisis integration.*

Here are some of the parameters to be considered in the clinical assessment:

10.8.1 Before the crisis

The pre-morbid personality should be assessed: there are individuals who since childhood have experienced a lack of sense of self, repeated thoughts that question their existence, leading to social withdrawal and inability to work; people who have never developed their individual and individuative potential as others have. In these cases, energetic activation could be both cause and consequence of a further loss of contact with a separate identity.

In the SE, on the contrary, the more advanced evolutionary level allows for a systematic thinning of the ego, which enables the individual consciousness to merge with the universal consciousness. This is seen as a process of transcendence rather than a breakdown of the personality.

10.8.2 During the crisis

The difference between an SE and a psychosis depends above all *on the subject's attitude* towards the process and the way he experiences it.

In SEs, the patient, while experiencing unusual phenomena, often maintains a certain narrative coherence and desire for understanding, is well-disposed towards experimentation; during the crisis he then goes through a "holotropic" experience and recognizes that what is happening is an inner experience.

Symptoms: *delusions* in SE often have symbolic content, messages interpreted as inner guidance or connection with the divine; they are often consistent with the subject's religious background, e.g., identification or encounters with mythical figures, benevolent figures such as angels, spiritual guides, feeling of cosmic unity. The experiences are embedded in a framework of personal growth or awakening.

In psychosis, by contrast, fragmented and ego-dystonic contents (e.g., persecution, paranoid grandiosity), beliefs inconsistent with the cultural context (e.g., control by secret services, conspiracies), are more likely to occur.

Visual and auditory *hallucinations* in SE tend to be structured (e.g., lights, guide voices), and integrated into a growth narrative, with maintenance of social functioning.

In psychosis hallucinations are intrusive, destabilizing, and indicate a loss of contact with reality; they are usually chaotic perceptions (e.g., fragmented and disorganized), with distressing content (e.g., threatening or demonic figures), often hostile, threatening, critical, or we may have persecutory voices (e.g., insults, commands).

The nature of the experiences: in SE, explicit spiritual themes prevail: experiences of symbolic death and rebirth, feelings of cosmic union, perception of subtle energies, encounters with spiritual or mythological entities, and memories that seem to belong to previous lives, often included within a religious or spiritual context (his own beliefs and those of the people around him).

In psychosis, themes of persecution, hostile external control, and fragmentation of the self are more common.

Emotional impact and functioning: in SE, *emotions are positive or neutral*, perceptions are experienced with curiosity, serenity, or a sense of unity, eventually integrating and enriching identity by enhancing well-being and social connectedness.

In psychosis, hallucinations generate fear, paranoia, or agitation, disorganization, interfering with daily life. There is a disintegration of the ego, with loss of identity, confusion, and deterioration of social relationships.

Insight and relationship with reality: in SE there is partial insight, a recognition of the symbolic or inner character of perceptions, with the possibility to doubt or discuss them. The subject recognizes the irrationality of phenomena but attributes them to a process of growth, is aware at least in part of a direction towards greater integration or expansion of consciousness. The patient tends to attribute the cause of these perceptions to divine forces, archetypes, or metaphysical dimensions. Perceptual alterations are experienced as transitory and aimed at a higher adaptation. The patient responds to psychotherapeutic content integration through symbolic practices (e.g., journaling, art) and emotional support.

In psychosis we find an absence of insight, with absolute conviction of the reality of hallucinations and delusions, even in the face of contrary evidence. A sense of threat and disintegration prevails. Patients may interpret their psychotic experience as a disease, either of the brain or the soul. There is often a loss of egoic boundaries: voices or visions are perceived as external and uncontrollable, patients tend to attribute the voices to concrete entities (e.g., enemies, technological devices). There is generally a greater disorganization of social and work functioning. The patient is unreceptive to integrative intervention and requires the use of sedative psychotropic drugs.

Importance of Context: SE often occur in conjunction with intense spiritual practices,[24] near-death experiences, significant emotional traumas, or during periods of existential transition, whereas psychoses often lack such a condition.

ES tend to evolve positively when they receive appropriate support, whereas psychosis generally requires more structured and sometimes pharmacological interventions.

10.8.3 After the crisis: Evolution

In this approach, therefore, *some NOSC would be more pathological* than others: some would be pathological and psychiatric, others not; there would then exist *intermediate conditions,* a grey and treacherous zone where the TP view seems not to know quite how to move.

The prevailing orientation in TP is that there is a clear difference between these clinical conditions, and that it is important to distinguish them clearly because of the different prognosis and treatment.

However, in practice, it is by no means easy (and perhaps impossible) to clearly distinguish NOSCs that have a weak or strong psychotic component from pure SE.

It is probably rather a continuum, due to the complex interaction of multiple factors.

Let us therefore take summarize the diversity of CPs and their evolution:

- *It depends on the crisis*: not all CP are the same in terms of intensity and nature; some are very rapid and intense, others unfold over time, even throughout life, in a continuous or discontinuous manner. Some relate more to the identity component, others more to the energetic component. Awakening, let us remember, does not follow the rules of the ego: life, God, does as it pleases; and this imponderable factor pervades the whole clinic, even the egoic reaction.

    - According to James (1902),[25] there are *two general types of spiritual or mystical experiences*: *the educational type*, which occurs gradually over time, and the *sudden type*.
    - In the case of *the gradual spiritual emergence*, the educational type, the transformation does not occur immediately but over time; in this case, there may be more opportunities for a more conscious spiritual experience.
    - *Sudden and dramatic spiritual awakenings* can occur in two main ways: with the *dissolution of the ego* (what we have called identity crises) and with an *explosive energetic awakening* (what we have called energy activations, i.e. of *Kundalini*).[26]
    - James concludes that "It is important to note that these sudden awakenings, especially energetic ones, can sometimes be interpreted as psychiatric disorders, even though the individual perceives them as an intense experience of spiritual awakening."

- *It depends on the patient:* on the person's conscious attitude, their purity, willingness or resistance, which will condition how much they will accept or reject the process, how much they can understand it, or are curious about it. Some patients will be able to observe, rather than identify with, the images and visions that arise, and may feel danger or curiosity rather than being overwhelmed. This will depend on the *evolutionary* level of *the patient*. How the crisis will go will also depend on many other factors, such as the degree of adaptation, in work, in relationships, before the awakening, the presence of any previous psychiatric crises. It will depend also on the *resilience of the ego, the characteristics of his personality, his emotional and intellectual resources*; the reaction will finally depend on his capacity to endure suffering, his view of the world and of death, and, for those who believe in it, on their horoscope and destiny.

One should not fall into the trap, Wilber argues, of aiding a deconstruction of the ego in a patient who has yet to consolidate the ego, the so-called *pre-trans fallacy*: the *fallacy* would be to believe that every psychosis corresponds to an evolution.

Table 10.1 Differential diagnosis of Spiritual Emergencies vs Psychosis

Aspect	*Spiritual Emergencies*	*Psychosis*
Premorbid functioning	Often good, no prior psychiatric history Typically stronger ego, higher functional integration, capacity to observe without identification.	Often impaired: Ego may be underdeveloped or fragmented, leading to overwhelm and identification with content.
Onset	Often sudden, invasive, unrelated to conscious existential processes; no perceived meaning in symptoms.	May be gradual (educational type) or sudden (e.g., ego dissolution, *Kundalini* activation); often meaning-oriented.
Triggering factor	Transformative event, spiritual practice, use of psychedelics.	Not always identifiable, often absent.
Attitude toward the experience	Sense of meaning, growth, openness, perceived as transformative.	Fear, alienation, perceived as threatening.
Insight	Partial insight maintained; phenomena may be doubted or explored symbolically.	Lack of insight; delusions and hallucinations perceived as objective reality.
Functional Impact	Often preserved or temporarily impaired; possibility to maintain therapeutic alliance.	Severe and persistent impairment of social and functional domains; disruption of daily life.
Relationship with reality	Perceptions linked to inner transformation; capacity to reflect on their symbolic meaning.	Loss of boundaries, danger of coherent perception of external reality; externalization of perceptions.
Origin of disorder	Spiritually based; often linked to spiritual practices or transformative events.	Supposedly organically based, linked to predisposition; often related to developmental, biological, and environmental factors.
Nature of symptoms	Often experienced as transformative, positive, part of a personal growth process. Mystical experiences, cosmic union, visions of spiritual entities, previous lives. Symbolic content. Often culturally congruent.	Persecution, control, fragmentation of the self. Experiences perceived as intrusive, chaotic, ego-dystonic: threatening hallucinations, social withdrawal, poor spiritual content. Often lack symbolic or existential context, bizarre or culturally incongruent.

(*Continued*)

Table 10.1 (Continue)

Aspect	*Spiritual Emergencies*	*Psychosis*
Hallucinations	Structured, meaningful, integrated into self-understanding (e.g., voices of guidance, visions of light).	Intrusive, chaotic, persecutory or threatening in nature (e.g., demonic voices, hostile figures).
Perception of the crisis	Awareness of a light at the end of the tunnel, seen as a transformative experience.	Experienced tragically, as a threat to life or loss of control.
Energetic symptoms	Present: perception of energy, warmth along the spine, transformative bodily experiences.	Absent or nonspecific; bodily symptoms related to anxiety or medication.
Evolution over time	Alternating phases of peak and integration, progressive improvement.	Tends to worsen and become chronic.
Therapeutic approach, and Response to treatment	Psychospiritual support, emotional containment, pharmacological if necessary. Requires containment and meaning-making. Variable response, often better with psycho-spiritual support, receptive to symbolic integration (e.g., journaling, dialogue, art therapy.	Frequently requires pharmacological and psychiatric containment. Requires stabilization and often pharmacological intervention; Often resistant to symbolic approaches; focus on restoring boundaries and function.
Prognosis	Frequently transitory (weeks–months); potential for spiritual growth and identity integration, positive resolution with appropriate support.	Tends to become chronic without adequate treatment. Prone to relapse, cognitive decline, and social withdrawal if untreated.

Patients with an ego that is not yet well constituted, built up, would have a worse prognosis also because of the greater difficulty in processing and integrating the accelerated evolution of consciousness that the crisis imposes. When the person *has never reached (or regresses* for various reasons) the levels of functioning of the lower *Chakras*, we are more likely to be faced with traditional psychiatric situations, which sometimes also require pharmacological and/or restraining psychiatric interventions. In *evolved* people, on the contrary, who have had time and the opportunity to build up and stabilize a strong ego, capable of relating in a healthy way to the inner and outer world, i.e., in people who have attained a consciousness of the higher *Chakras*, we will much more easily have NOSC of a spiritual kind.[27]

It depends also on circumstances: the expression and management of a CP will also depend on the environment, the dedicated care, the experience of the caregiver, i.e. what is around the patient, factors that are independent of the patient. Among these patient-independent factors will be the type of approach to the crisis, which will condition the type of pharmacological and psychological intervention, and its timeliness, the social and emotional support network, and thus the prognosis.

Evolution and outcome: in SE, the duration is often transitory (weeks–months), and while they may be intense and sometimes destabilizing, they would instead have evolutionary potential, resulting in spiritual growth and greater integration. Often a certain integrity of the personality structure is preserved, with the ability to maintain a relationship with the therapist and a certain awareness of the extraordinary nature of the experience.

Psychotic episodes, on the contrary, impose themselves without warning, completely dominating consciousness. They tend towards chronicity, and generally lead to impaired psychological functioning, cognitive decline if left untreated, isolation and distress.

Notes

1 V. Harner: *The Way of the Shaman* (Harner 1980). Michael Harner was an American anthropologist with good academic credentials, who experienced, in his fieldwork in the Amazon, a powerful shamanic initiation. I paraphrase the text.

2 v. Franz Alexander (1931) psychoanalyst physician (Budapest 1891–USA 1964), considered one of the founding fathers of psychosomatics and psychoanalytic criminology.

3 The psychologist generally does not treat psychotic cases, so that he is rarely called upon except for supportive psychotherapy.

4 One example is the modern world's favor for extractive pharmacology, and the banning of natural medicines, including natural herbal remedies. It almost seems that natural is synonymous with anti-scientific, when exactly the opposite is true. An active ingredient in a plant acts together with all the other

vital components of the plant, it is alive and integrated; when extracted, due to the power that man wants to exercise over nature, it becomes dead and potentially dangerous.

5 As we know, *the doctor is the first medicine.*

6 We will see more in the final chapter on training.

7 Roberto Assagioli, *Psychosynthesis.*

8 We must also take into account the type of treatment that has been given to psychiatric patients up to now, so we cannot exclude that, especially in the past, asylum environments first, and the biological vision of the disorder as pathological and irreversible later, had a significant impact in leading to situations that seem very different from those of an evolutionary crisis. However, there is no doubt that these processes are different from one another, and as we shall see, they must be carefully evaluated in order to bring differentiated and appropriate help to individual situations.

9 In 1994, the DSM-IV included "religious and spiritual problems" as a non-pathological diagnostic category.

In DSM-5, this category has been retained. This represents the official recognition that not all intense spiritual experiences are symptoms of mental illness.

10 In these cases, we will see the gifts of these experiences emerge over time, due to the transcendent function, and the ability to contain and integrate the crisis by transforming.

11 As an Italian spiritual teacher (Salvatore Brizzi) puts it, we must distinguish: "on one side there are the enlightened, and on the other those who have been struck by lightning."

12 See S. and C. Grof, *Spiritual Emergency,* Tarcher Putnam ed. (1989). Drawn and expanded from Bertagni's fine site, www.gianfrancobertagni.it/materiali/psiche/variet%C3%A0.htm.

13 "In that light my spirit saw through everything, in and beyond all creatures, even in plants and grass, it knew God, who he is, how he is, and what his will is ..." (Jacob Bhome – Aurore Naissant). The basic characteristics of a typical peak experience, according to W. *Pahnke*, would be: *Unity* (internal and external), *Intense positive emotion; Transcendence of space–time; Sense of the Sacred* (numinosity); *Paradoxical nature; Objectivity and reality of the insights gained; Ineffability.*

14 As we saw in the section discussing the Physio-*Kundalini* syndrome, numerous psychic, physiological, consciousness-expanding symptoms manifest here.

15 "It is my opinion that the pathology of a psychotic state is not in the 'mental content': in fact, *images and symbolic sequences seem to be the natural psychic process operating in all of us.* The problem lies in bringing to light the life of passion; and nature gives its answer in the form of a *turbulent ordeal, a trial* by immersion in the source of the passions" (John. W. Perry-La dimensione nascosta della follia. Liguori editor).

16 Ex: "Suddenly I am renewed, I am changed, I am immersed in ineffable peace, my mind is full of joy, all past sorrows and unhappiness is forgotten. My soul exults, my intellect is enlightened, my heart is inflamed, my desires are kind and gentle, I do not know where I am because my Love has embraced me" (Hugh of St Victor).

17 "Then I looked again, there was something wrong: this wall had no windows, doors and no furniture was leaning against it. It was not a wall in my bedroom. Yet there was something familiar about it. Suddenly I realized: it was not a

wall, it was the ceiling. I was floating on the ceiling, swaying slightly with every movement I made. I turned in the air, stunned, looked down.

There in the dim light below me lay the bed. And on the bed lay two figures, on the right was my wife; next to her was another person. Both seemed to be asleep. It was a very strange dream, I thought. I became curious. Who did I dream about as my wife's bed partner? I looked closer and the shock was intense: I was the other person in the bed" (Robert Monroe – Journeys Out of the Body).

18 *Mediumship* has played an important role in human history. Among the spiritual teachings transmitted in such a form are many scriptures of enormous cultural importance, such as the *Vedas of the ancient Indians (Rishi), The Koran,* and *The Book of Mormon. Many passages from the sacred text of Zoroaster, the Avesta,* and *the Bible* itself originate in experiences of this kind. Among the important mediumistic sources of the 20th century is an identity that has called itself the *Tibetan*; *Alice Bailey* and *Elena Petrovna Blavatsky* have referred to him as the source of their spiritual writings. *Roberto Assagioli* pointed to him as the true author of his psychological system called Psychosynthesis. During his lifetime C. G. Jung had many transpersonal experiences, particularly dramatic was the one in which he medianically transmitted his famous text "septem sermones ad mortuos"; the entity that inspired him presented himself to him as the Gnostic Basilides. Jung also had powerful experiences with the spirit guide Philemon. One of the best known contemporary mediumistic texts is A Courses in Miracles, transmitted by Helen Schucman and dictated by an entity who called himself Christ.

19 "The patient was increasingly overwhelmed by the phenomenon and told of taking part in a terrible battle in ancient Persia. Suddenly she felt a sharp pain in her chest: she had been pierced by an arrow. She lay on the ground, where she died in the dust of a sun-baked day. She watched as vultures made wide circles in the blue sky above her head, and came closer and closer. Then they landed around her, awaiting her death. She was still alive when some of them began to tear chunks of flesh from her. Screaming and struggling, the woman fought desperately with the pecking birds in a battle she had lost at the start. Finally, she gave up and died. When she emerged from this experience, she was free of the bird and feather phobia that had plagued her for many years." Hypnotic regression described in: *The Adventure of Self-Discovery*, by Stanislav Grof.

20 "Memories of past lives can be a source of other problems; when they are close to consciousness, but not close enough to surface, they can cause emotional and physical discomfort.

The person concerned may experience strange feelings and sensations in different parts of the body that do not originate in ordinary reality, unmotivated fears, unexplained and compulsive attractions to certain people, situations or places, acute pains in the body and feeling suffocated without a definite cause.

An image of an unknown face, landscape, or object may recurrently emerge in his consciousness. ... Other problems may occur when a strong karmic experience begins to emerge from the unconscious in the midst of daily life, deeply disturbing its normal course. The person concerned may feel compelled to enact certain elements of the underlying karmic theme before it has fully come to consciousness and been understood or brought to an end." Excerpts from *The Stormy Search for the Self* RED editions (1995), by Cristina and Stanislav Grof).

21 "Suddenly Flora began to say that the facial cramps were causing her unbearable pain. Before my eyes the spasms became grotesquely accentuated and her

face became fixed in what could be described as a mask of pain. Flora began to speak in a deep masculine voice, everything in her had changed so much that there was nothing left between her present and previous appearance. Her eyes had an unspeakably painful expression and her hands were like claws contracted in spasm. The foreign energy that had taken possession of her body and voice presented itself as the Devil, 'He' addressed me directly, ordering me to stay away from Flora and abandon all attempts to help her. She belonged to him and he would punish anyone who tried to invade his territory. This was followed by explicit intimidation, a series of fearful threats of what would happen to me, my colleagues and the research project if I did not obey." (Stanislav Grof, *The Adventure of Self-Discovery*).

22 Individuals in this difficult situation experience a *deep real night of the soul*: they feel evil, abominable, cut off from the world, and abandoned by God; relatives, friends, and often even psychotherapists tend to ostracize them. In many cases, the alien energy remains latent and causes a wide range of problems as long as its true nature remains hidden.

It can be the cause of serious pathologies, various forms of antisocial and even criminal behavior, suicidal depression, and aggression that can reach homicide and self-destruction, promiscuous or deviant sexual impulses, alcoholism and drug addiction.

In the most extreme and dangerous form, defense mechanisms fail and the problem manifests itself uncontrollably in the midst of everyday life.

However, when approached in the right therapeutic context, these spiritual experiences can be transformative and healing.

23 When we speak of *spirituality*, for the avoidance of misunderstanding, we mean to express that *which characterizes an individual's relationship with the universe*; it is a disposition, which does not necessarily require a formalized official structure, a collective ritual or the mediation of a priest or religious person. The modern term we use to refer to the direct experience of spiritual realities *is* "*transpersonal*": the transpersonal experience is that which transcends the usual way of perceiving and interpreting the world from a separate ego position (from "Holotropic Breathing", by S. Grof, in www.respirazioneolotropica.com/emergence.htm); See also in https://integraltranspersonallife.com/wp-content/uploads/2016/06/VS-38-Emergenze_sett-2021_web-1.pdf

24 See, e.g., search:

"Kundalini-like Experience as Psychopathology: Case Series and Brief Review", (Suchandra et al., 2021, India), on the risks of *Kundalini* awakening for mental health.

25 William James: *The Various Forms of Religious Experience: A Study of Human Nature*, Milan, Fratelli Bocca (1945; published in 1902 in New York)

26 James elaborates his reasoning in a manner very similar to the account we have presented in our classification of PCs: "The dissolution of the ego involves a sudden collapse of the ego system; in some cases, this may follow a long period of gradual spiritual development, during which a 'humiliation or deconstruction of the ego' occurs. Intense experiences such as bereavement, depression, addiction and intense stress can induce this type of awakening. The dissolution of the ego releases the energy normally spent on the ego's activity and the maintenance of its structure. Explosive energetic awakening is related to the release of an inner energy or vitality, similar to the yogic and tantric concept of Kundalini ... This energy, traditionally associated with sexuality, awakens and can manifest in intense sensations and physical and emotional transformations

... This type of sudden awakening also appears to be frequently induced by intense forms of psychological disturbance."

27 This theory is questionable though; see Steve Taylor, "Beyond the Pre/Trans Fallacy: The Validity of Pre-Egoic Spiritual Experience", in *The Journal of Transpersonal Psychology* (2009). Taylor challenges Ken Wilber's "pre/trans fallacy," which holds that childhood (pre-egoic) spiritual experiences are not true transpersonal experiences, but merely primitive states of consciousness, different from those of adult mystics. Taylor argues instead that children's pre-egoic spirituality is authentic and valid, even if different from adult spirituality, and that both derive from the same deep "source" of the psyche.

Chapter 11

Awakenings

Let us now look at some examples of successful awakenings from spiritual masters of the past (East and West), while leaving out countless others.[1]

The foundational myth of our *Christian tradition*, the *Resurrection*, describes this process of dying and being reborn, transformed on another, immortal plane of existence.

Similar examples exist in all religions.

In addition, other great souls have also conveyed similar experiences; for example, Dante Alighieri in his *Divine Comedy*, as well as many spiritual masters who recount, for teaching purposes, the experiences through which they passed in order to go beyond ego identification.

Awakening, moreover, has occurred in people who are still alive, but that are often less publicly known, in whom, however, the awakening has entailed a radical transformation, and has led them to then express their new state of consciousness in healing, teaching, writing, and art.

In these cases, one can speak, as with Dante, of an individual consciousness that is purified (meaning is without stain, i.e. ego identification), and is now *ready to ascend to the stars*: thus also *willing*, i.e. disposed to do so.[2]

In other words, individual consciousness is willing and capable to experience the partial or complete ascent of the Kundalini along the Chakras, without manifesting relevant or permanent psychiatric symptoms, with the result of eventually identifying with a higher state of consciousness.

A true inner revolution. This is how one becomes a master: at that point, the awakened "Self" is fully expressed in the "me," with no more filters or obstacles.

The experience of awakening and of the absolute, witnessed by all these stories, is essentially the same: that is, the realization that we are the manifestation of cosmic consciousness, that we are the divine in human form.

And yet each of these testimonials emphasizes a different aspect of the teaching as well as of the initiatory experience and the way to reach it.

DOI: 10.4324/9781003676461-11

This section is intended to help us better understand the underlying thesis of the book, namely that these awakening processes can, in their own time, have a strongly positive and transformative outcome if understood, accepted, and helped in the right way, and to provide the basis for a new psychiatry, for what we called a *Conscious Psychiatry*.

These are always, as we shall see, identity crises and testimonies of ascending *Kundalini*, in various proportions, with scarce or absent reactions.

11.1 Ramakrishna[3]

According to *Ramakrishna*, an Indian saint and enlightened sage of the last century, the yoga tradition distinguishes between *partial and total awakening* of the *Kundalini* energy.[4]

While partial awakening can lead to various manifestations, both physical and mental, the complete ascension of our potential energy towards the seventh *Chakra* (*Sahasrara*) will awaken the true impulse towards God-realization (or spiritual liberation).

The awakening of the *Kundalini is accompanied by different sensations and experiences.*

A strong feeling of *warmth* appears if the *Kundalini* awakens by ascending through *Pingala Nadi*, or a feeling of *coolness* if it ascends through *Ida Nadi*, first along the back and then throughout the body.

The entrance of the *Kundalini* into the central spinal canal, called *Sushumna*, is accompanied by a *specific feeling of unification*, which is experienced throughout our entire being, often accompanied by a brief suspension of the breath.

When the *Kundalini* reaches *Anahata Chakra*, heart palpitations may occur. We may have tingling sensations in the fingers, and sometimes the whole body begins to tremble.

And as tradition states, the ascent perceived from the back up to the top of the head may be like *the slow progress of* ants, or like *the sinuous movement* of a snake; at other times like *the flight* from one point to another of birds, or like the slow pacing of a fish through placid waters, or even like the leaps of a monkey from one branch to another. These are all described in the traditional texts of Hinduism, particularly those of yoga and tantrism.[5]

11.2 Swami Satyananda Saraswati

Continuing on with the experience of the awakening of the *Kundalini* and the consciousness in the Indian tradition, let us listen to this experience of a yogi.

Swami Satyananda Saraswati (1923–2009) was a *Sanyasi*,[6] yoga teacher and guru both in his native India and in the West. He was a student of Sivananda Saraswati, the founder of the *Divine Life Society*, and founded the *Bihar School of Yoga* in 1964.

> *The most singular and common experience is the release of energy, like an electric shock from the base of the spine, just as if it were connected to an outlet. This experience may be accompanied by a burning sensation in muladhara Chakra and energy flowing up and down sushumna.*
>
> *Sometimes you hear the sound of drums, flutes, bells, birds, celestial music or you may even hear peacocks singing. You may have the momentary sensation of sitting outside in the middle of a monsoon rain and there may also be the sensation of dark clouds constantly moving over your head and the sound of thunder. Sometimes you can feel your body so light and even visualize your spinal cord as a fluorescent light. The sensation of internal illumination is also common, as if hundreds of tiny lights are lit inside your body. Another aspect connected with the actual awakening is the emergence of all the anger, passions and everything that has been repressed. Sometimes you are so full of fear that you cannot sleep, sometimes for many days in a row you have nothing on your mind but sex, sometimes you cannot think of anything else but food.*
>
> *However, all these symptoms pass within a few days or weeks.*
>
> *Some people acquire psychic powers, develop clairvoyance, telepathy, clairaudience, psychotelokinesis, the ability to heal, etc., and this brings many temptations.*
>
> *Another possible symptom is a feeling of nervous depression: one only feels like sitting, or one has the feeling of being limited and closed off. There is detachment from the normal emotions of life, it can happen that for many days in a row one is prey to total discouragement. One has no interest in life and everything seems as barren as the desert, but at the same time the mind becomes very dynamic and seems formless.*
>
> *Other sensations, poetic emotions and artistic perceptions also take place, such as visions of angels and gods.*
>
> *Anything can emerge from the depths of the mind.*
>
> *These are just some of the symptoms one can experience, all of which, however, disappear quickly. The storm sooner or later subsides, and then the yogi lives a very normal life. Outwardly his life seems the same as any other person's, but the inner awareness is infinitely greater.*[7]

11.3 U. G. Krishnamurti

Uppaluri Gopala Krishnamurti (1918–2007), better known as *U. G. Krishnamurti* or just U. G., was an Indian philosopher and lecturer, recognized as an awakened master by all. Krishnamurti had a sudden enlightenment experience, which he called "the calamity": he spoke of it as an internal explosion, which brought him into a state of both pain and ecstasy that lasted for several days.

He later said that his life story can be separated into two parts, *before and after the calamity*. In the description that follows, the identity component seems to prevail.

Describing his post-calamity life, he claimed to function permanently in what he called "*the natural state*": a state of spontaneous, purely physical, sensory existence characterized by the discontinuity—though not the absence—of *thought. Krishnamurti* also argued that, being in the "natural state," he had lost all acquired knowledge and memories, and had to learn everything again, *as if* "... the slate had been wiped clean."

The first signs began with a strong migraine, then he had dissociative experiences.

> *I went through tremendous physical torture. There were days, a week of preparation... the changes began, every day a change.*
>
> *First I discovered the softness of the skin and that I no longer blinked and there were changes in touch, smell and hearing....*
>
> *On the seventh day I was lying on the sofa relaxing and enjoying that disconnected state .... When I felt that something was accessing my inner self; vital energy from different parts of my body became concentrated in a focal point. I said to myself:* "The end of your life has come, you are going to die" ...
>
> *At a certain point it was as if the shutter of a camera was closing. So the opening was trying to close itself, and there was something trying to keep it open. Then after a moment there was nothing left, not even the will to prevent the opening from closing. Then suddenly it closed and I don't know what happened next. The whole process lasted 49 minutes. It was like physical death.* [8]
>
> *Then on the eighth day I was sitting on the couch and suddenly there was an explosion of tremendous energy—tremendous energy that shook the whole body, and together with the body, the couch, the chalet and the whole universe, so to speak—shaking, vibrating. It is not possible to create that movement. It was sudden. Whether it came from outside or inside, from below or above, I don't know—I couldn't locate the place; it was the end of everything. It lasted for hours and hours. I couldn't bear it, but there was nothing I could do to stop it; there was total helplessness. This went on and on, day after day after day.*
>
> *I call it "calamity" because from the point of view of someone who thinks it is something fantastic and full of bliss, love or ecstasy, this is physical torture; this is a calamity from that point of view. It is not*

a calamity for me, but a calamity for those who have an image that something wonderful is about to happen[9] *. The energy operating there does not feel the limits of the body; it is not affected; it has its own momentum. It is a very painful thing. It is not that ecstatic, blissful bliss and all that rubbish and nonsense!; it is really a painful thing. It's like a nuclear explosion, you see—it shatters the whole body. It's not an easy thing; it's the end of man—a* 'destruction' *that blows up every cell, every nerve, in your body.*

Krishnamurti, *The Mystique of Enlightenment*, 1982

11.4 Sri Govinda

Sri Govinda is a spiritual master who insisted on the necessity for the awakening of the direct transmission of Kundalini from the Master to the disciple who has come to be ready to receive it (called *Shaktipat*).[10]

The Kundalini does not awaken for meditation. It awakens during meditation by the grace of the Master. The awakening of the Kundalini is not a psychic process, it is a spiritual process, that is why it requires the grace of the Master. The sleeping Kundalini is not conscious of its sleeping state. That is why it does not awaken on its own. The unconsciousness of the Kundalini is man's spiritual ignorance of lying dormant in another Individual. The purest Divine energy cannot unfold if it is surrounded by impurities. The purpose of meditative practice is to purify the inner self and create the right condition for awakening, to achieve the required degree of purification. It awakens automatically by the grace of the Master. It is the awakened Kundalini of the Master that awakens the dormant Kundalini of the disciple. In this consists the Master's grace, his power of Shaktipat.[11]

11.5 Gopi Krishna

Gopi Krishna (1903–1984) was an Indian yogi, author, and mystic known for his studies and writings on *Kundalini*.[12] In them he recounts how unbalancing the initial period of his awakening was, leading to symptoms close to madness, which required much effort to integrate and overcome.

He emphasizes the risks of sudden awakening without preparation (as was his case) compared to gradual methods under guidance.

In 1937, during a meditation session, he had a *Kundalini* awakening experience that radically changed his life:

Suddenly, with a roar like that of a waterfall, I felt a river of liquid light entering my brain through the spinal cord. Completely unprepared for such a development, I was taken completely by surprise; but instantly recovering self-control, I sat in the same posture, keeping my mind at the point of concentration. The illumination grew brighter and brighter, the roar louder, and I perceived a swinging sensation and immediately felt myself slipping out of my body, completely enveloped in a halo of light.

His awakening was not immediately complete; years of hell followed, periods in which he was severely challenged by the changes occurring in his nervous system, which caused excruciating pain, constant malaise, even the thought that he was no longer sane.

The reason for the imbalance, in his opinion, was an initially distorted path of the life force along the *Pingala* solar channel, which burnt the subtle body with its fire.

Even after rebalancing, it took him several years to regain his equilibrium, paying great attention to his lifestyle, such as sleep patterns and limiting periods of intense concentration.

A great deal of attention had to be paid to his diet; as soon as he got out of a rigid routine, his energy and consciousness changed markedly and he became very ill.[13]

His transformation included the spontaneous appearance of psychic, intellectual, and literary powers. He produced entire books of poetry, the result of inspiration due to his transformation.

Gopi Krishna was also very socially committed, intervening for the rights of women and widows in India in his time, and even ending up in jail for it.

His writings influenced western interest in *Kundalini* yoga; he also described the symbols of the *Kundalini* in every culture in the world (from ancient Egypt, to the Aztec world, to the Mercurial Caduceus). He believed that *Kundalini* awakening experiences, initiated as personal revelations, were the basis of all (or most) religions.

11.6 Sri Aurobindo

Sri Aurobindo (1872–1950) was an Indian yogi and philosopher who asserted that the *Kundalini* would not induce psychosis per se in people who are healthy and not predisposed (to emotional imbalance or illness); however, in individuals with a constitutionally weak nervous system, predisposed to emotional problems, a decompensation may occur under the impact of the awakening of this energy, especially if appropriate precautionary measures are not taken.

His own awakening is described as seeing the divine presence (*Vasudeva/Krishna*) in everything; this non-dual vision, where separation dissolves into unity, marks the essence of his awakening.[14] He then went through a progressive transformation from initial scepticism, to an expansion of consciousness, to the final realization of unity with the divine that permeates all existence.[15]

Sri Aurobindo, in his works and conversations (such as "Letters on Yoga") spoke extensively *about the ascent and descent of Kundalini* through the *Chakras*, emphasizing that *while in the Tantric tradition the Chakras open from the bottom upwards, in his yogic approach the opening occurs from the top down.* This method involves the higher centers opening first, allowing the higher consciousness to descend and transform the lower levels of being. In addition, Sri Aurobindo points out that while in traditional yogic practice the ascent of the awakened inner consciousness (*Kundalini*) up to the brahmarandhra (seventh *Chakra*) is clearly perceived, often, on the contrary, the descent of this higher consciousness is not perceived as clearly. In his yoga, emphasis is placed on both the ascent and descent in the process facilitating an integral transformation of being.[16]

11.7 El Collie

El Collie is a North American woman who died at the age of 55 of brain cancer and recounted her experience of a very troubled, though successful, awakening. From her awakening, a *mutual aid network* was born, composed of people who had already gone through and overcome similar experiences, in order to help those who would go through it after her."[17]

Here are some extracts from her story:

> *I knew nothing about the Kundalini when it awakened in me and I was in no way prepared for what was to come.*
>
> *To tell my story briefly, in 1971, after about two years of formal meditation, a powerful white light lit up my being like the sun, and from then on the energy flowed down my spine uninterruptedly as it still does today.*
>
> *Subsequently, I realized that I could no longer concentrate much on studying without waking up during the night; therefore I could not complete college. Prolonged concentration caused copious and overwhelming amounts of Kundalini to enter my head, giving me severe headaches.*
>
> *Once the Kundalini is awakened, it is no longer possible to make it descend, to go back.*
>
> *Today my condition has relatively improved; my only problem is sleep disturbance when I go beyond certain limits, physically, mentally or spiritually. On the positive side, I am blessed with the lightness of being, and I look younger than my years and have experienced a quantum leap in compassion. I have realized that compassion and love are fundamental in the school of life and beyond.*

Basically, I simply surrender my heart to the Absolute (God, Christ, the Tao or whatever one chooses to call it) and ask for guidance at the heart center.

Kundalini energy has literally paralysed me mentally; it has destroyed some people. Everyone wants spiritual experiences until they get them. Very often we see that those who have been caught up in this process have had serious problems.

Kundalini seems attractive to many people because of the powers it can bring. Few are aware of the prolonged and sometimes arduous process that follows the activation of Kundalini.

I believe it is best not to try to awaken the Kundalini directly. If it is meant to happen, it will happen; trying to speed up the process can entail risks.[18]

In the first period of the process, I felt extremely tired. An enormous weight weighed down on my chest, I struggled to breathe. I seemed to lack oxygen; I felt dizzy and light-headed. My symptoms multiplied and worsened. ...

Afterwards, I felt worse and worse; I felt an enormous weight on all my limbs. My head felt enormous, and I was in an altered state; my whole body felt drugged or poisoned.

I began to sink into terrible anxiety and suicidal depression.

I kept getting worse; I began to be unable to lift my legs, to do any exercise, especially if it required effort. I found myself in bed an invalid, barely able to use my hands even to dress or feed myself.

I was in and out of hospital as new symptoms developed. Small, painless muscle contractions developed all over my body. I felt a growing fear. I started to suffer from muscle cramps and a terrible systemic burning sensation. The spasms affected every part of my body. The symptoms changed and became stranger and stranger. For several months I remained in a state of near-paralysis.

The physical pain reached a crescendo in the middle of one night when I woke up in agony. Every muscle in my body, from the soles of my feet to the top of my scalp, was writhing as if trying to detach itself from my skeleton. Moreover, I was burning inside.

Soon after, I began to experience more classical and full manifestations of Kundalini. Suspended in an etheric, oceanic energy, I remained in an altered state for months.[19]

My sensitivity—physical, emotional and psychic—was amplified, colours were extraordinarily bright and my hearing became so acute that I shuddered at every noise. I had full-blown convulsions, with energy powerfully rising from the base of my spine and pouring out the top of my head.

I saw spectacular lights... I could feel a disconcerting electricity circulating within me... I felt unbearable heat. All the while I was experiencing elaborate, involuntary body movements (they are called Kriyas and Mudras.

For several months I was flooded with mystical experiences. I had visions, inwardly heard and saw guides who instructed and helped me through the process, and had vivid clairvoyant dreams.[20] *Sometimes I saw an aura of golden light radiating from my fingertips.*

During all this, I was overwhelmed by a flood of ever-changing physical symptoms, being torn apart and recreated at every level. I was constantly pushed to the limit of my possibilities.[21]

11.8 Anonymous[22]

Here is a case of awakening associated with mediumistic faculties:

In 2006 after a long period of meditation, often also channelling spiritual guides, I involuntarily awakened her.

At that time I had no idea what I had done; I immediately thought I was possessed.

For more than a month I didn't sleep at night, and I started to rest on the floor moving continuously because I was "burning all the time."

On those days I had difficulty working because the mind was constantly wandering. My third eye was wide open, and I was often outside my body, and I could see myself from dozens of metres away. This was the most difficult part where the Kundalini made its way through the Chakras out of the seventh.

Soon after, this dimension took shape through communication with higher entities; it made me find that extra "something" I was seeking. Now I talk about it very calmly, but I can assure you that in the early years I thought I was dying on a daily basis.

These contacts continued for another eight years where, by meditating daily, I had to direct this energy to dissolve and burn away all the blocks I had accumulated in this life, and in others, or simply in some layer of my consciousness.

Reflecting over time, I have deduced that there are several types of Kundalini, and the one I have experienced is the strongest, called the "fire type."

There are lighter ones, which still lead to expansion of consciousness, but sometimes they are meant to prepare the body for the stronger one.

But what is this Kundalini? I would call it a spirit energy (she knows exactly what to do, and it is not we who command her, as is often said), which has the task of dissolving everything that is not pure, to make us realize that we are only the spiritual part. Initially this is traumatic because, from one day to the next, parts of our personality with which we identify may disappear. Afterwards, little by little, one gets used to it; and the more parts one loses, the more one has the feeling of being whole. It can also happen that the awakening occurs only at the base of the spine, and it stays there silently, until at the appropriate moment, this energy decides to ascend all the Chakras. Obviously, there is no single, identical experience for everyone.[23]

personal account

11.9 Suzanne Segal

Suzanne Segal (1955–1997) was an American writer and teacher who had a sudden experience of self-realization that she wrote about in one of her popular books, "Clash with Infinity."[24]

The account of her awakening is interesting for the debate it provoked on the depersonalization and awakening, where identity symptoms are prominent; despite the great difficulties she encountered, Segal then enjoyed the fruits of this labor by offering them to the world. Let us listen to her account of her awakening (Segal 1996):

One day, taking the bus, I lifted my right foot to board the bus and collided head-on with an invisible force that entered my consciousness like a stick of dynamite silently exploding, opening and blowing open the door of my usual consciousness, splitting me in two.

In the open space that appeared, what I had previously called "me" *was forcefully pushed out of its usual position within me, into a new position that was about a foot behind and to the left of my head.* "I" *was now behind my body looking at the world without using my body's eyes.*

This episode was tremendously unpleasant for her, full of anxiety and fear:

The moment my eyes opened the next morning, my mind exploded with worry. Is this madness? Psychosis? Schizophrenia? Is this what people call nervous breakdown? Depression? What happened? And would it ever stop? ... The mind was in agony as I tried valiantly to make sense of something I could never understand.

In the first few years after her "break-up" *(or opening)* Segal continued to function in life and social life with apparent normalcy, completing a doctorate in psychology at the Wright Institute. She continued to feel completely *depersonalized*, literally as if her name referred to no one. She described it as if her

> *... body, mind, speech, thoughts and emotions were all empty; they had no property, no person behind them. I was completely deprived of all my previous notions of reality.*

Twelve years after her initial awakening, Segal went through *another dramatic phase of* her experience, centered on perceiving a sense of unity between herself and the world[25]:

> *In the middle of a particularly eventful week, I was driving north to meet some friends when I suddenly realized that I was driving through myself. For years there had been no self, yet here on this road everything was me: I was driving through myself to get where I was already. In essence, I was going nowhere because I was already everywhere. The infinite void that I knew I was now was as evident as the infinite substance of everything I saw.*

In addition to being known in the spiritual community, Segal became a model case of the dissociative condition known as *depersonalization disorder (DPD)*.

During her spiritual "journey" some therapists formally diagnosed her with DPD, while others had no clear explanation.[26]

11.10 Modern awakenings, Neo-Advaita

For those who would like to explore a larger number of accounts from our contemporary awakenings and the rise of the *Kundalini*, and its consequences (difficult or not but generally positive), I recommend, among others, the *Batgap* site,[27] also present on Facebook.[28]

In this site numerous interviews with people who have experienced an awakening process that then continued over time are collected.

The thesis proposed on the site is that awakening happens much more frequently than one would think from reading the ancient scriptures, and that it is important to recognize it in our lives when it manifests itself because of the characteristics that the interviewees have in common.

Moreover, awakening is believed to be something that *continues throughout life*: these are interviews with *spiritually awakening people.*

The interviewer, *Rick Archer,* has interviewed more than 700 people of all kinds, with depth, irony, and lightness.

Each interview lasts an average of two hours, and is sometimes even repeated at a later date, to check the development of the process.

In these live dialogues, these people recount with great sincerity and detail about how this transformation took place in them, how the emergence of a new form of consciousness radically different from the ordinary one manifested in them (that is, of NOSC, Non-Ordinary States of Consciousness), and about the related energetic manifestations were, which were often very intense and difficult to manage and integrate.

The interviews generally concern people who are relatively well prepared to sustain this process. After the awakening, many report having been radically transformed, becoming spiritual guides, or recognized as genius artists; others teach, write books, travel, do anything.[29]

Another interesting site is *Conscious TV*, by *Iain and Renate McNay,* which since 2016 has been collecting similar testimonies, each lasting an hour.[30]

Elsewhere on the internet, we find contributions on *Kundalini* awakening or rebirth; unfortunately, the level of these contributions is very uneven, and there is generally a lack of a systematic framing of these experiences, such as the one we have tried to provide in this book.

Notes

1 To name but a few of the spiritual masters of the past in the East: *Jesus Christ, Lao Tze, Shankara, Rumi, Ibn El Arabi, Abinavagupta, Ramana Maharshi, Nisargadatta, Yogananda and his masters (Yukteswar, Lahiri, Babaji); and in the West: Dante Alighieri, St Catherine, St Teresa of Avila, St John of the Cross, Meister Eckhart William Blake, St Hildegard of Bingen, etc.*

2 At the end of Purgatory, once completed the purification process, Dante says he was "pure and disposed" *to ascend to the stars*.

3 I give the following examples not so much because they are *greater* or "*better*" (for I would not know how to evaluate, and I only know a few of the many examples that have appeared in the history of the world); I only give a few to exemplify clinically, or because I have come across them, or because they emphasize different aspects; the list is by no means exhaustive in my intentions.

4 Taken from www.yogaesoteric.net. And in particular see www.yoga-integrale.it/il-risveglio-della-Kundalini-secondo-ramakrishna/

5 "In addition to the different ways in which a soul ascends to perfect unity, you must also know the planes of consciousness it must pass through. No matter who it is that meditates—whether it is Buddha or an ordinary man—it must take it through six different valleys—six distinct planes of consciousness—in order to reach the seventh, the ultimate. Whether your soul's intuition leaps like a frog or flies like a bird, it has to pass through the seven valleys. No matter how the soul reaches it, the experience of each of these valleys is always the same."

6 A *sannyasin* (or sannyasi, a Sanskrit word that literally means "renunciation" *or* "surrender") is, in the Hindu tradition, a person who has embraced the path of *sannyasa*, that is, the total renunciation of material possessions and worldly attachments in order to devote oneself entirely to the spiritual quest and the attainment of mokṣa, liberation from the cycle of reincarnations and union with Brahman. In the contemporary context, the term has also been taken up by spiritual movements such as Osho's, where the "neo-sannyasin" is one who consciously chooses to live life with mindfulness, meditation and inner freedom, regardless of outward rules and religious affiliations.

7 From *Kundalini Tantra,* Swami Satyananda Saraswati, Satyananda Ashram Italia editions, 1984.

8 "Even now it happens to me: the hands and feet become cold, the body stiffens, the heartbeat and breathing slow down, then the breathing ceases. Up to a certain point you are there, you take your last breath, so to speak, and then you are no longer there. What happens after, is that there is no one left to know. I can't say anything about that moment because the experiencing entity was finished, so there was no one to experience that death". As Buddha puts it, "one reaches the limit of perceptibility".

9 *Krishnamurti* also claimed that the *calamity* had nothing to do with his life up to that moment, or his upbringing. He repeatedly described the calamity happening to him by accident, and insisted that he could not, in any way, transmit that experience to anyone else. However, he was certainly someone close to being able to receive it, having done meditation for years, followed spiritual masters etc.

10 From the book *Cosmic Consciousness* by Shri Govinda, quoted by V. Salles.

11 "It is as if a person is under anaesthesia. You can shake him or cut his body, but you cannot awaken him. Awakening is not a physical and external process that coincides with the material act of shaking, but a mental process that takes place within the individual. If there is no such psychic, inner process, awakening from sleep is impossible. The awakening of the Kundalini is not due to thought concentration and pranayama techniques, which are mental processes external to the Kundalini, in this case physical, but is due in a spiritual process that takes place within the Kundalini itself.

The Divine energy of the Lord is one throughout the universe; the Kundalini that is awakened in the master is the same Kundalini that sleeps in the disciple. There are not as many Kundalinis as there are human beings, but only one spiritual energy which in some is active and conscious, while in most people it is in the passive, unconscious state."

12 Gopi Krishna is known for *Kundalini: The Evolutionary Energy in Man*, (Shambhala Publications, varie ristampe, orig. 1967), based on his first awakening in 1937, in which he described in detail his experiences of the initial awakening of *Kundalini* and his reflections. J. Hillman wrote a preface-psychological commentary to this first work of his, which was also translated into Italian by Ubaldini. Later on (in 1967, at the age of 64) he published *Living with Kundalini: The Autobiography of Gopi Krishna*, Shambhala Publications (1993), based on the original core of the first book, where he recounts his lifelong experience with *Kundalini.*

He has also written several other books on the subject: *Kundalini: Empowering Human Evolution*, Institute for Consciousness Research ed (1997), *The Awakening of Kundalini, Kundalini: Path to Higher Consciousness, Kundalini: The Secret of Yoga, The Biological Basis of Religion and Genius,*

Serpent of Fire: A Modern View of Kundalini, Higher Consciousness and Kundalini, The Wonder of the Brain, Ancient Secrets of Kundalini, Initiation into Kundalini (in Italian), The Secret of Yoga Kundalini (in Italian)

13 This may provide us with a new key to understanding anorexia nervosa.

14 This first happened while he was in prison in Alipore, in 1908–9, for his political activism; on that occasion he felt that the prison walls, the garden tree, even the bars and the door were the divine itself protecting him and embracing him on the cell bed (from *Sri Aurobindo, Tales of Prison Life).* Hence. "The feeling of liberation, as if you had been released from prison, always accompanies the emergence of the psychic being or the realization of the higher Self. That is why we speak of liberation, mukti. It is a liberation in peace, in happiness, in the freedom of the soul no longer bound by the thousand bonds and cares of ignorant outer existence." (Sri Aurobindo, *Letters on Yoga*)

15 Spiritual evolution, for Aurobindo, follows a natural progression, where "consciousness appears in everything that seemed unconscious before, and once it appears it progresses on its own to become greater and greater and at the same time enlarges and develops towards greater and greater perfection."

16 "The force you felt must evidently have been an ascent of the Kundalini rising to unite with the Force Above and bringing down the energy needed to relieve depression and then rising again to strengthen the connection between that which is Above and the lower centers. The apparent expansion of the head is due to the union of the mind with the consciousness of the Self or Divine above. That consciousness is wide and unlimited and, when one rises into it, the individual consciousness breaks its limits and feels wide and unlimited."

On the descent of the higher consciousness, Sri Aurobindo explained:

"Correspondingly, the experience of descent occurs when the higher consciousness pours down through the body via the Kundalini, making its way through the head (mental sheath), flooding the vital sheath, bringing peace and bliss, until it reaches the last Chakra at the base of the spine (i.e. the physical sheath)."

17 *Shared Transformation* (1993). See also her book *Branded by the Spirit*, at https://elcollie.wordpress.com/the-history; there are more sites about his life. See for instance: https://espirited.com/wp-content/uploads/2014/01/branded-by-the-spirit_by-el-collie.pdf

18 "If I had the choice I would have opted for a path without Kundalini. That said, it may be that Kundalini awakenings are inevitable for some of us. And if this is the case—or if one is determined to awaken the Serpent—then I would strongly recommend a path that focuses on the heart or has a Master known for compassion."

19 "Once awakened, it transports us to 'a world that is totally different from our world: it is a world of eternity,' as Jung put it. Nothing could have prepared me for the wonder of this experience, not even my past adventures with LSD. Yet, it would be equally true to say that everything in my life had led to this."

20 Others see complete auras around people and other living beings. Seeing auras or trails of light around living beings and so-called inanimate objects are common *Kundalini* experiences.

21 "Many months later, I finally came across Sannella and Greenwell's writings on the Kundalini experience, two of the most comprehensive Western texts on the subject. Also of great help was an ES support group and SEN (Spiritual Emergency Network, founded by Cristina Grof).

I thus understood that what had happened to me was a 'dynamic' awakening, as Swami Muktananda would call it, my mind finally saw a glimmer of hope in the fear."

22 http://conversarecongliangeli.com/riflessioni-sulla-Kundalini/

23 "The Sufis have the knowledge to awaken it, and also some sects like the Rosicrucians, but there is very little information about them (very nice book 'The Abyss of Fire'). Other texts are the Divine Comedy, which shows the path of purification through Hell, Purgatory and Paradise, or Gurdjieff talks about it in 'Tales of Beelzebub to his Nephew' talking about reopening the Kundabuffer organ. Better known, however, is the book of the Curandera, where there is some information. True Tantra uses it, but even here the knowledge is handed down from master to pupil". (the book *Tantric Ecstasy* is very special and nice).

24 *Collision With the Infinite: A Life Beyond the Personal Sel* (1966) ed. Blue Dove.

25 This recurrence of a new acute and even more transformative phase years later, when the person and his nervous system are more advanced, is not at all rare.

26 Let's see: awakening? That is, "a shift from the conventional sense of self to the uninvolved witness, and / or to the all-pervasive presence, and / or pure awareness, and / or Being, and / or emptiness / emptiness, and / or the Self, and / or the simple recognition of non-separateness." Those who have commented on these episodes confirm that this was indeed the case for Segal. Others, however, remarked that perhaps it was depersonalization, dissociation. Then of course came the fear, followed finally by a return to normality. But the urge to do the same thing again and again returned in Suzanne. Many people with depersonalization disorder have cited similar episodes in the course of their disorder.

27 Batgap is an acronym, made up of the initials of the phrase "Buddha at the gas pump"; *it* is intended to emphasize that nowadays we should not look far away for an awakened master, for example, in a cave on a high mountain; we could rather easily meet them in our daily lives, even at the gas pump or in the supermarket. Batgap: https://batgap.com/

28 www.facebook.com/BuddhaAtTheGasPump

29 See, for example, among the many who tell of their post-awakening state and how it happened, the likes of *Tony Parsons*, *Bonnie Greenwell*, *Jack O Keefe*, *Caterina Maggi*, *Igor Kufayev*, *Adyashanti*, *Neumann*, *Halliday*, and many others. On the Batgap site, therapists' interviews (there is an option to have the list by category) are here: https://batgap.com/interviews/categorical-index-guests/page/2/?el_dbe_page

Outside Batgap, plenty of testimonies of awakening processes are found in the field of music and poetry: e.g., *Kirtana*, *De Gregori*, *Lucio Dalla*, and others through their songs, if one knows how to read them.

30 https://conscious.tv/index.php

Chapter 12

Therapy

12.1 Which therapy?

The plurality of existing therapeutic approaches stems from the fact that each is based on different conceptions of mental disorders and is implemented by professionals with often heterogeneous training backgrounds.

It is necessary to examine the characteristics and limitations of these interventions in order to better understand how a different kind of therapy, a TP-based therapy, and a different training could depart significantly from traditional approaches and pave the way to a renewed psychiatry.[1]

12.1.1 What happens when a psychiatrist intervenes

Psychiatric training in Italy with a six-year degree in medicine and surgery, followed by a four-year specialization in psychiatry—which is considered a medical discipline focused mainly on the biological aspects of mental illness.

Across European countries, medical and psychiatry training follow a similar pattern, but postgraduate psychiatry lasts a median of 5 years, with wide variation. Worldwide, high-income countries are shifting toward competence_based curricula with more psychotherapy, neuroscience and relational skills. In the United States, the standard pathway totals 12 years after high school (4 years of college, 4 of medical school and 4 of psychiatry residency), while in Russia psychiatry follows 6 years of general medical training plus a 2 year residency, and in China 5 years of undergraduate medical education plus a 3 year standardized psychiatry residency.

Typical psychiatric intervention focuses on *diagnostic classification*, often using manuals such as DSM-5, and *anti-symptomatic drug therapy*. Follow-up visits are generally spaced out in time, with a prognosis that often assumes the condition will become chronic, according to the "once psychotic, always psychotic" paradigm.

From a TP perspective, the administration of psychotropic medication has an effect similar to regulating the energetic flow in the subtle body and

DOI: 10.4324/9781003676461-12

can decisively support the recognition and rediscovery of oneself as consciousness, thereby reducing the confusion and disorientation that accompany CP. In fact, reactions to discomfort usually quite rapidly (within days or weeks) relieving the patient of suffering sometimes to a great extent, thus creating more favourable conditions for psychotherapy to take place.[2]

When the approach is primarily biological, the use of medication implicitly conveys and reinforces an interpretative model of suffering as *endogenous*, *biological*, *pessimistic*, and *passive*. This can be potentially stigmatizing for the patient, who may begin to identify with the image of a chronically ill person

The real challenge for a patient seeking genuine healing is precisely to question (but not to deny that identification), move beyond this identification.

12.1.2 What happens when a psychotherapist intervenes

The figure of the psychotherapist, in Italy, includes graduates in psychology (five-year non-medical degree course), or in medicine.

In order to practise psychotherapy, specific post-graduate training in a *recognized school of psychotherapy* lasting at least four years is required, which includes adequate theoretical and practical training. Registration on the psychotherapists' register, which has been established in Italy since 1989, confirms professional qualification.[3]

Psychotherapeutic intervention generally relies on *interview-based approaches,* aiming to understand and address suffering through psychological, rather than pharmacological, means.

Often, the objective is symptom control, this time through the mind.

Cognitive-behavioral psychotherapies are those most frequently recommended by mainstream psychiatry guidelines, and focus on symptom control. *This approach tends to disregard the unconscious,* focusing on behavior modification through specific techniques.

There are numerous other psychotherapeutic approaches that are not derived from a psychoanalytic basis, such as *Rogerian therapy, transactional analysis, and EMDR*. Despite the variety, mainstream psychiatry tends to favor more interventionist approaches to symptoms, aimed at a *reconstruction of the personality and a return to a socially accepted sense of normality.* Sometimes, the psychotherapist may recommend concurrent *psychiatric support* for pharmacological management. If the psychotherapist is also a psychiatrist, they may directly oversee the pharmacological aspect as well.

12.1.3 What happens when a psychoanalyst intervenes

The psychoanalytic approach is distinguished by its focus on *the unconscious origin of the psychic crisis* and the search for a deeper sense of

distress. To work as a psychoanalyst, one must be a doctor, psychiatrist, or psychologist with specific psychoanalytic training (which includes personal analysis). Therapy consists of trying to understand past and present psychological dynamics together with the patient, bringing unconscious drives and ego defenses to consciousness, through analysis of transference and counter-transference, interpretation of dream symbolism, work on relationships and past or present traumas. *The aim is to unravel the root causes of the crisis* through a therapeutic relationship based on dialogue, with a potential duration of several years and a variable focus (child psychogenesis, trauma, spiritual aspects, family, etc.) depending on the analytical approach (Freudian, Jungian, Lacanian, Reichian, group analysis, bioenergetics).

12.1.4 What happens when a transpersonal psychotherapist intervenes

As we have seen, transpersonal psychotherapy (TPPT) differs by *considering spirituality and transcendence as essential therapeutic components*, and by interpreting *Non-Ordinary States of Consciousness* (NOSC) *as potentially evolutionary*

A fundamental aspect of this therapy is the therapist's own level of consciousness, derived from personal direct experience of the transcendent.

Unlike approaches that aim to "solve" and eliminate symptoms, TPPT seeks to participate in and understand the psychological dynamics from a perspective of transforming states of consciousness. The object of treatment is not just the "me" in crisis to be medicated, but the patient's soul. The TP approach aims to understand the necessity, intelligence, and teleology of psychotic deconstruction brought on by the crisis.

In the acute phases of a psychosis, it is generally considered ineffective and unimportant to intervene with psychotherapy, except for generic ego support. However, in the TP approach, on the contrary, considers these acute and destructuring phases of the crisis as privileged moments in which to propose a TPPT intervention, concurrently aided by an adequate use of psychopharmaceuticals, in order to contain, and not abate, the acute crisis, and avoid a neurotic chronification or a "default" recovery.

In conclusion, different types of therapy depend on different views of mental suffering, but also on the fact that there are different needs for different patients.

Different psychotherapeutic approaches can be justified by the *different evolutionary levels of people and their consciousness*. For example, *Wilber* proposes a progression of different interventions over time according to the integration and transcendence of the patient's consciousness. The early stages in individual development are constructive for the strengthening of the ego, while the later stages imply a progressive abandonment of identification with it.

For example, according to this author, supportive *psychological counseling* will be sufficient to deal with contingent difficulties, while confronting the shadow and integrating unconscious parts will require psychodynamic psychotherapy. To foster mind-body integration, the use of psycho-body techniques such as bioenergetics, *IBP* (*Integrative Body Psychotherapy*)[4], and yoga are probably more suitable. If the aim is instead to accompany the patient towards a transcendence of the personal self and access to transpersonal states, to the perception of subtle realities, Jungian analysis will be indicated, but also tantric yoga techniques and shamanism. The ultimate goal of the dissolution of the individual self in consciousness will require an approach such as those employed in Tantrism and Vedanta.

The transition between these levels is not linear, and different interventions may be used in sequence, bearing in mind that too rapid an expansion of consciousness can be destabilizing. Each stage therefore has its own function and value, and practitioners working on different levels may tend to downplay interventions that apply to evolutionary phases other than the one they are dealing with.

12.2 The TP psychotherapy method

In the next section, we will examine in detail how a TP psychotherapy session is conducted.

In order to understand the clinical rationale of this way of proceeding, and for the techniques proposed, it is necessary to expound some fundamental concepts here. Only after having seen the session in detail will we be able to resume and conclude our reflections on TP therapies.

12.2.1 There is method and method

We have to distinguish the traditional conception of method, based on systematic and repeatable procedures, from the "method not method" proposed by Jung and adopted by TPPT.

The method in TPPT is *fluid, non-systematic or repeatable.* It will proceed differently depending on the therapeutic phase, reassuring or deconstructing, analyzing or favoring psychosynthesis, more attentive to the psychological level, to favor the integration of experiences and give a profound meaning to existence, or at other times more directed towards the spiritual, to favor the expansion of consciousness and the recognition of what lies beyond the mind. The method is constantly evolving, alive and adaptable to each individual.

TP psychotherapeutic intervention does not exclude, but *includes analytical work.*[5] This means that the TP therapist also works with dialogue, pauses, intuitions, listening, and verification, touching various aspects of the patient's life, past and above all present; they take into account what happens in the session (at the level of transference and counter-transference), and maintains a basic focus on processes of associations, lapsus, memories, traumas; they also work with dreams (analyzed first symbolically but also anagogically), or with Active Imagination. The focus is on inner dynamics, but also on interpersonal relations, that is, on understanding projective and interactive dynamics.

Sessions may include an educational, light, episodic contribution of information on the energetic, spiritual, or archetypal dimension.

However, what truly characterizes the TP method is the therapist's constant attention and residence in a *state of consciousness not identified with the ego*: they must remain in a centered and present state of consciousness, in contact with the energetic perception in one's own *Chakras*, thus helping the patient to do the same, by internal imitation, or rather by *induction* of that state *that is one in all*. We could call this action a *direct introduction*.

The therapist thus helps the patient to enter and remain in that state, and give their *indications* about it: they guide the patient in real time to realize, to listen and recognize what is happening in their state of consciousness; they help them to realize when they come out of the state.

In other words, they accompany them not only to temporarily experience but to *remain in the state*, to take residence in it, to choose it.

The patient *learns* how the *mind lies,* how not to be fooled by its own spell, *not to remain in doubt*, which is one of the main defensive strategies of the ego to paralyze the evolutionary process.

This will enable the patient to acquire the tools to *operate on their own* during the interval between sessions, and to stabilize this ability to move into a higher state of consciousness.

The goal is liberation from suffering, care, and the caregiver.

The essence of the method is *deep listening,* which goes beyond identification with mental states, perceived as internal objects by the percipient consciousness.

This method is similar to, but differs from, *Autogenic Training* or *"Focusing"*, or is even similar at times to *Yoga Nidra* techniques.

The therapist is therefore *highly attentive to the energy:* they direct their own *attention* (and the patient's) *to whatever is happening in real time at the energetic level, in the Chakras, and in the energy flow* in the session, welcoming any NOSC that may emerge.

The patient is *instructed on how to support their own energy*, to recognize, manage, and support the transformation process.

Practical exercises, such as *Guided Deep Relaxation*, or the *Holotropic Breathing* Technique, can be proposed in this direction.[6]

The TP method is natural, it does not force processes or manipulate timing, but adapts to them: this is because listening acts as a guide for action;

it is therefore a matter of taking orders from the process and not giving them.[7] *The method can be learned, but not taught in the traditional sense,* as it requires the development of the subtle perceptive capacity that must be awakened, rediscovered. *However, it can be induced and activated in the patient in the course of therapy.*

12.2.2 Therapy and the non-dual field

The TP method is aimed at facilitating the *shift of* identity from the usual personal self (small s), preoccupied, tense, to the Self (capital S) that is already present, which is who we really are.

The method helps one to reside in this larger space of consciousness, in which all this is observed and contained, which is aware and stable, which is already in peace: it helps one to rediscover oneself, to realize that one is "the same but different," *to accompany awakening*. The patient is therefore invited to "look towards what is looking," to return to the pure consciousness that precedes phenomena.

> *You know the joke of those two psychiatrists, one young and one old, who argue with each other at the end of the working day.*
>
> *The young man complains:* "How tired I am! I've been listening to patients all day, I can't take it any more! They have sucked all my energy!
>
> But I don't understand, how can you, after listening to so many patients all day, still be so fresh and rested and calm in the evening?"
>
> *And the elderly one, after a moment's pause, replies:*
>
> "Yes, but ... who listens?"

With this question, the elderly psychiatrist invites reflection on *who is really listening* during therapy. If what listens is the image of the therapist identified with the role of the one who must strive to help, this can lead to exhaustion. If, on the other hand, what listens is a *consciousness free of* this identification, a vast and neutral space that welcomes without attachment and without defense, then the experience becomes light.

Here, this is where psychiatry ends: when the interpretative mind vanishes and only the "percipient subject" remains, without separation and without the suffering of a specific "someone." Suffering is then seen in this process as a painful sensation that does not only happen *to* "you, character," but rather happens "in" *you,* "consciousness," without memory and without desire, like a wave in the sea.

The *therapeutic* field is generated by the *therapeutic couple*,[8] by the intention to help and co-operate, and this is the subtle and sensitive reality that allows one to perceive and intervene in the field.[9] The therapeutic couple, united by intention, acts *in and on the* field, in turn moved and transformed by it. *The perception and observation of the therapeutic field*, the field of the relationship, is essential to operate in the therapeutic vessel, the alchemical "*Athanor*".

The *real actor and driver of the process, however, is*, the *therapeutic field, generated by the therapeutic alliance:*

A *unified* "field" is thus activated—an energetic or morphogenetic field,[10] endowed with memory and information—in which emotions and psychological dynamics are transmitted and transformed

The concept of a "collective memory" within morphogenetic fields parallels the transpersonal idea of a *shared unconscious, or a field of consciousness* that connects all human beings.

This morphogenetic field *is an activity of the* same *creative consciousness*, the same one that operates beyond the space–time concept.[11]

In religious terms, we speak of this activity of the creative consciousness in terms of "Love," in the profound sense of *a-mors*, deathless, hence *love*.[12] It is that energy-consciousness, that timeless (eternal) reality operating in time, in becoming, that transpersonal principle at work in our lives.[13]

This field is generated by the Self, and is not comprehensible and perceivable until we die to identification with the individual ego.

This is why TP therapy, although carried out through the therapist, uses the field and the therapist together, for the relief of suffering, for liberation: the *therapist is the pencil of the field*.[14]

12.3 Guided deep relaxation

This is a technique of self-treatment of the *Chakras*, implemented by the patient under the guidance of the therapist, who applies it within themselves during the listening phase.

To do this, the therapist does not start from an ordinary but from a transpersonal state of consciousness, relying on their own inner perception: they listen to the state and quality of their own energies, their own *Chakras*, asking the patient to do the same in their own *Chakras*.

The therapist perceives changes in the patient's *Chakras* through their own *Chakras*, thanks to the presence of the unified field of consciousness. *Chakra* conditions can be perceived, transformed, accompanied, and resolved. This procedure aims to lead the patient towards a state of openness from which they can better examine all phenomena emerging within themselves.

A first effect of this guided deep-relaxation *exercise is to promote the resumption of the internal circulation of* energy, a beneficial, therapeutic, direct effect, and this is already of no little importance; the patient generally and easily succeeds in overcoming suffering in the course of the session, while at the same time learning a method that can also be useful to them later on.

A second and more important result, however, is that this exercise brings consciousness closer to the threshold of self-recognition, it helps to perceive directly that there is something perceiving, to *look at the beholder*: thus that recognition of who we really are (I found myself), the true Self, consciousness, could happen in an instant.

12.3.1 Part one: Connecting

In the first part of this exercise, the *patient is seated* in front of the therapist; they are guided to shift attention from thoughts to bodily sensations, *from thinking to feeling*, to let go of thoughts and bring attention to sensations in the body.

To help the patient, they are advised to *close their eyes and listen inside*, and is shown, as we shall see, what to listen for, and how to identify and evaluate the intensity and quality of the sensation. The aim is to favor a direct perception of the inner space, reducing the attention we usually pay to mental activity, and favoring listening to the subtle body.[15] The patient is encouraged to keep their muscles relaxed and to listen to their natural breath.

The hands are placed on specific energy points: one hand on the *third Chakra* (mouth of the stomach) and the other hand on the *second Chakra* (bladder-genital area). Contact with one's own body is fundamental in this perception exercise: it is a bit like hugging oneself, but it does not require any physical contact on the part of the therapist; patients work on their own *Chakras*.

The patient is then invited to bring their attention to their body regions, naming them and gradually going through them from the feet to the head, identifying any tensions or poorly perceived areas and gradually relaxing them.[16]

The patient is then invited to bring attention to the sensation of heat in the hands, the subtle *heat, the heat one* "feels" in the hands; and to identify the hottest hand of the two. Generally, listening amplifies the sensation, which in turn tends to increase.

The patient is then asked to rate the variations in intensity and quality of heat, using a *subjective scale from* "0" *to* "10," where "0" stands for "no feeling" and "10" stands for "the strongest feeling ever."

12.3.2 Part two: Getting inside

One is then asked to perceive *whether the warmth of the hottest hand* trasfers itself *to* the body surface underneath the hand; and then whether it is felt to *penetrate deeper inside*, and how much.

The same procedure will be applied with the second hand.

Often this perception inside the body is quickly detected, other times it takes longer.

The patient is then asked to observe whether the internal heat is limited to the region of the hand, or tends to spread, expand, move, and how this happens in the surrounding areas.

This phase fosters greater awareness of energy distribution in the body, preparing for the subsequent experience of connecting with the *Chakras* and main energy channels.

The hands are still placed over the second and third *Chakras*; at this point, if it is felt that the opening is sufficient or complete and stable, the patient is asked to *bring the hand placed on the third Chakra, slowly, over the fourth chalra.*

The patient is also asked to become aware of the quality of *the sensation*, which changes in quality as it rises.

Listening now to the sensation under the hand placed on the heart *Chakra*, one will be able to perceive the change in the quantity and gradual diffusion of the warmth in the chest; one will be able to observe that the quality of the sensation also changes, and to perceive different feelings, tensions, fears, and emotions.

From this position, one will sometimes be able to better perceive sensations pertinent to the upper *Chakras*, such as the fifth (which often signals a tension compensatory to the opening of the fourth), or the sixth (sensations in the head of dizziness, euphoria, confusion, tinnitus). In listening to the heart, one could perceive the condition of the posterior part of the heart *Chakra*, which has a different quality; Finally, one could perceive the *flow of* energy ascending along the *Chakras*, in the form of shivers, of heat ascending, of flow in the subtle channels.

12.3.3 *Part three: Abiding in the state* (evolution *and* stabilization)

One can now shift attention from the *Chakras* and the flow in the channels to the natural breath, to the prana flowing there. This may help to amplify the state of relaxation, recalling pranayama practices and the Taoist *small heavenly circulation.*[17] One can thus perceive a continuity and amplification of the energy circulation, listening to and accompanying the rising of the energy in inspiration, as well as its descent from the seventh to the first during exhalation.[18]

One thus arrives, to a more or less complete extent and each at one's own pace, without effort (only by accepting and observing the increase in intensity and the greater diffusion of the energy, just by listening) *at a stable background state of diffusion of the warmth, sense of well-being and harmony, and deep energy relaxation.*[19]

To help the patient realize the transitions and the final state, they are asked to *evaluate with a score* (always between 0 and 10) the warmth, its diffusion, pleasantness, overall relaxation.

This will help them realize, perceive in real time, together with the therapist, the quality of the energies they are listening to and their transformations.[20]

If the patient is able to remain present to the sensation without identifying with distracting thoughts, they can *perceive clearly the* internal energy *circulation* and a state of *meditation that tends to grow or deepen*, of deep contact with themselves. The therapist guides the timing of the individual phases according to their own perception.

The overall effect is an expansion and stabilization of energy, a global spreading of relaxation and wellbeing.

This state, once recognized and stabilized, promotes *the direct perception of the background* in which all this is perceived, i.e., the Self. Its nature is Sat Chit Ananda, i.e. *consciousness, wellbeing, joy*,[21] and abiding in that one experiences a sense of inner peace, of Holy Peace, a true medicine.

By repeating the experience a few times (even a few, 3–5), the patient develops a *growing awareness of* the energy body and the *Chakras*, which fosters a *learning process* in the patient: they learn to listen to the subtle body, to observe phenomena on the energy level and becoming aware of consciousness itself. From there, they learn how to change and reshape their inner state. The patient gradually becomes more aware of the condition of the astral and causal body and the influence of thought on energy.

12.4 A session of TP psychotherapy (TPPT) and comment

I will now detail a session carried out with this TPPT approach, and some excerpts from later sessions to show the evolution, in order to better illustrate what has been said.

I will first expound on the first part of the session, and then comment on it; afterwards I will expound on the second part, where the patient recounts a dream, in order to comment there too on the method used.

Some more general methodological principles will be taken up in the next section.

The patient, a woman of about 50, a psychologist, who, had sought help for a period of intense depression and anxiety, partly due to a difficult family situation.

12.4.1 The session

P: Here we are.

Then she falls silent and looks at me.

I immediately perceive a feeling of uneasiness coming from her (an impression based maybe on how she was sitting in the chair) I feel it in her internal state, and I perceive a deep pain in her heart. So I say:

T: What happened to you?

She transmits to me a heavy feeling, a pain she carries, I feel it in my heart; I feel her heavy heart. I also feel that she is immediately a little relieved by the very fact of having been seen and understood. She almost cries. I say:

T: Leave these thoughts alone, which seem to justify your malaise, the sense of death that we feel: you could feel like this even without them.

I can sense that they are thoughts about the family situation, which shows no tendency to change; but the only place where anything can change is within you now: if you do not intervene now in your inner world, you will not be able to intervene at home either. Let's listen more deeply to what you are feeling.

Pause

P: In fact, this week my family members told me just that: that my anxious worrying about them stresses them out; that I have to accept it.
T: OK. But what do you feel now?

Pause

P: An intense, unpleasant burning, here at stomach level,

I also listen, and I feel that her second and first Chakras are not very open: there is a slight tension, and scarce activity, and a little discomfort in that region; I *do not feel much activity in the third Chakra, in contrast to what the patient was saying. So I tell her:*

T: Let's listen better; put your hands on the second and third *Chakras*, and don't follow your thoughts; what do you feel?

She puts her hands where I told her to, and concentrate by closing her eyes.

As soon as she does this, I could immediately feel that the energy at the bottom began to open up, increase in intensity and spread out, unifying the legs, belly and back.

T: Do you feel yourself relaxing? And do you feel this state spreading?

She confirms by nodding. I listen, and in the meantime I talk a little, to help her pay attention to these internal changes, so that she is aware of them.

She starts to move her shoulders a little, rolling them, as if to release the muscles and the feeling of tension, which she only now perceives is still present in that region. I insist:

T: Are you feeling the state of relaxation spreading, is it pleasant?

Even before she answers, as we continue listening, I perceive that at my saying the word "pleasant," *a pleasant feeling is activated and grows in her, and this happens in the region of the heart.*

One feels a lightening of the heart; the feeling that emerges is love, and a light joy.

As soon as I perceive this, I consider it as a development, a track to follow, to become aware of, and so I ask her straight away:

T: And what do you feel now?
P: I feel the lower *Chakras* much more now, and a growing pleasant flow through them and around them.
T: All right, though that had already started before now. Listen better: besides that, do you also feel something new, in other parts, that wasn't there before?
Look, to help you, tell me if you perceived something when I told you that something "was spreading"; at that moment there was a change.
P: Yes, it's true, I felt something new ... in my heart, which I didn't feel before; maybe a slight pressure, or maybe an opening.
T: And what would you call that feeling?
P: Peace, serenity ...

I see that she didn't immediately grasp what I was talking about, and she's still referring to the previous sensation, relaxation; she hasn't yet recognized the more active element, of love, joy, that I perceived.

In the meantime, moreover, this complex sensation has opened up more, and I feel it flowing upwards, and towards the back.

So I continue, pointing:

T: And in the heart, behind, what do you feel?

P: I feel a more pleasant state, an increasing sensation of opening, and now I also feel a flow of energy in the back.
T: Good, let's listen more.

As we listen, we feel the flow of energy in the fourth Chakra, on the back side, intensify: we perceive a flow that tends to continue and mature and open upwards, higher up.

One also perceives, however, that this flow does not expand and pervade the fifth Chakra region as well, more specifically the region of the jaws and ears.

As I observe this process, I perceive that the intensity of the energy flow in all these regions expands, and evolves towards a wider integration and diffusion in the body, a more homogenous diffusion.

Shortly afterwards I also perceive a fading of the intensity of the overall sensation, as often happens when the energy evolves into a "steady state", *when it becomes integrated, normalizes, stabilizes. The difference in flow between the supra-diaphragmatic Chakras, and the sub-diaphragmatic ones that we had observed before, is also reduced.*

Pause.

The activity in the Chakras and channels continues, stabilizes, is considered by both. I perceive that the patient now is aware not only of the sensations but also of observing them.

That is why I use a resource, the reading of a wisdom passage, as a support and mirror:

T: I read you a short passage from a Taoist text.[22]

Silence.

She absorbs; I feel that she has understood what the text is about.

I feel that she is aware of these internal processes,

that she is aware and welcomes them and follows and facilitates them.

This is one of the moments, repeatedly experienced throughout the session, in which I perceive that her mind is still: it does not come and go;

I feel that in this "other" *space-time, in which she is suspended, the mind has no importance, no influence, and there is no sense of separation.*

After a while then I say to her:

T: Now you are at peace, and that is why you could now be able to bring this state into your relationship with your daughter, who gives you so much anxiety.

This is the medicine for your loved ones; because in the state you are in now, the one you are now perceiving, there is no one defending or offending: you are in the pure perception of what is there, without judgement.

You are free: you have freed ourselves, perhaps briefly, of all problems, and of the problem factory. This is the method. And you are seeing it at work, you are perceiving the energetic release, you are looking at it from another point of view.

This release from personal identification—and therefore from personal problems—represents the true medicine, for the sense of death that you feel in your daughter's heart, to really accompany her, and you cannot offer it to her unless you have first recognized it.

We are again in that suspended state.

She absorbs, nods.

She remains open, at peace, and in the perception of the flow circulating within her and between us, which stabilises.

After a while, I ask:

T: Were there any dreams during the week that you remember?

12.4.2 Reflections on the session

Before continuing with the second part of the session, in which we examine a dream the patient brings, let us take a break to reflect on some points of the session so far. We believe we have shown here, at least in part, how the transpersonal method is implemented in the treatment of mental suffering in psychology and psychiatry.

This method does not exclude different forms of treatment, but rather offers a distinctive characteristic compared to other forms of psychotherapy lack.

The TP approach to therapy as reminded, is a radical process of cure: it aims *not so much at the liberation* "of" "me" *from suffering as liberation* "from" *identification with* "me."

As we have seen, the method of active listening to the *Chakras* and energy and consciousness transformations was implemented in the session, managing the patient's resistance according to the TP method. But let us go into more detail.

12.4.3 There is what there is

In the session I start from what is there, from what the patient presents to me, from her present condition: I listen to the field that is created every time I meet with a patient, and it is the field that indicates about what, how, and when to intervene. I therefore proceed in my diagnosis and therapy not according to what the patient tells me, but according to what the field tells me.

It can rarely happen, as can be seen here, that I do not even let the patient speak. Usually, however, I wait for the patient to start, or if this does not happen, instead of waiting a long time, I ask how it is going.

If the patient is more advanced in the transpersonal work, they understand that by that I mean "how is the energy in the Chakras going now"; meanwhile, I perceive directly the Chakra's condition.

Often, however, the patient decodes my question in a dualistic way, interpreting my question as related to how life is going outside, what has happened during the week, or what has happened psychologically; but even so, during the narration I listen to how the energy flowed (inside and outside) in those narrated episodes, or in a reported dream; this is possible because the energetic diagnosis is delocalized in time and space, and is carried out with the same clarity online.

It is an exercise in subtle, impersonal perception.[23]

I therefore perceive what is there:

> *the* "what"; *the* "where" *and* "when" are simplified to "here and now," in both, in the "field."

When I do not interfere in the field, what I perceive is really there; *if I am truly transparent*, what I see *in the me*, is what is happening *in the you at* the same time.

Of course, and also *to corroborate my inner perceptions*, I do not forget what I have learnt in many years of clinical practice, namely to also observe the face, behavior, posture, tone of voice, hesitations, dreams, the account of intervening psychological dynamics, memories of the past and so on.

However, I mostly listen "inside."

We could say that I perceive *out of empathy, out of identification*.

But the discourse is more radical: more correctly I would say that *I feel what happens in his Chakras through my Chakras*.[24] In fact, we are not actually two (although we are also two distinct persons): it is a non-dual method of psychotherapy. In this method of therapeutic intervention one *goes* "beyond" *the roles* of one who helps and one who is helped.[25]

It is therefore about "going into One."

It is about overcoming the separation, the sleep of consciousness, thanks to the *awakening* in the therapist: then all happens both in the individual and in the field; in the field of miracles, where things just happen.[26]

12.4.4 Opening the Chakras

We have described above the technique of opening the *Chakras* in general; in this session this exercise was applied at the moments indicated by the field, according to the principles of respect, neutrality, TP accompanying.

In the unified energy intervention, there is not an active and a passive agent, acting; rather, there is a therapeutic action, restoring the energy circulation, operated by the non-dual, unified field, guided by the therapist's awareness. The therapist does not operate alone, they do not substitute the patient, they do not impose truths, they only indicate possible steps, doors. The therapist supports possible efforts, and comfort possible discouragements, and stimulate possible intuitions. During th sessions, the therapist invites the patient to cross the bridge that keeps them divided from themselves, respecting the fact that it is the patient, however, who needs and wants to cross that distance.

For example, in the session, after my intervention (and for the mere fact that I have indicated it to her, and she is willing to do it, to be guided as I tell her), she promptly *changes* her internal *attitude*: she listens. *And, contextually, immediately, as always*, she *transforms what she perceives*. And I too then, with her, immediately perceive that her *Chakras* are perceived more.

In particular, one feels the tension in that specific *Chakra* transforming, dissolving, transforming into a pleasant relaxation; one feels the beginning of the blossoming of the flower, of the flow of energy.

It is interesting that what has been set in motion after the intervention also *continues its* therapeutic action in time and space: its action progressively and increasingly *transmits and manifests itself also in* the *surrounding Chakras*, and then in the channel between the *Chakras*, and even in the area surrounding the channel connecting them, where "resident" tensions often reside, tensions that arise and persist due to the presence of inhibiting thought forms, which condition happiness and security.

As the tension in the region *melts* away, transforming itself into a state of relaxation, of warmth that expands, one perceives at the same time *the reactivation of the* energetic *circulation* characterized by wellbeing and which goes to include, relax, bring back lifeblood and wellbeing to the whole region.

This energetic expansion has its own dynamic, which proceeds to its completion and then becomes integrated and silent.

The expansion can *still develop,* with a sinusoidal pattern, which directly indicates where and how the process is still going on, when it reaches *its peak*, and when it is completing. The process progressively and gradually comes to a steady state in a globalization, a homogenization throughout the body of this sensation, stabilizing in a *plateau*, and finally fading into a state of stable peace and harmony.

12.4.5 Action, not reaction

In the session, my first intervention might seem rather unorthodox: *I immediately make the first move, I speak first*; as if I knew where we are, and what is best to do.

This is already the first move, the fact that I move first. This first *move is actually the second move*, because it follows, it responds to what I encounter in the relational field: consequently, *I proceed following the flow* that I perceive.[27] This state is the *background to everything said and perceived* in the session, by me or by the patient.

The implicit message that reaches the patient is that when I move I am taking it for granted, witnessing and communicating that I know how and what they feel, that I am feeling their desires and frustrations, their joys and sorrows, in the here and now, and in which *Chakra*; *the patient realizes that we are therefore already speaking from within.*[28]

By doing this I overcome the problems of communication, adequacy, understanding each other, etc. in one single step, and directly convey the experience that we are in contact on a different plane than the mental and linguistic and dualistic plane: a plane that precedes the mental, separation, doubt.

During the session we are in fact already immersed in a common field, we are connected in experiencing and understanding that we are One, and I witness and utilize this truth, I do not explain it in words. I do not make it personal.

> However, as can be seen in the subsequent development of the session, *language is still used*; however, it no longer has the function of producing change, it is no longer a tool for transformation, as is generally argued in psychology: words and symbols are rather just *the words that express it.* They have the function of *bearing witness to* this *cum-prehension* (that is, taking together), they are the manifestation emanating from the psychic and relational space of the "therapeutic arena": they are rather an "ornament" of the transforming state, and are sometimes also a *stimulus and support for* the alchemical process.
>
> Here is a clinical example from another patient's dream: "I dreamt that I was in a room, which could have been the one in the session, but it was strange... not really like the real one; and there were other people, a somewhat unreal atmosphere, not people I knew.
>
> The strange thing was that one communicated in a strange way, with images, which one exchanged; or with words, a key word, for example one word instead of a whole sentence, and one understood each other like that, almost telepathically. Then it was strange how one moved around in that place, sometimes levitating and remaining suspended, other times walking around, and it was strange to move like that."

12.4.6 The way is not a constant way

One can see in the following passages of the session how *I proceed by letting myself be guided by the intelligent sequence of sensations that change and emerge in succession:* sensations can in fact be listened to and understood.

They speak to us, and respond to us according to how we respond to them.

For example, at the beginning of the session *I had a first sensation of the fourth Chakra,* the heart: heavy, pained, tired. I remember it well.

However, as the session continued, during the exercise of self-perception of the *Chakras,* and after the first sensation had been recognized and accepted by the patient, *a second sensation emerged in me.* This one was initially very faint, it did not speak, it was not perceptible; but as it emerged and now demanded new attention, I was able to welcome it, to give it more attention, which caused it to further emerge in the foreground; the right moment to do so, however, was indicated to me by the dynamics taking place in the field, it was the sensation itself which indicated to me that this was the right and opportune moment to do so.

So we see that depending on how one proceeds (pay attention, don't superimpose onself to the process, but rather be guided by it), whether or not new phenomena occur, new perceptions emerge in the *Chakras.* The medicine emerging from this field and operating on it, at the same time, is this awareness, becoming self aware.

> *Let's see it in the session:* the patient had stated that she perceived a strong and painful activity of the *third Chakra.*[29] Listening to her *Chakras,* on the other hand, disagreed partially because I had perceived that the third *Chakra* was not very disturbed, and that instead the first *Chakra* was contracted, reduced, silent, while in the second there was an unpleasant feeling. All this indicated displeasure and insecurity respectively.[30]
>
> Thus my intervention had the function of inviting the patient to check whether her perception was correct, and to correct the corresponding energy in this new attention; it would seem that this did indeed happen, judging by her confirmation.
>
> The question could be raised as to whether the patient had convinced herself of my perception as her own, whether it was plagiarism, my superimposition. This, however, could only happen if I were operating from my egoic centred consciousness and purpose, whereas it could not happen if I were abiding in a state of non-dual consciousness, "without memory and without desire," as Bion would say: and this only the session can say, or leave it in the shade.

What is of interest here is to indicate how my proceeding in the session changes recectively in keeping with what is unfolding.

In this method, *the way follows the feeling*; and does not follow constant guidelines; it is always a new art. The intervention in the session changes according to the different conditions, to the different degree of consciousness of the person, to the different capacity to accept and assimilate what emerges, with different timing for each person and each moment of the session.

The intention is to help the natural flow of things, to paddle with the current. Life wants to flow, the flow is always changing, and the TP therapist accompanies this loosening, opening, becoming, subsiding.

It is a method that *cannot be* taught, because it is the therapist who teaches you, *but it can be learned* easily, once *you talk less and listen more.*[31]

12.4.7 Rectification

In the session, I invite the patient to consider what she perceives directly in the present moment, to give importance and value to her "seeing"; sometimes it happens, as in this case, that the patient realizes the gap between *what she* "believes" *and what* she experiences, *that she* "sees."

The consequence of my intervention helped the patient to shift her attention from mental representations, to the energy underlying them and preceding and originating them.

This delicate passage is described in the session, which took place with my "*falsification*" intervention: I stated that what she said she was feeling was not corresponding, wasn't true; this was, based on my perception, which was different from hers.

Here again, my intervention was unorthodox to say the least, something that would be discouraged and criticised in the light of the theoretical teachings of any school of psychotherapy.

Specifically, here is the sequence:

- *I see-feel within myself that* what she is telling me is *not true* (the patient was saying: "I feel a strong burning sensation in the third Chakra"), or at least that that is only part of the truth of the subtle facts.
- *I feel and believe* my perception to be clinically correct instead (even though the patient is not yet aware of this).
- *I step in for her to verify.* I defend her truth, against the mind that lies,[32] and also indicate when, how, and where she betrays her feeling, when she believes what the mind tells her. With this conscious procedure, I bring a direct attack to her egoic assumption, I unmask the deception: I make the patient aware of the egoic game, which plays the old game: "It is true but I do not believe it, it is not true but I believe it." Thus this work of verification allows one to get out of mental stories,

which only become powerful and influential if they are believed to be true. *A thought believed to be true* can move a war, a *thought not believed* has no efficacy.[33]

As can be seen in the session, I rectify her perceptions and interpretations directly, not by substituting myself for the patient, but by guiding her to verify for herself, to do it herself. This intervention proves to be correct in the clinical verification: one could feel in the session a change in energy and consciousness immediately after my intervention, the flow reactivated in real time, and one can perceive the relief of being able to recognize oneself. This verification allows the patient to return to reality, it is itself already a healing process.[34]

12.4.8 Consensual validation

When I say something true, the energy responds, and opens up; if I say something false, or at the wrong moment, nothing happens, or the energy closes down.[35]

External and internal confirmation reactions can be observed.

Sometimes, this inner response is accompanied more or less consciously by an explicit confirmation, expressed verbally, or with gestures. This in therapy is called *consensual validation*, and its modality (the readiness, the enthusiastic movement of response, emotional openings, Joy, further material emerging, evolutionary dreams in the following days) confirms the truth of what has been observed and shared.

In this specific session, the patient heartily approved of what I was indicating to her, adding other congruous material in confirmation: for example, she recalls how during the week her family members had already pointed out to her her neurotic resistances, and how this generated further difficulties and suffering, to her and to others.

At that point she shares that she is now able to clearly identify the dynamic we are talking about in the session, and smiles gratefully.

12.4.9 Consciousness and transformation

In the session, I do not merely perceive (and rectify) the relationship between her feeling and thinking, but go a step further: *I also perceive whether and when she realises that she is not realising, when she sees that she does not see.*

In the example of the session, I realize that she does not go down and listen to the lower *Chakras*. So I take a step in that direction, explicitly asking her *to pay attention there.*

When I help her see that she does not see, I am actually accompanying her to realize this inner blindness.

The effect of this perceiving that she does not perceive is surprising; as we see in the session, she immediately regains contact with herself, she wakes up. Sometimes it is not even necessary to verbalize it, the essential thing is that the therapist becomes aware of it, that this perception and awareness arise in her consciousness.

12.4.10 There is no two without three

In short, *in the session there are always three of us*: she, myself, and the field, which is both perceived and perceiving us. We dwell in that space-non-space of the subtle world, in the time-without-time of the actual present, which does not usually coincide with the virtual and mental present.

The patient continues to be connected with me, as I am with her, or even better "not separate, and inseparable," while at the same time we dialogue from two different banks of the river, *separate*.

So the session goes on, always changing the point of support, and this serves to work through different materials, and yet always keeping the focus on the union that exists within separation, both inwardly and in the transference-counter transference relationship, which serves as the container for this work of elaboration.

At each turning point of the flowing session, like a river, both participants recognize, verbalize and integrate in real time what is happening in the consciousness and its energy.

They can also recognize where this happens, and how, and also, therefore, why it happens. In short, one becomes aware of the relationship between all that moves in the inner world, of the intelligence of motion, one becomes aware of its quantitative and qualitative change, perceived by the still awareness.

12.4.11 With skill and art

We have stated that in the session one should follow the indication of what is presented, be receptive, and only respond accordingly.

However, sometimes it is also necessary to act in reverse.

In the session it can happen that I become active, actively directing the psychic material.

For example, while investigating a subtle change (perceived by both of us) I often *point or direct the listening work, the attention, towards new sensations* that emerge, trusting my anticipatory perceptions.

In these cases, *I do not follow the session but direct it;* I therefore act sometimes by moving autonomously in one direction, and other times in the opposite direction, not following one that the patient indicates to me.

It also happens that I urge, actively support, or even sometimes cautiously determine or force certain steps, always ready, however, to listen to the ensuing response, and to evaluate its appropriateness and clinical utility at that particular moment, so as to always avoid potentially harmful movements.

Sometimes I intervene *at crucial points of the session, to temper or reinforce, to deviate, to suggest, to challenge*; I intervene on points that I consider crucial, according to my feeling, at specific moments in *my-her* consciousness, in *my-her* energy: moments that are in progress, or that are to come, or that have already passed but are still alive in the therapeutic field.

In doing so, I become an active element in the process, and not just a participant who records and replays, in order to recognize the events that occur.[36]

12.4.12 The map

In this session (but this happens also on other occasions) *I explain some steps of the method we are following by referring to a map of the subtle world and consciousness*. Sometimes I use the map of the subtle body as described in yoga and astrology, or in myths. Sometimes I use the map of the Divine Comedy, because I work with Italian patients, and this map is masterfully complete, exhaustive, and detailed, and if you understand it well, it illustrates and explains and unfolds every psychic and psychiatric aspect of the transformation very well; it perfectly connects the process of revelation with every psychic and relational manifestation that is more or less obscured or in the process of purification, of illumination.

I believe that these interventions *do not stand in the way of* the alchemy of the process.

On the contrary, as in the Comedy, they can serve as points of reference, as encouragement, as clarification of steps and techniques.

Moreover, these interventions can also be *useful, along with others, to manage the regime of fire,* to temper and cool it, or to activate it. If used consciously, dosed appropriately, they can help regulate the temperature of the ongoing process.

For example, by talking more, abstracting myself more or from the specific, personal story, the patient and I move away from an excessively empathic involvement in the clinical moment and the process underway, to consider a possible understanding; however, while the patient moves away, while we talk, and explain, while we dialogue, and linger, I am aware that the process is continuing.

By listening and perceiving the ongoing fire, I can regulate how and how much to speak, and then re-enter the field at the right moment without explanations and plans.

So I talk more or less, depending on whether the patient needs to understand better intellectually; or I explain just to pause, or to shift the focus from the therapist guide (lower-case G) to the Guide (with a capital G), the Inner Master.

Of course one has to be aware of the *risk that* the patient or even the therapist might use these contributions to move to the mental plane and avoid the ongoing transformation by rationalizing it.

12.4.13 The dream in the session

In the course of the session, the patient then recounts a dream. Do you remember my question? We continue from there.

T: Do you remember any dreams from this past week?
P: Yes, various, but I mainly remember one dream from this night:

> *I was in a big crowded room, like an American party, there were also black people there; it also looked like a disco.*
>
> *I realise that something serious is about to happen, a massacre, where everyone kills everyone;*
>
> *I feel I have to participate, but I also want to leave.*
>
> *Then the shooting starts.*
>
> *I try to protect myself, and I see that the gunshots, also directed at the floor, which looks like plastic, tear it apart.*
>
> *At this point I see myself almost at the entrance to this room, and I see that under the opening in the floor there is another room, where there is a care room for these people who are dying.*
>
> *Then a small, wrinkled old woman arrives, like the ones in the mangas (which are a bit crazy cartoons in my opinion), moving with surprising agility, which scares me, and I retreat.*
>
> *Scene change.*
>
> *I find myself on an avenue where there are many restaurants; I was in one of them, with my parents and my current family.*
>
> *They are worried about making me eat vegetarian, as I am, because it seems that there is only barbecued stuff there.*
>
> *So they ask the waiter, who says that there is a dish suitable for me: a kind of risotto; however I see on top of the risotto like some telline (wedge clams).*
>
> *He reassures me that it's OK for me, but my family is worried.*
>
> *However, I trust the waiter, although he also seemed a bit shady, and I accept to eat the dish.*
>
> *I wake up.*

Again that suspended state emerges and lingers.

After a while, I feel that we can proceed to interpret the symbols that appear and the energetic dynamics of the dream, precisely because we do so from this suspended state.

T: Let us see the symbols that appear:

The opening of the dream is in a *room which could represent a room-world,* the psychic space; a wild party takes place there. There is the true risk that everything falls apart, and you are blown up.

That's why you worry.

P: Yes, it resonates with me; I remember that when I was young I went through such a psychological crisis that I was afraid of making "the big bang", to blow up. Then I got married, with this depressed husband, I found in my role as mother and wife a reassuring stability, and I took care of others, with my job. But this fear of breaking down inside remained, for example with my daughter, who I fear will explode.

T: The *youth identity crisis*, which occurred then, can often occur regardless of the conditions in which it occurs: we could also envision that great bang, as a beginning, a *glimpse* of awakening, which however leads to the crisis of what was there before: it proposes the psychological death, of the identity that was there before.

P: In fact, even with my husband it happened several times that we went into crisis, because of his problems; but I chose him again and again, knowing that he is a nice person, after all.

T: The choice of the depressed husband, however, was perhaps both for the good, *(the love between the two of you), but also* for the pathology he carried: this too you chose; and this speaks of you. It is not only your husband who does not change, you also don't.

Your daughter's labor also speaks of you, of what you had not fully explored at the time of the first crisis: perhaps the daughter experiences a painful crisis, which her mother also experienced.

Recognising the process in yourself would thus free the two of them from having to re-enact these dynamics to you, to be able to recognise them as projections, to see in the two of them a mirror.

Pause

Let us go on to interpret the dream:

In the dream the *massacre* does not seem so bad: you are in and out of the situation.

On the one hand all this happens *to* the main character, whom you believes yourself to be, while dreaming; but all this happens, at the same time, *in you*-consciousness, in the dreamer.

From the waking point of view, she become aware of the dynamics, you do not just live and act them; you can then see them, process them, integrate them.

Thus, you are outside and inside; she stand *on the threshold,* as in the dream.

We see other aspects and symbols in the dream: *the little old woman, disturbing and agile*, could correspond to your madness and wisdom, to your strength, of which you are afraid; an ancient force, still active and present, the same force that gripped her then, and grips her daughter now.

She could represent for these symbolic aspects your archetypal feminine *energy*, *the activated Kundalini energy*, which wreaks havoc but also takes care of everything, and which is transpersonal. It is *in general* the driving force behind all movement and transformation of the dream and psyche, thus also of the firing, and of the opening of the floor and consciousness. *Specifically*, in the continuation of the dream, you find yourself for example eating: this can represent the growth of nutritive energy, and also stands for psychotherapy.

P: Yes; you should know that I had become vegetarian at the time of that initial crisis, because I saw that it helped me to feel better, not to have that "big bang"; however, in the dream, I remember that I was no longer rigid about it.

T: Yes, but now perhaps it's time to go through that crisis, rather than only contain it, because it's still happening and it's already happening; but it's happening, now you see it well, within your consciousness; and happens imbalance outside, without noise, because you, today, can handle it.

You can handle it because you are experiencing that you remain the same and centered in the void. This remaining in the steady state of pure consciousness and energy balance also happens more and more often during the sessions, and in your everyday life.

In the dream, in fact, it appears that you basically accept, trust the state; this is an important point, there is a change in your attitude towards the crisis.

It seems that you are now ready to go through, or at least begin to go through.

In the past, though, you were following the policy of control, so as not to be sick, remaining in the egoic separation.

12.4.14 Reflections on dreams

The first part of the session is generally dedicated to working on the present, and how one can relate those recent events reflect into the session. This is also true when we discuss about the more distant past, e.g., childhood.

We always try, however, *to leave some space for the interpretation of any dreams*, where we can often clearly see how it correlates with previous dreams and with the dynamics we uncovered in the first part of the session, as these are "transferred" into the field and interact with it.

Let us now look at some characteristics of dream interpretation in a TP key.

The dream work does not consist only in a psychological, mental, academic interpretation of symbols and explanations, but continues the alchemical work begun and active in the first part of the session. Dreams can be analyzed in a literal, symbolic, and anagogic key.

1. Literal

We can observe how in this session the symbols are associated with the patient's biographical events; in this I accept their *literal meaning*.

In the dream in question, for example, the figure of the daughter or the husband, at the restaurant, is interpreted "at the level of the object," as it really represents the real person who appears in the dream; this has its own importance, as it gives us deeper insights into these people in the patient's world of relationships.

2. Symbolic

The dream contents are examined in their symbolic aspect, as identity self-representations of the patient's psychological world; the figures that appear are interpreted "at the level of the subject," i.e. as parts of the patient's Self, i.e. as parts of the patient's Self.

We analyze the resistance and suffering generated by the rigid identification with these roles, observing how they manifest themselves in the dream material.

All this helps the patient to become aware of her inner thater, of the identity game with which she identifies.

For example, we will look at how her roles (as a wife, mother, daughter, therapist) manipulate her inner world. We examine what use she makes of these roles, what facilitating or resisting actions they enact.

3. Anagogical

All this psychological work is helpful in introducing, highlighting and supporting the *anagogic* interpretation of dream contents.

By this term[37] I mean a level that is operative in the present of the session, since it concerns the alchemical process itself.

Here we try to focus on the *here-and-now* of the session. We interpret the symbols as "photographs" of the here-and-now state of the relationship between the ego and the unconscious, in line with the Jungian perspective, and of the condition of the *Chakras* and energy channels and their blockages, symbolized in different ways in the dream material. From this perspective, archetypal figures (e.g., that of the "special woman") can be read as active transforming powerful energies (*Kundalini*) that guide the resolution of crises.

This level of interpretation fosters awareness of how these energies operate, of their wisdom, and of how to accompany them, - of what the process requires at that moment, - instead of reassuringly confirming the patient's ego. One thus gains access to a form of seeing, that is, one becomes aware of where, when, how, and in what forms phenomena occur that bear witness to this process, recognizing the symbols as the best expression at that moment of the ongoing process.[38]

This is precisely the most transformative aspect of dream analysis in my opinion, the entering into the true life of the symbol, in its operating transformations and allowing oneself to be transformed; this is what makes this practice useful. One can thus see how even in the world of the dream one can find the same truth we uncovered working on conscious material.

The dream material is dynamically correlated with *three elements: the events of the week analyzed in the first part of the session, the energetic perceptions in the Chakras that emerged during the listening, and the transferential-counter transferential processes active in the relational field.*

This integration is not a mere theoretical exercise: the interpretation concretely continues the alchemical work begun in the listening of the *Chakras*, facilitating the awareness of energy dynamics, the integration of psychological resistances, and the regulation of the transformative "fire regime."

An *active neutrality* is maintained, under which the therapist conveys an *implicit teaching,* about how to "attune to" the transformation, on how to recognize its intrinsic intelligence. This approach transforms the dream from an object of analysis into an active partner in the therapeutic process.

What is most interesting is to show and make the patient aware of the awakening of consciousness, rather than the energetic-affective and dynamic aspects that are symbolically expressed in the dream.

The dream material lends itself very well to the psychological work of co-operating with the process of awakening, since from the dream, which is only one of the states of consciousness, we naturally and repeatedly awaken each day into wakefulness.

There is a physiological step between the dream state of consciousness and the waking state of consciousness, which is precisely waking from the dream.

The dream functions as a privileged observatory of the awakening of consciousness: the physiological transition from sleep to wakefulness becomes a model for recognizing the transition to pure consciousness. The continuity between waking and dreaming dynamics reveals the unity of the transformative process, which can be observed from multiple temporal perspectives – biographical, dream and soul.

12.4.15 Reflections on the dream in the session

Entering now into the specifics of the dream reported in the session, let us consider the symbols that appear.

The scene opens with a room; this could represent the space of consciousness, a room-world. Here, there are so many people, they can be interpreted at the level of the subject, as so many parts of the Self, and their association in a party or event indicate an activation, (so much energy converging, expressing a force in activation). Shortly afterwards, in fact, its expression is seen in the explosion of this force.

The massacre that follows has to do with the collapse of the internal world, of identity construction; and this happens in the present, because the time is ripe, thus it should not be interpreted psycho genetically.

One can see here, in how I proceed in my interpretation, how important it is to clarify what the patient is identified with, from what point of view they are looking:

- *From the point of view of the individual ego*, i.e. the character who undergoes death-rebirth, in its various phases, the transformative process is often ego dystonic; this is why we have that little voice in the head (we all know that little voice well) that says that things are not right, that they are not as they should be, that it would be better if they did not happen.

The patient could interpret the dream from this point of view by saying that it is a bad dream, a nightmare, because dangerous things happen (actually, for ego and its defenses).

- *On the other hand, from the point of view of the Self,* which awakens and evolves, the dream acquires another perspective meaning in view of a transformation; this key seems to explain more and better the events that occurred, and in this sense can be considered more valid. In this vision, death should be understood symbolically as the end of a psychological self representation; this can be endured and accepted with the awareness that it is not only happening to the character, but also in the space of consciousness, which is therefore able to contain and support it.

The prosecution of the shows, this interpretation is correct, as does the ability of the patient, once awakened, to elaborate and integrate the dream.

- *In this sense therefore are interpreted the protagonist's participation and non-participation, her standing on the threshold, and opening of the underlying therapeutic space.*

As one can easily observe, in the interpretation I give in the session there is no attempt to refer it to past personal traumatic experiences, or external present events. Moreover, I do not express compassion or solidarity for the difficulties the protagonist encounters in the dream.

Although, as a person, I empathize with the patient, I am nonetheless aware that the drama portrayed in the dream is describing the modes and phases of a transformation process, of death and rebirth. This drama is therefore not understood as a tragedy but viewed in a positive light; nor, for that matter, does the patient appear overly disturbed by the drama in which she takes part.

The fact that the dream recounts facts must be considered, in this view, as the best possible visible translation into symbols of the mysterious invisible underlying process; it is taken as the spontaneous phenomenological expression of the process underway, to be accepted even in the midst of a thousand difficulties that the consciousness encounters and represents. *What is happening in the dream is what must happen*, and our task is to help as best we can, not to judge or oppose or avoid.[39] The interpretative attention goes to the anagogic, energetic, and transformative, healing meaning: the crisis is seen as the beginning of a healing.

This basic position helps the patient to observe what is happening with another eye, and indicates, teaches a method, a way, to go through her crisis.

It shows in practice how to go along with the transformation of the caterpillar into a butterfly (while understanding and accepting that this is a misfortune for the caterpillar), how to "die and be reborn" really.

- In this sense also *the special woman who arrives*, ancient and agile, mad and wise, disturbing, because she is endowed with superpowers, can represent the activating and resolving feminine energy which brings the dream to a turning point; the whole movement of energy represented in the dream and also personified by this female figure could be said to represent the activated *Kundalini*, the Shakti which makes people gather, shots explode, kill, and heal everyone, the force capable of opening separating floors.

All this is seen and integrated by the patient who in fact moves literally to a true threshold of consciousness in order to "see":

As the account of the session shows, the transformative alchemy expressed in the dream's symbolic material mirrors that of the first part of the session.

Thus, after having interpreted the dream, I observe and interpret how there is no solution of continuity between waking and dream dynamics; when seen together they help us to see even more clearly the process underway and how it troubles us.

Specifically, I point out to the patient how the events of her daily life are aligned with the dream dynamics; furthermore, these energies, their flow or impediment, emerge and can be felt *in the corresponding Chakras.*

The dream thus helps us to see the same thing from another point of view: we find in it again the process of transformation, this time from another point of view, in another time, that of the soul.

12.4.16 Conclusion of the session

We continue the story of the session, which comes to a close harmonizing on a plane of clear consciousness and inner calm. It is reconnection that brings strength and calm: *union is strength, and calm is the virtue of the strong.*

Silence: openness stability, peace.

P: Yes, I resonate with this interpretation, and also with this method of psychotherapy, which I had not encountered before; I like it. And I feel better, and supported in this difficult period.

The session is ending, the heart and the energy are now open; I feel that some thoughts of doubt are passing, or that the rethinking itself of some points of the session involve small variations in the energy flow in her Chakras; however, I sense that they are not of great magnitude and importance, they are transitory. I decide not to mention it for now; we will return to it later.

T: Well, we'll stop here; see you next week.

We leave each other in this silence that has already emerged and been recognised several times during the session; a pause at the center of the movement, in which one stops, listens; there is openness, the mind is silent, one just lives.

And this can be felt, and can be seen: in fact, as I look at her on the computer screen, I am struck by the slow circular motion of the fan blades in her room, reflected in the glass just above her head, which had been there all along, though I had not yet noticed it.

Above her seventh Chakra that regular, indifferent, undisturbed motion, seems to correspond to my –our –feeling that this perception expresses the final outcome of the process: of moving and not moving, of her being centered and open.

P: She smiles, greets with joined hands.

I close Skype, she disappears from the screen

12.4.17 Follow-up

Let us now briefly report some follow-up considerations,[40] referring to the *developments* in the two sessions following the one described here.[41]

12.4.17.1 Follow-up one week later

"I was calmer this week, as if I saw things a little less involved, participating but without manipulating, pushing and pulling, to make things go the way I want them to. I felt more at peace, and I saw and understood more things, I don't know how to explain it, it was like I saw more of my own and others' dynamics, like I had a key to understand.

I followed things a little bit as they come, without saying they were good or bad; I have the impression that I have to go *a little slow*, without saying too much "*what I want is this*" ... When things happen I try to just listen.

I feel more relaxed than last time: always the stomach that sometimes makes that knot, and I try to breathe, to stop, and I try not to do anything, not to follow the thoughts, which then I can't control; I feel less at odds with what is around me.

What do I feel at this moment? ... as if there was ... a kind of flat sea, I don't feel movement. But maybe I wasn't listening deeply enough.

Actually, I notice that when we have crises in the family I am able to let it go *sooner; and at the same time, in the family too, they stop the fighting sooner.*

I feel that I have more fully accepted what is there, that I am learning not to run away.

Even with my husband I've noticed that this week I've reacted differently; for example, this morning he had made a commitment and then he didn't fulfil it, and once I would have reacted a lot, I would have made him pay for it, and instead this time I just did it, without a lot of fuss, without reacting too much, I have come to terms with it.

... I realized that it's not so much a matter of letting go but of having a broader view of what's in front of you, while before you could only see one perspective, and maybe you get stubborn ... maybe I have been very self-centred, always wanting to be the one in control of everything ... sometimes I look at myself from the outside, almost as if in a mirror..."

One can see how the patient continued the work of the session in the following days, practising and learning from the experience of this new approach.

She reacts less, sees more deeply in herself and in others, listens to the energy.

12.4.17.2 Follow-up two weeks later

"How do I feel? I feel a particular sensation in the pit of my stomach, like a flickering, a burning sensation, but a pleasant one; perhaps because I felt a little ready for this meeting; because it gives me pleasure, I feel pleasure in short, to confront, to talk.

This week some things have happened that could have worried me; but in fact I have begun to feel what we do in the session, to feel the sensations in the body (when you tell me to pay attention to the Chakras), and it's also beginning to happen automatically for me during the day, when I'm faced with a situation that's a bit challenging, or that could worry me.

This work on relaxing, breathing, calming the mind, is triggering me more automatically. For example, yesterday I had a difficult family situation, but I kept calm, I spoke calmly, and instinctively said and did the right things, and everything took the direction it was supposed to take without letting myself get caught up in anxiety about what comes next, in doubts about whether I was doing things right. I did what felt most humanly right to do, because I had managed not to go, as I did before, into opposition or helplessness, or doubt or judgement. I didn't feel as agitated as the other times.

After the last time I came out of the session, I was thinking about it, *I seem to dwell less on my thoughts;* even if something happens to me, even if it's important, even if I think about it. And I process it between head and heart, *only the sensation remains*, it happens that, if you then ask me about it, *I no longer remember it. Whereas before, my brain was always working, and it would linger a lot on certain situations that filled my head, and almost blocked any other sensation, even pleasant ones throughout the day*: because there was always this thing that stayed there.

-*It seems to me as if I do not remember things*: which is strange for me, since I have always had a constant memory of details; now I don't remember them. It's a bit of a strange feeling for me, that since childhood I was very attached to my thoughts, and now I'm a bit like in dementia.

The passage of time also seems different to me these days; I plan because I have to plan, and of course I do it, but I do not have that heavy feeling. It is more that I do things as and when I have to do them. With my husband as well, two situations of conflict came up, but I 'moved beyond' them: I did not take it all that badly, I just said what I had to say and that was.

I feel that while we are talking we are also partly in another space ... that's the feeling I had at the beginning! ... it seems from this experience that I no longer remain attached to things.

I am hopeful, I am a little afraid, but I feel that life is moving towards something greater ..."

This second follow-up also shows that the patient is rapidly making the working method her own, and finds it satisfying, applies it creatively, and her maturation is evident in the session in both her energetic and her consciousness state.

12.5 Characteristics of TPPT

Having now examined the method as it is used in the session, we can return, as previously planned, to some further general considerations on PTT psychotherapies.

12.5.1 Aims of TPPT

We can state that the ultimate aim of therapy is to help, to cure, to go beyond suffering.

But since suffering derives from the fundamental separation from being, from origin, here *therapy's ultimate aim is to heal this disconnection*, this separation.

That is why *cure means yoga*, i.e. reconnection, reconnection of the current in the *Chakras*, baptism into the inner river, which restores life.

The aim of all therapeutic work is to rediscover happiness: that is, a state of non-contrast and free internal flow of energy: a state free of the me, not a liberation of the me.

The ultimate goal of therapy is, to help the person return to their Earthly Paradise, where everything flows without more friction, without more opposition.

To summarize: the most important aim in therapy is:

1. To *cure* means to bring back the person to a state of well-being, of peace, of joy, of serenity, in which they can feel active yet calm, without causing harm (*primum non nocere is a basic rule in therapy*). To cure means to take care, thus to get the patient to take care of *themselves*.[42]
2. *To offer clinical tools to the patient to make them autonomous*

   Once transmitted and experienced, the technique of internal relaxation *can be practised independently* by the patient, without risk, as a tool for rebalancing and returning to inner stillness, to a greater connection with one's own deep perceptive dimension.[43]

The consequence is a rediscovery of inner circulation, a sense of relaxation and a calming of the mind, a resting in being

3. *To provide theoretical tools, taken from tradition and the modern world*, as a background against which to place the clinical experiences that are made and repeated in clinical observation. It offers a different perspective on psychology, psychopathology and treatment, proposing an alternative theory of mental functioning.
4. *Learn about the connection between energy and the mind*: see the link between *energy and consciousness* and the *psyche*, that is, all mental phenomena, thus understanding how and why hey are generated, interact, transform.

   The patient can in this way reconnect, recognize, understand in a new way psychic life, made of dreams, transference, interpersonal relations, because they understand the dance of energy in consciousness. This will foster a different view of all *psychic phenomena.*[44] For example, the patient can more easily see the connection between certain sudden thoughts of death and a condition of spontaneous or provoked energetic activation.[45]
5. *Liberation from the limits of a psychocentric view* to open up to a spiritual, consciousness-centred view. Through inner, direct listening, the patient becomes aware of mind's illusions (the mind lies!) but also of its cooperation in liberation. The symbols and their transformations, the director and the actor, are now seen, explained. When one understands mind's strategies and prison, the way opens to go beyond.

12.5.2 Reactions

Three possible reactions to the evolutionary process can be observed:

1. **Rejection:** *opposition to* the loss of identity and the rebirth process, with the development of symptoms of resistance, flight or control. In the identity crisis, the *ego-dystonic attitude* contributes largely to suffering, paving the way to the most severe psychiatric conditions.

   I am reminded of dreams of patients in which people are faceless, or the subjects themselves are, indicating this loss of the identity of the other or of oneself. When waking up from such a dream is not acceptable for the conscious personality, anguish arises out of resistance.

   A similar process, in a less pronounced form, is when the dreamer loses a loved one, and feels lost themselves, or does not find their documents, their bag, his mobile, or their car, etc. Negative reactions basically emerge from impraparedness of the ego to let go of himself.

2. **Ambivalence:** we have here *acceptance and resistance* together, with rationalization and psychologization.

   In the patient there is an unconscious conflict about identity loss: to disappear or not to disappear; to be or not to be, that is the dilemma.

   A transpersonal therapy should take into account the fear of the ego but also the emergence of awakening, preparing the patient to relocate the process in a larger, impersonal space of consciousness, in the consciousness of the Self.

   Most traditional psychotherapies welcome the ego's request not to succumb, as the ultimate goal of help, and not only as a competing and temporary phase necessary to support the ego during its dissolution, to help it die in peace.

   TPPTs, by contrast, help the patient to recognize the states of expansion, even ecstasy at times, or peace, that pertain to a larger and impersonal space of consciousness, which supports and contains the transformation.

3. **Acceptance**: in other cases, finally, it seems that *the experience can be welcomed*: *the patient* clearly *feels* that this whole process is happening for the greater good, that it will end well after all. The patient knows that it is not tragedy after all, but something incomprehensible that can nevertheless be accepted: in spite of all the suffering there is trust, in the unknown, in our deepest nature.

   In this case, the condition is less ego-dystonic, and with the passage of time it may even become *ego-syntonic*, even being perceived as a blessing, a grace, a path to a happy ending; even if one must first cross the desert, pass though a psychological death.

   Not much psychotherapy is needed here; sometimes healing happens gradually, sometimes suddenly, like an enlightenment: sometimes because of an indication, like a Koan, a: "Aha! I saw! I have understood," liberation.

12.5.3 Duration

The duration of therapy depends on the ego's reactions to change.

Some patients since the beginning report an *immediate beneficial effect*: at the end of the session they feel lighter, with a clearer mind, less depressed, anxious, or confused. The effect is similar to that of an effective medication, offering temporary relief and a sense of renewal.

The stability of these results over time, though, more complex and varies from person to person, as in the Gospel parable of the sower: the therapy takes root according to individual predisposition. However, *significant progress is observed over time*: the patient enters the therapeutic state more quickly, reaches greater depth and develops a better associative flow during the session.

In the long term, the state of wellbeing is prolonged, and the patient becomes more active in bringing this awareness into daily life, spreading a transformed energy. This does not generally generate emotional detachment, rather a *greater capacity to participate, understand, and love.* The process, if understood and integrated, leads to *stable and lasting change*, as confirmed by feedback received years later.

How much time, then, is needed for a TP psychotherapy? Time is needed for:

- *Time needed to transmit the method,* so that the patient can make it their own: experience it, understand it, internalize it and begin to apply it.

  We can be satisfied when the message gets through, when the seed is planted, and the patient dedicates themselves to cultivating it, because this will be of great help to them on their journey.
- *Time to metabolize* what has been received: time to *welcome, understand, activate, accompany, support, and make* the individuative evolution *blossom.*

  There is a time for everything. The success and end of a TP therapy depends on the patient's openness to cooperating with the ongoing spiritual process, and the deep understanding of the path, not on an abstract time factor.

  Besides, Time is a "natural" *factor:* it *takes as long as it* takes, i.e., the *time* needed to bring about and especially stabilize this new state of awareness.
- In the end, depending on the case, it will take a *variable amount* of time *to stabilize the patient's autonomous capacity to proceed*, the new condition of consciousness.[46]

Finally, *Time depends mainly* on the *patient's capacity*, i.e., on the *level of consciousness* of both the patient, and, of course, of the therapist.

TP therapies can be very short, in those clinical situations that are already ready to evolve; here one could see a very rapid healing process, as in the reported session; they are "*very short therapies.*"

However, for those patients who are still far from this awareness, less ready to see the essence of what is being proposed, *it may take more time to tune in.* The patient will then need time to experience in the sessions and repeatedly see in detail the practical demonstration of this operating, traversing, transforming; patients will have to take their own time (and not follow ours) to recognize and integrate the clinical material into the session.

Let us not forget that therapy and the process of healing from suffering are in place from *the very beginning*, even before the first meeting, in the energies leading up to that meeting, and certainly already in the first phone call.

It is in place from when the patient is sick, and from their call for help.[47]

Since the opening of "crisis and cure," a battlefield in consciousness and therapy has been activated, a field of confrontation and growth, a *therapeutic field*, an alchemical pot.

It is this field, non-dual, that transcends division, that sustains and is therapy, that *underlies*, that "lies beneath" transmission, transmutation.

Therapy, on the one hand, is always present, at the beginning, during, and at the end of the sessions, it has *no duration*; and yet, it unfolds gradually amidst obstacles, victories, dialogue, the gradual unfolding over time, until healing. and needs the right time to develop and complete.

This changes the approach to the time factor: therapy happens in "real time,": only in the present changes occur in the subtle system, energy starts flowing again, the system opens up and relaxes, and more light passes through.

12.5.4 Outcomes of TPPT

As time goes by, patients increasingly succeed in *tuning* into the therapeutic field, to enter it and stay there, and to deepen the healing state of consciousness of the egoic symptomatology. The patient *maintains* states of wellbeing for longer periods, becomes more active in daily life, more aware and centered, moving around with a different energy. The patient acquires greater detachment (not indifference), with an increasing capacity to participate, love, and understand. In the long term, all this leads to a stable inner and outer evolution.

Let's look at some clinical examples of this condition of openness and positive energy stability, in session or in dreams:

> In sessions:
> "Normally in the sessions I feel very good, it is difficult to explain; previously, I wasn't aware of the condition of the body, how I feel; I wasn't not aware of the parts, it is as if I had a form but not well defined. Today, however, I felt everything, I was very lucid, my mind was free and quiet but different from usual: not light and floating, but crystal clear."

Dreams:
"I knew I was dreaming in the dream, I could see my body suspended in the dark, but he was illuminated, as if he had a light around him, and was suspended in the air; the sensation of well-being was greater than the one we experiment during the relaxation we usually do in the session, the peak had been exceeded, I was not as light-headed as usual, but I was aware of the whole body, and the mind was free."

"I was sleeping and I was relaxed, as in the session; at a certain point someone took me and made me sink deeper, as if into a deeper, softer bed; and I was also sinking into a much deeper wellbeing, I couldn't understand how I could feel so good; and I felt at the same time a presence in the room, as of a non-material, non-human being, who was like this wellbeing, that is, cuddling me, protecting me."

12.5.4.1 Negative transference

Some people, while experiencing benefits, do not choose deeply to follow the path of relaxation and change, withdrawing from out-of-session work or even discontinuing therapy. The speed and effectiveness of the method can discourage those who are anchored in an inner life of resistance and control. Even when the opportunity presents itself, the patient might choose not to take it.

Certain pathologies may not be suitable for using this approach.

This method seems more suitable for people who are already quite advanced and healthy, who have perhaps already done traditional analyses and are familiar with the ego's defense mechanisms.

A careful anamnesis and assessment are always therefore necessary to evaluate prognosis and choose the best treatment for each and every patient. Not all patients can undertake this type of therapy.

Clinical Examples of Negative Reactions

Case No. 1: Patient I have been seeing for a long time, and who takes steps forward and backward, although less intense and frequent than before: in a moment of despair she accuses me of deceiving her by telling her that it was possible to change, when in fact she so often seems to be at the same point as before, if not going backwards.

My reflections: Perhaps the deception does not come from me, however, but from her not being sincerely firm in not going back, and for this not taking responsibility she blames the outside.

Case No 2: "I want to stop therapy because after almost a year I don't agree with your harshness. I don't discuss your method but to me it creates discomfort and not improvement. I don't believe in the energy-only Kundalini method... I don't see results. I'll stop this Chakra Kundalini bioenergetic therapy. ... I would not have approached a psychiatrist and psychotherapist like you if I had only known... Your behavior, besides violating deontology, is a narcissistic act of a healing guru who only knows how to punish and shut up. You deceived me and above all took advantage of my weakness and fragility."

Reflections of my own: The patient had started to persecute me with numerous messages for every problem he had, requesting psychological or pharmacological assistance for any small problem and malaise. In the past, he had manifested explosive outbursts of anger, states of bipolarism not well diagnosed and defined, psychopathic, obsessive aspects, resistant and marked insomnia, problems with family members. A typical feature of these negative reactions is that the ego attributes a harmful intention to the therapist, when in fact it is the ego itself that refuses to cooperate, attacks, and cannot tolerate not being supported.

Case No. 3: Patient who had been suffering from panic attacks for some time; recently, they were more frequent and intense, probably also sustained by the active season (spring).

I proposed drug therapy, which she refused, wanting to resolve things with psychotherapy alone. So we started sessions with TP approach, that rapidly immediately had a positive effect: there was good understanding, trust, and a good response of the unconscious; she was better, experienced states of peace in the midst of her torment, and she was pleased about it.

One day, however, without warning, she did not come to the appointment.

When I called her back she told me in a very resentful tone that she was very angry with me, that I was an irresponsible doctor because I had put her in touch with things and at times that were not suitable for her, that I had made her feel very bad after the last session and that she wouldn't come again.

Of course I felt sorry because she had been ill, but it struck me because I had not expected such a marked reaction; in fact, from my point of view, she was beginning to unblock the energy and experience the positive stages that follow.

However, on deeper reflection, this could have been the point: the negative transference reaction was precisely because things were moving towards a resolution, but the patient had not made the choice to heal. Healing included the choice to heal, to recognize the fundamental error: that is, to take as true what the reactive mind was saying, namely that this therapy was hurting her (the mind). It was precisely the egoic reaction that had considered rather dangerous, negative, this opening and unblocking of life energy we witnessed. Or, as Jung put it, what is a medicine for one patient, may be a poison for another. So she had projected all these negative feelings onto me, holding me responsible for all this malaise of hers that stemmed instead from her resistance to proceed in that way at that time.

12.5.5 Difference with traditional interventions

The TP view of mental illness departs radically from the *organicist biomedical model*, which sees the cause in the brain and biochemistry. However, psychiatric pharmacological intervention is recognized as important for crisis containment and the management of specific symptoms.

It also differs from *psychogenetic orientations*, which look for the cause in childhood relationships or society (exogenous).

It also differs *from shamanism and magic*, where the egoic, masculine, active component attributes the merit of change to its own male will, to its own action, albeit with varying degrees of collaboration with natural laws.

In the method we are going to describe, on the other hand, the personal will is completely secondary, and subordinate to cooperation in the process itself; here it is rather a matter of a more feminine, receptive attitude, rather like the Socratic, obstetrical attitude of helping to emerge what already wants to be born.

Finally, this is not a *method of suggestion*, in which one might see changes, which might however be *ephemeral*; in the method we describe here, on the contrary, the main point is to make the change stable. This is possible because the ability to ride the process becomes a *stable* and natural part of the new way of being, based on awareness.[48]

12.6 Training of TP therapists

It will be clear by now that a transpersonal therapist will have to be a different therapist, and this requires a *different professional training* from the traditional figures: they need to be a medical doctor, a psychotherapist, as well as a guide to navigate in non-ordinary states of consciousness.

The training of a therapist, in general, requires a lot of time, study commitment, extensive clinical practice, and a substantial investment by a civilized society. For the training of a TP therapist this is even more true, although in this case the cost falls mainly on the shoulders of the therapist themselves.

Let's take a closer look at the requirements of a TP therapist.

There are conditions before, during and after, that overlap over time.

12.6.1 Motivation

The basic prerequisite for any helping profession is a *starting disposition, a motivated choice, and a vocation.*

Personal qualities that lean towards a "helping profession", ego stability, and qualities like sensitivity, and intelligence should be present.[49] The person should also be quite "healthy" (a concept that goes far beyond the lack of psychiatric pathologies).[50]

The decision, the choice to devote oneself to this type of helping profession should be *matured and conscious*; in fact, it is not enough to have inclination, one must also consciously choose to take on this type of life.

However, the selection that introduces to these training courses (first of all in the case of the traditional degree course, medicine or psychology, but then also for specialization courses in a specific psychotherapy specialization) should in my opinion be based in the first place on the student's motivation, willingness, and ability to love and understand one's neighbor. Motivation to do this job should be a fundamental prerequisite, and evaluation of the candidates should include the level of maturity and sanity, and their developmental level.

The selection, moreover, should take place spontaneously, in the inner recognition of this calling: one *self-applies* for this "impossible profession". In a way, one is "born a therapist", but this gift then has to be recognised and accepted, and one "becomes a therapist" by learning the work through dedicated, specific training.

This job requires a passion, a fire of dedication, a spirit of service capable of sustaining the often long and difficult process of training; it will be this passion that will drive the next inner and outer steps, enabling him to devote themselves to their work, having put their ego aside.

12.6.2 Traditional routes

An academic education will always be necessary to acquire the specific culture of the field (medicine, psychology, nursing, etc.).

A long and difficult course of study is also a test of intellectual maturity and forces one to develop a solid traditional education.

Traditional university knowledge specific to the field must be acquired, such as knowledge of ego structure, defense mechanisms, transference and counter-transference, family and group dynamics.

In my opinion, the therapist should have a much more solid and critical preparation in the *social side of psychology*, i.e. on conditioning, history, and geopolitics. These training aspects should be included in university training programs, for they are as essential as knowledge of the mind for learning and working in this field.

The therapist must then be trained in *some school of psychotherapy* that provides theoretical and clinical preparation in a specific orientation, so as to be able to work with competence and creativity for the benefit of the patient. These training programs come in many types and levels, but almost always include at least three or more years of theoretical training, and often but not always, some form of supervised clinical practice and/or personal experience in that same clinical orientation.[51]

12.6.3 Other paths

The roads to becoming a psychiatrist or psychologist can be *disappointing and frustratingly incomplete.*

To complete their training, a TP therapist must open up to a *broader cultural and human enrichment, to additional forms of knowledge and experience* that complement *academic training.*

In their specific training, a TP therapist must develop *other areas of experience, not only academic*, in order to become a complete person and work with altered states of consciousness, as well as prepare to go through themselves.

They should also have had experience in *the personal maturational area*, regarding intimate relationships, child-rearing, friendships.

I am referring to *inner work through different avenues*, such as several years of deep analytic work in order to see one's personal issues clearly, or through other paths, such as *family constellations*, with *body-oriented techniques*, etc.

In order to broaden their human psychic and spiritual capacities, it would be advisable for the TP therapist to venture and travel through the territories *of Meditation,* in which they should sustain a *constant practice.*

They should be curious and willing to delve into *Astrology,* preferably Vedic, in its spiritual and liberating form.

They should have an interest or, better, some reale involvement in *the arts,* know at least a little *about alternative medicine.*

For example, it would be helpful if they had some *experience* with *martial arts*, had *travelled extensively* and had studied many *languages.*

In all these areas *the person who will then venture, let us say, in deep waters should have already traveled a long way, should have a curriculum that cannot be prescribed and cannot be predicted,* since they will be required to go beyond the ordinary level of consciousness.

12.6.4 Awakening experience

However, *all* this will *still* not be enough: *everything has yet to begin.*

The therapist will necessarily have to go *through an initiation into the non-ordinary states of consciousness* that they will have to deal with, and that no external training can ever provide.

A TP therapist should possess a truly transpersonal vision and experience of their own: having experienced NOSCs themselves, they really know what they are about. They will have to have encountered to some extent the experience of awakening: (at least a *glimpse* of it), of opening the roof of the house, and at least some deconstruction.[52]

And they will also then have to have sufficiently *integrated* this into the new condition of consciousness.[53]

Having navigated this experience will constitute an essential foundation of their qualification, the only one truly able to guarantee the depth of their work, the level of depth they have reached, and the extent of its integration.

The transpersonal therapist should therefore *know their own* "madness." They should have known "death" and "wounding": only the wounded doctor heals.

They should have gone at least a little bit into madness, but not too much: they should be a "sane madman."

However, having had a crisis does not mean that they have overcome it. They must re-emerge from their initiation an expert in these "things of the other world," but also capable of moving well in "this world," balanced and able to love and understand. Only those who have truly passed through their own hell will be able to lead someone else there.[54] Only someone who has gone through their own crisis and come out of it with a new state of consciousness will be able to act as a guide.

This therapist will and can be a guide, a Virgil through the stormy journey of transformation, aware of what is happening in consciousness and energy.

12.6.5 Purification practice

Awakening in the therapist requires an integration that passes through a gradual transformation of their individual consciousness, an illumination of every internal and external aspect.

This will be possible if one goes along with an overall, progressive rectification through a progressive *purification process,* as described in the Divine Comedy, so as to allow the consciousness to truly go beyond egoic identification.

At this point, the motivation of such a therapist will no longer be based (as it was before the awakening) on personal motivation, however evolved and healthy. Motivation will become in this purification and maturation a "motivation-beyond-motivation," a force beyond personal good will.

Individual motivation will have to mature in the fire of the great change.

The training of the TP therapist matures over the years, thanks mainly to the patients.

One learns to live by living, and one learns to be a psychotherapist by practising psychotherapy. Clinical work is fundamental for the therapist's purification, for learning humility, love, for becoming familiar with suffering.

Many take side paths or stop along the way. The therapist's *resistances* may express themselves in *rationalizing or projecting* the crisis outwards.

One may want to take care of others to avoid facing one's own identity "identity death"; anyone engaged in this work should be aware of this.

These are sometimes forms of resistance with respect to death, madness, disappearance, that every human being knows; however, in the case of a TP therapist, these can be dressed up in much more sophisticated strategies.

You may know the joke where a psychiatrist meets another psychiatrist and says

"*Hi! You're fine, how am I doing?*"

We laugh it off, but behind the psychiatrist's identity, there is often a sense of the very madness, which we sometimes try to cure in others.

From what has been said so far, it might seem that the qualifications for good training are indeed many, perhaps too many; only a few could really claim to possess them.

And yet, it is not necessary to be a genius or a saint, or a rare exception: even *without being a spiritual master*, *one can acquire mastery* by awakening the awareness of transpersonal consciousness embodied in everyday life and within ourselves.

Today many patients are going through partial awakenings, and new therapists, though still imperfect, could perfectly well dedicate themselves to helping them, because they know this path at least in part.

Many of them walked this road of death and rebirth themselves, and because of this they can help others.

Some degree of realisation is nevertheless required: one cannot teach others to fly without ever having done so. Psychiatrists and psychologists who are dissatisfied with traditional training because it is limited and limiting, can move towards the new figure of TP therapist precisely by working closely with and in dialogue with these attempts at evolution on the part of their bolder colleagues.

The fundamental condition for flying are the "*wings of great longing*": the availability and inner capacity that arise in the heart of those who are willing to help cross that territory and accompany the patient in their transformation.

Notes

1 *Care* refers to global and responsible attention to the person, embracing every aspect of well-being. *Therapy* is a more circumscribed clinical process, intended for the diagnosis and treatment (medical or psychological) of a specific condition, carried out by personnel qualified for this. Treatment goes beyond therapy, including the dimension of relationship, daily support, listening, and continuous presence.
2 We will not go into detail here on the types of drugs used, the doses, and the time of the therapies. We will only mention here that they are intended to symptomatically medicate mood in affective disorders, thought disorders in psychosis, or sleep disorders and anxiety, which are transversal to the various syndromic pictures.
3 In the UK, clinical and counseling psychologists (and psychiatrists) are fully regulated professions with protected titles and mandatory registration. Counselors and psychotherapists instead rely on voluntary registers (such as BACP and UKCP), which set training and ethical standards but do not have statutory power. In the *United States*, psychotherapy is delivered by several licensed professions (clinical psychologists, psychiatrists, social workers, counselors and others), each with its own long doctoral or medical-specialty pathway. *In Russia*, psychotherapy has traditionally been the domain of psychiatrists, who pursue additional and only partly standardised psychotherapy training, while clinical psychologists are emerging mainly as "medical psychologists" within health services. *In China*, the profession of psychotherapist is still consolidating: most psychotherapy in hospitals is provided by psychiatrists, and psychologists work mainly in urban specialist and university settings, with training programmes and licensing criteria that are not yet unified nationwide.
4 IBP is a psycho-body integration technique developed in the United States by Jack Lee Rosenberg. It is a holistic therapeutic approach that aims to integrate mind, body, emotions, and spirit.
5 Generally, patients come on a weekly basis; this rhythm can become fortnightly after a short time; rarely are single sessions involved. We usually meet for months or sometimes a few years (two, or three generally), for sessions of about 50 minutes.
6 It will be up to the art of the therapist to see "how and when and how much" to introduce these techniques into the session, so that these interventions are important contributions and not interventions dissociated from the background work described above (i.e., analyzing the therapeutic relationship, dreams, or otherwise).
7 There is a saying in medicine that "you cannot overcome nature if you are not with nature."
8 Jesus says "For where two or three are gathered in my name, there am I in the midst of them" (Matthew 18:20).
9 For Jung, the archetypes of the collective unconscious give form to transpersonal and individual experiences in common with other human beings, This conception is quite close, in my opinion, to that of the morphogenetic field. The fields of group therapy, gestalt therapy, and family constellations are also the main actors in the therapeutic process.
10 *Sheldrake*'s morphogenetic field theory can be used as a metaphor to interpret certain psychological and relational phenomena. This British scientist and

writer suggests the existence of *invisible fields that guide the formation and development of living organisms, but which can also guide, influence, and transmit* "habits" *or behavioral and structural patterns within a species.* According to Sheldrake, these fields contain *a kind of* "collective memory" *that influences growth.*

11 Recently, neuroscience has provided us with *studies on* "mirror neurons" that support this vision of a unified field in psychotherapy. Mirror neurons represent one of the most significant discoveries in cognitive neuroscience in recent decades. These neurons are mainly found in the premotor cortex and inferior parietal lobe of the human brain, areas involved in motor programming and sensorimotor integration. They are activated both when an individual performs an action and by just observing another individual perform the same action. Their involvement is not limited to the motor domain, as they also participate in emotion processing, suggesting their role in the capacity for empathy.

In the human brain, therefore, there would exist neural mechanisms through which we "feel" *the experience of others and are thus able to understand their emotions*, thus being able to understand the mental states of others intuitively and immediately.

In psychopathology, it has been hypothesized that dysfunctions in this system may underlie disorders such as autism, characterized by difficulties in understanding the emotions and intentions of others.

12 Of that "love that moves the Sun and the other stars."

13 Some experiments or experiences induced in transpersonal practices (deep meditation, experiences of transcendence) have been *interpreted in a* "quantum" *or* "energetic" *key*, suggesting that consciousness can operate in a non-linear way and not limited to traditional space-time. Strange things happen in therapy, connections we do not understand, insights, and miracles. To be honest with ourselves, even when we believe we find some logic between our therapeutic action and the result of a change in the patient, we should admit that it may have played a part but that in part what we observe happened in an incomprehensible way, according to a law other than that of cause and effect, perhaps of synchronicity, perhaps spiritual, perhaps due to chaos, which as they say is after all only God's second name: therefore chance exists, since God exists.

14 To be able to do this the therapist must have reached a level of purification such that their perception is no longer subjective and ego-bound. We are well aware of the *risk of projections* by therapists who are still identified and unaware of operating from a dualistic state of consciousness; only after overcoming the separation between ego and true Self can he truly operate within the separation that is still present in the patient. Hence the need for long and deep *preparation*, and complete dedication, at least within the therapy itself: indeed, love for the patient and the potential of the therapeutic field can raise the therapist's level of consciousness almost beyond him, and help transcend egoic identification.

15 Remember the proverb: "Speak little and listen much, you will never go wrong."

16 The rhythm can and should vary: the therapist feels through their body, or rather the field, when it is time to move from one region to another, and what condition of tension or relaxation is present in those regions of the patient.

17 Generally, I do not recommend *imagining*, because the mind loves objects, and this distracts from the source; however, specific techniques are recommended in meditation texts to accompany this energetic circulation, e.g., in VBT a visualization of a luminous point is described which, following inhalation and exhalation, rises and falls along the astral spine.

18 Sometimes paying attention to the breath may help a patient who cannot easily perceive tension or openness in the *Chakra*. For example, to unblock the first *Chakra*, which feels tense and does not change, one could imagine that the inhalation starts from the first *Chakra*, from the perineum, and travels up the *Chakra* to the crown and imagining the contrary path during exhalation, back to the perineum. One will observe that within a few thoughtless breaths the *Chakra* not only opens but offers its energy in the circle that is being reactivated and then remains open and sensitive.

19 If regions of tension and non-diffusion still remain, the patient can locate them, or be guided to them by the therapist who perceives them; bringing non-judgmental attention to these tensions in the Chakras is usually sufficient to locally induce their dissolution into the general relaxed state.

20 The patient not only benefits from the alchemical miracle of the transformation in the vessel, but at the same time becomes master of this gentle conducting of their own energy towards a fuller free and conscious state. Now the patient realizes *in* real time, *in corpore vili*, that they are vase and operator, alchemist and raw material together, that they are witnessing a miracle, simple, present always and, everywhere. They have found the fountain of happiness, the medicine, the elixir.

21 It is the state of the *I am*, always present without effort, from which we are always distracted by identification with mental objects. To return home we need only not leave home. In Hinduism it is called *Sat Chit Ananda*, being-consciousness-joy.

22 The passage says how healthy and easy it is to circulate light:

> *When the light circulates, the powers of the whole body stand before his throne, just as a holy king manages a capital, lays down his rules and collects tribute. You only have to circulate the light, which is the deepest and most wonderful secret. Light is easy to move, and if it moves sufficiently in a circle, it crystallises. This is said to be the condition for you to fly* "silently high in the morning"
>
> From the secret of the golden flower, Wilhelm

23 It is the identification with "me" that makes it *personal*, "mine," *and limited*. The child learns "me and mine" very early on, but before that moment she/he also lives in an enlarged perception.

24 The method outlined here is therefore based on the individually recognized, and otherwise unprovable, assumption that perceived reality is One, and not divided into the manifold; and that it is correct and appropriate to start from this point of view. It is a method suited to people who fly, but who do not yet fly well; thus these fallen angels must be rescued and directed.

In Paradise, for example, Dante asks a blissful spirit how it is possible for him to know what he wants to ask, even before the question is expressed; to which the blessed soul replies that this is possible because he sees question and answer in the mirror of God, which reflects both of them. Dante often uses new expressions in Paradise to indicate this state of non-separation (e.g., *"if I was in you as you are in me..."*). This "mirror" is God the creator, (i.e., Cosmic Consciousness, which also lives in each and every man, which when re-discovered has no temporal-spatial limits), who creates and perceives both; we could say: the *field*. Indeed, in a dream, our creative consciousness *perceives what it conceives*, in the time-without-time of the present.

25 *Ramana Maharshi*, a non-dual Indian spiritual master, says with a simple example how everything happens in the One: "If my hand feeds my mouth, shall I say thanks to my hand?"

26 It is, as in the rite of the Mass, about *communion*. In the rite of the Mass, communion symbolically and substantially corresponds to the process of complete reunification with Christ Consciousness, signifying living in it, just as She lives in us.

Communion represents in a ritual form the end of separation, the healing of the ancient and fundamental separation, of the ego from the Self, from the One-and-All, from God.

27 There is a saying: *if anyone forces you to go one mile, go with him two miles.* This, however, is only possible if the patient also feels and validates and desires this, which is different from following a disconnected personal movement, which could easily be driven more by ego needs, anxieties or blind spots rather than the movement of individual consciousness in the direction of the Self. This is why we clarified in the previous point how this method is based on a non-dualistic condition of consciousness.

28 "Knock, knock!," *I knock on the door. The door opens. I was knocking from inside!* (Rumi).

29 That however indicated how her ego was concentrated in the activation of her third *Chakra,* the *Chakra* of self-assertion, and anger (the third *Chakra* in astrology is represented by Mars)

30 The psychic representation of energies and psychological functions is set out *extensively* in my book "Astrology and Yoga."

31 It is a proverb that can be understood, like all proverbs, at various levels; here we would like to insist on its alchemical, operative meaning: it is a matter of not listening to the mind, of "speaking" little to it, and listening instead to sensations, to perceptions.

What is often done in psychology, on the contrary, is to superimpose one's own method, made up of words, concepts, visions, on top of what emerges, while listening very little to what does not fit into the scheme. In this way, pseudo-psychological, pseudo-scientific theories are superimposed on the wisdom of nature, on knowing God.

32 There may be *various reasons* why she is not perceiving correctly what I think is happening. A first hypothesis could be that she *is perhaps not really listening to what is happening to her,* and instead to what speaks in her head; she *believes* the thoughts of the mind instead of *perceiving* present sensations and tells herself a story instead of really listening. My disallowing her and inviting her to listen thus leads us to operate before the mental translation and interpretation, in the real here and now; it serves to bring her, to welcome her, into the real world! A second hypothesis is that perhaps the sensations I am feeling have not yet emerged in her space – time and experience but are already perceivable in mine; it is in this way that they can be perceived in her, because she still is in a state of consciousness affected by separation.

33 Gandhi said that *men often become what they think they are.*

34 Another example with *an obsessive, patient,* who tells me that he feels very anxious about the beginning of the session. Listening to him, and seeing him

smile, I perceive that it is not true that he is really very anxious; and yet I have to acknowledge, I have to listen to what he thinks he feels and wants to communicate to me. However, I must also always discriminate: who is talking in his head?

I then invite him to listen to whether or not it is true that he is really anxious at that moment; I invite him to listen inside, to see where he feels it and how intense it is. Quickly the patient realizes that what he believed to be true does not correspond to what is his present perception.

35 The very fact of rectifying and falsifying the egoic belief may often not be well received by the patient; this though may become a diagnostic element, as to how much the obsessive identification with the ego still predominates or is ready to recede.

36 For example, in the session I point to the moment when I began to perceive an energetic shift, and as a *tactic* I often point to the time, or sometimes the location, but usually wait for her to recognize, to call by name, what I had already perceived and recognized.

37 Dante argues that one must look for different levels of meaning, for example, in the Commedia: the literal, from which one must always start, the symbolic, allegorical, and anagogical, or higher-sense. Even in the sapiential tradition, e.g., the Jewish, it is maintained that the (inner) garden of Pardes is accessed through the four gates of knowledge; the term PRDS (hence garden, and our term Paradise) in fact stands for the four meanings, from the first, the literal (first letter, Pshat, simple), to the fourth, the last (last letter, Sod, secret).

38 From this point of view, Jung argues that dream symbols represent, photograph the real condition, in the moment of the dream and often in the present moment, of the relationship between the ego and the unconscious.

39 A clever joke tells of one who dreams of a monster who wants to eat him. He then begs the monster not to do so, and heartily explains to him many reasons, that he is young, that he must raise his children. The monster, however, is perplexed, and replies that he does not know if he can fulfil him, "because," he tells him, "you know, this dream is yours!"

40 In clinical practice, the term catamnesis refers to the follow-up or long-term monitoring of a patient after the conclusion of a treatment, therapy, or acute phase of a disease. It makes it possible to assess the evolution of the patient's clinical condition over time, to check the effectiveness of treatment and the possible occurrence of relapses or complications.

41 To assess the effectiveness of an intervention, we can discuss the procedure and the results with colleagues. In the TP method, however, we cannot make use of this aid, since in order to be able to compare the clinical procedure, they would have to apply the same method with similar patients, but this comparative element is lost when the very concept of separation is overcome.

42 "Primum non nocere"; and this method can do no harm because it comes from listening to what nature wants to do.

43 Teaching the patient to activate the *Chakras* of the hands, to become aware of energetic activation, and to use the hands as energy-sensors for their main *Chakras* is a form of *initiation*. The sentient, operating, and creative capacity is already present in the consciousness and only needs to be rediscovered. *This experience is only welcomed by those who are ready to receive it*; however, to varying degrees, almost all patients can benefit and learn by consciously following the instructions.

44 The patient in the session, for example, was immediately invited to review and reinterpret the meaning of her symptoms as related to the local consciousness and energy conditions of that moment, or of the her family system.

45 An example: a patient became alarmed at strange sensations – for him – at the level of the heart, and on the occasion of these perceptions repeatedly rushed to the emergency ward in a panic in fear of having a heart attack. After our sessions, he was more willing to reinterpret those sensations as signs of an opening at the level of the heart *Chakra,* which signaled his energetic and spiritual advancement; and he was able to do this because he was now in possession of a technique to help his own energy, and because he gave a different value to those phenomena were, until then, only occasions of fear and alarm.

46 Every therapist knows that some processes happen in a short time. Or, at least, that some crucial psychic knots can dissolve quickly, even instantaneously.

However, they also know that the whole therapeutic process takes much longer and often needs time to stabilize, deepen, start again.

47 I remember a patient I once asked how long she had been ill; and she replied: "Since I have been coming to you, doctor!"

48 Moreover, in this view, the crisis is irreversible, irrevocable, and therefore can only proceed in the direction of death rebirth.

49 Astrology may provide indications of ego stability and disposition to service, but it does not determine the choice to become a therapist.

50 In the case of training in a school of psychoanalysis, this evaluation is guaranteed by personal analysis and the analyst's presentation to the committee that accepts the candidate.

51 This is especially true for psychoanalytic training schools, where the minimum hours of perosnal analysis, didactic analysis, and supervision of clinical cases are defined.

52 Patient – "Doc! "Did your brain ever break down?" Doctor – "Well, break down, not really, I don't think so." Patient – "There, you see, I knew it; so what can you understand about me? ..."

53 Dr. Grof, in the early days of experimentation with LSD, thought a different training of young psychiatrists could be achieved by the intake of psychedelic substances, so as to overcome a purely mental understanding of what it might mean to be out of one's mind; e.g., the perception of unity with the cosmos, visions, the perception of opening of the *Chakras*, etc.

54 As Jung said, "no therapist can lead a patient further than he has gone himself". See C.G. Jung, *The Practice of Psychotherapy*, Collected Works vol. 16, §179.

Conclusion

We have explored how psychiatric disorders can be reconsidered, from a TP point of view, as processess accompanying the awakening of consciousness in the individual.

Awakening is almost always accompanied by mental suffering, which largely arises from the individual consciousness being unprepared to accept and accompany this process that mysteriously arises.

Not finding sufficient physical, psychic, or relational justifications to explain the onset of psychiatric disorders, some researchers, such as Dante and Jung, suggest that the responsive factor is the awakening of consciousness and the energetic activation in the system, i.e., the re-discovery of oneself, meaning Consciousness, our true Self, in the Divine Comedy of life. The psychological, emotional disorders that we see as mental disorders would in this view be an expression of awakening and its labor.

Therefore in this view psychiatry is to be related to an *endogenous process* of transformation (death and rebirth) *of spiritual nature, a transformation of consciousness.*

Since the process involves suffering, for the process activates resistance, the need arises to help patients to go through this *no man's land*, this "dark night of the soul." This process—if properly assisted—can lead to the birth of a new being, a new consciousness.

From this vision arises a *new hope* for psychiatry, which finds a new key to understanding the genesis and developmental patterns of psychiatric disorders, and the need also arises *to include and transcend the biological medical psychiatric practice, and the traditional psychological practice* that have developed so far, but which in their effort to help they are mainly trying to bring the patient back to their previous self-balance.

Hence the need for psychiatry to *open up to new horizons, to a transpersonal psychology and psychiatry, a psychiatry* of the future, a *conscious psychiatry*, an *alchemic psychiatry*, in which suffering is included as an important component of the primary process:

DOI: 10.4324/9781003676461-13

anguish is joy dressed in black—lead that must be transformed into gold.

Hence also *the need for a different training for therapists* intervening in psychiatric crises, to help them accompany these suffering souls through the three realms of the Divine Comedy of life. The new therapists need not only bring help and relief to these *people who go to sea* to support them in the process, but also need to have sight of the other shore: they must help the patient to cooperate, to die and be reborn. I am confident that some or perhaps many therapists will take this path: for "the times are a-changing."

Proposing and practising this method requires loving and understanding. It is a way that cannot be taught, but that can be learned: for *therapy responds to love*, which is *true knowledge*, and which can lead "Deo concedente" (*God willing*) to liberation.

Bibliography

Adler, A.
The Meaning of Life, Astrolabio Ubaldini, 1933
The Physician as Educator, Rivista di Psicologia Individuale, 1904

Alighieri, Dante
All Works, Mursia, 1965
La Divina Commedia, Sansoni ed., Bologna, 1957, Commentary by A. Momigliano
See the beautiful commentary in Italian by V. Sermonti, *Dante's Inferno, Purgatorio and Paradiso*, Rizzoli, 1990
See also *Il metodo Dante*, Schaub R. and B.G., ed., Piemme 2004

Apuleius
The Metamorphoses, or *The Golden Ass*, BUR, 1955, 1981

Assagioli R., (1973)
Principles and Methods of Therapeutic Psychosynthesis, Astrolabio, Ubaldini, Rome
Psychosynthesis, ed. Astrolabio
L'atto di volontà, ed. Astrolabio, 1998 *(The Act of Will)*

Avalon, A.
The Serpent Power (1919), *Il potere del Seroente*, Mediterranee, 1968

Basaglia, F.
What is Psychiatry? 1967, edited in the volume:
The Denied Institution. Report from a Psychiatric Hospital, 1968

Bhagavadgita, Feltrinelli, 2007

Jerusalem Bible, ed. Paoline, 1971

Blackwell, S.
Am I Bipolar or Waking Up?
on his website, www.bipolarawakenings.com

Boggio Gilot, L.
Transpersonal Psychology, 2009, Raffaello Cortina Editore
Spiritual Healing, 2011, Raffaello Cortina Editore

Mind and Consciousness. New Perspectives in Transpersonal Psychology, 2013 – Laura Boggio Gilot (ed.), FrancoAngeli

Spirit and Person. Psychospiritual Integration in Psychotherapy, 2016 – Laura Boggio Gilot and Piero Ferrucci, Raffaello Cortina Editore

Bolognini, S.

Il Mestiere Impossibile, 2002, Cortina Raffaello publisher

Brennan, B.

Hands of Light, Emerging Light, Longanesi ed.

Carroll, Lewis

Alice in Wonderland, Alice Through the Looking Glass, Bompiani, 1991

Collie, El

Shared Transformation, 1992

Branded by the Spirit, by Keepers of the Flame Foundation, 1995

Diagnostic and Statistical Manual of Mental Disorders (DSM-5)

American Psychiatric Association (2013)

An essential reference manual for the diagnosis and classification of mental disorders.

Edwards, L.

Awakening Kundalini, ed. Sounds true, 2013

Eisler, R.

The Chalice and the Blade, cited in *Awakening Kundalini*, L. Edwards, ed. Sounds true 2013

El-Mallakh, R. S., & Ghaemi, S. N. (2010)

Bipolar Disorder: A Clinician's Guide to Biological Treatments, Arlington: American Psychiatric Publishing

Eliade, M.

Yoga. Immortality and Freedom, 1954, BUR, 2010

Ellenberger H. F.

The Discovery of the Unconscious, 2 vols., Bollati Boringhieri, Turin, 1976 (1st Italian ed.)

Fenichel, O.

Treatise on Psychoanalysis, ed. Astrolabe, 1978

Foucault, M.

History of Madness in the Classical Age, Rizzoli, 1963

Frawley, D.

Astrology of the Seers, Motilal Banarsidass Publishing House, 1990

Freedman, Kaplan and Sadock

Kaplan & Sadock's Comprehensive Textbook of Psychiatry, USES Scientific Editions, 1982

Freud, S.

Massenpsychologie und Ich-Analyse (Mass Psychology and Ego Analysis), Published 1921

Das Ich und das Es (The Ego and the Es), Published 1923. *The Ego and the Es*, 1923, Bollati Boringhieri

The Interpretation of Dreams, Bollati Boringhieri, text of 1899

Three Essays on Sexual Theory, 1905, Bollati Boringhieri

Freud, A.

The Ego and the Mechanisms of Defence, 1936, ed. Hogarth Press, originally published in 1936, in Italian published in 1972 by Bollati Boringhieri

and also: *The Writings of Anna Freud* (7 volumes, 1973–1980), ed. International Universities Press

Friedmann, H., Hartelius, G.

The Wiley Backwell Handbook of Transpersonal Psychology, Wiley Blackwell, 2013

Gautama Buddha

The Discourses of Gotamo Buddho of the Majjhimanikayo (translated by G. De Lorenzo), Laterza, 1916, 3 volumes

Ghezzani, N. (2002)

Il male dell'anima: Le ferite narcisistiche e le illusioni del narcisismo, Milan: Franco Angeli ed.

Choa KoK Sui

Pranic Healing & Advanced Pranic Healing by the Institute for Inner Studies Publishing Foundation, 1987 and 1992

Gimbutas, M.

The Language of the Goddess, Feltrinelli, 2008

Goodman, L. S., & Gilman, A. (1975)

The Pharmacological Basis of Therapeutics (5th ed.), Macmillan

(Over the years, "G&G" has been acclaimed as the "blue bible" of pharmacology).

Gopi Krishna

Kundalini: The Evolutionary Energy in Man, Shambhala Publications, 1971, based on his first awakening, in 37; he published later (in 67, at the age of 64) *Living with Kundalini: The Autobiography of Gopi Krishna,* Shambhala Publications, 1993, a book based on the original core of the first book.

His other books are: *Kundalini: Empowering Human Evolution,* Institute for Consciousness Research ed., 1997, *The Awakening of Kundalini, Kundalini: Path to Higher Consciousness, Kundalini: The Secret of Yoga, The Biological Basis of Religion and Genius, Serpent of Fire: A Modern View of Kundalini, Higher Consciousness and Kundalini, The Wonder of the Brain, Ancient Secrets of Kundalini, Initiation into Kundalini (in Italian), The Secret of Kundalini Yoga (in Italian)*

Greenwell, B.
The Kundalini Guide: A Companion for the Inward Journey, Shakti River Press ed., 2014
The Awakening Guide: A Companion for the Inward Journey, Shakti River Press ed., 2014
When Spirit Leaps: Navigating the Process of Spiritual Awakening, Non-Duality Press

Grof, C. and Grof S.
The Stormy Search for the Self, TarcherPerigee ed., 2018

Grof S., (1988)
Beyond the Brain: Birth, Death, and Transcendence in Psychotherapy, 1985. In Italian, published under the title *Beyond the Brain, La Cittadella, Assisi*
Spiritual Emergency: When Personal Transformation Becomes a Crisis, published in 1989 by Jeremy P. Tarcher Inc. publishing house, which is a label of Penguin Random House
When the Impossible Happens: *Adventures in Non-Ordinary Realities*, 2006, ed. Sounds True
The Psychology of the Future: New Dimensions of the Human Spirit, 2000, ed. SUNY Press (State University of New York Press); in Italian *La psicologia del futuro: sviluppi nella ricerca sulla coscienza moderna*. Spaziointeriore, 2015
Realms of the Human Unconscious: Observations from LSD Research, 1979, (in Italian published as *LSD. L'innovativa ricerca psichedelica nei reami dell'inconscio. La nuova mappa della psiche*, ShaKe Edizioni, collana *Underground*, Milano, 2021, trad. di G. Gerboni). This book is the most detailed and systematic account of Grof's research in Prague.
The Adventure of Self-Discovery, 1988, State University of New York Press
The Holotropic Mind: The Three Levels of Human Consciousness and How They Shape Our Lives, 1992, HarperCollins
LSD: Doorway to the Numinous (1975) Publisher: Real People Press (Italian ed.: Edizioni Crisalide, 1996). Originally published in 1975 and later in expanded editions, this book collects and synthesises the results of 17 years of Grof's research with LSD, including the Prague years. Also on LSD work:
LSD Psychotherapy: The Healing Potential of Psychedelic Medicine, and
Stanislav Grof, LSD Pioneer: From Pharmacology to Archetypes (book-interview 2023).

Guénon, R.
The Great Triad, Adelphi 1980

Harner, M.
The Way of the Shaman, 1980

Hellinger, B.
The Orders of Love, F. Angeli ed., 2003

Hinsie, H., and Campbell, R.
Dictionary of Psychiatry, Astrolabe, 1979

Iannacone, M.
The Psychedelic Revolution, Ares editions, 2020

Corrado Tamburino
Rasarium. Medical Semeiotics, Giuseppe Di Maria, Idelson Gnocchi ed., 2023

James W., (1961)
The Varieties of Religious Experiences, Collier Books, New York,
transl. It: "Le varie forme della coscienza religiosa", Bocca, Turin, 1964

Jervis, G.
Critical Manual of Psychiatry, ed. Feltrinelli, 1975

Johannes, W.
Experiencing the Chakras, Macro editions, 2004

Johnson, G.
Non-dual Therapy, 2017, at www.iamhere.life, VeReCreations

Jung C.G., (1980)
Opera Omnia, Boringhieri publisher; i
In particular, Vol 11 (*Psychology and Religion)*, *Psychic Energetics* (1928), *Vol 8 (The Archetypes and the Collective Unconscious, 1944*), *Liber Novus* (The Red Book), 2010, 3 (*Psychogenesis of Mental Illnesses*)
Psychology of Kundalini-Yoga. (Seminar given in 1932, Boringhieri 2004, published posthumously, based on Jung's seminars and writings on the topics of kundalini yoga and intense spiritual experiences)
Symbols of Transformation, 1912, (vol 5), later expanded and reprinted, *Answer to Job* (1952)
Psychology of Translation, Opera Omnia, Boringhieri
Mysterium Coniunctionis, Opera Omnia, Boringhieri
The Symbolism of the Mass, in Vol. Psychology and Religion
Man and His Symbols, 1964, Longanesi
Psychological Types, 1921, Bollati Boringhieri
Also useful is reading Jung's autobiography, *(Memories, Dreams and Reflections of C. G. Jung*, collected by A. Jaffe, Bur ed. 1979)
Letters, Magi, 2006
See also Kirfel Barillà, Lioba*: Jung and Astrology*, from the epistolary, published in no. 6 (April 91) of "Ricerca '90" 1972)

C. G. Jung and R. Wilhelm,
"The Secret of the Golden Flower", Boringhieri, 2001

Kaplan and Sadock's Comprehensive Textbook of Psychiatry
Benjamin J. Sadock, Virginia A. Sadock, Pedro Ruiz (2017)
(Kaplan and Sadock's *Comprehensive Textbook of Psychiatry* is an encyclopaedic work covering all aspects of psychiatry. This work has been called "A university without walls", now in its 12th edition within 50 years of the first edition).

Kason, Y.
"Near Death Experiences and Kundalini Awakening: Exploring the Link", *Journal of Near-death Studies*, 1994 Human Sciences Press

Kahlshed, D.
The Inner World of Trauma: Archetypal Defences of the Personal Spirit, Routledge, 1996, and *Trauma and the Soul: A Psycho-Spiritual Approach to Human Development and its Interruption*, Routledge, 2013

Kerenyi, K.
Gli dei e gli eroi della grecia, Il saggiatore, 2015 (1st ed. 1963)

Klein, M.
Envy and Gratitude, 1957, Hogarth Press,
and also *The Writings of Melanie Klein* (4 volumes, 1975), Hogarth Press

Kowalski, R., Carpenter J.
The Only Way Out Is In, ed., 2001

Kraepelin, E. (1909–1915)
The German edition of his treatise came out in 1913 under the title
Psychiatrie: Ein Lehrbuch für Studierende und Ärzte (8th ed.). Leipzig: Barth
In Italy, this text was translated and published under the title: *Trattato di Psichiatria* in 1904 (Italian edition edited by F. Bonfiglio). Milan: Società Editrice Libraria

Kriyananda, Swami
The Art of Counselling, Ananda ed., 2016

Kurzweil, R. (2005)
The Singularity Is Near: When Humans Transcend Biology, New York: VikingPress, 2005; Italian edition: 2008, Mondadori ed.

Lacan,
Ecrits (Writings), 1974, Einaudi
Seminari (1953–1980), Einaudi (published between 2011 and 2016)

The Holy Bible, ed. Paoline, 2008

The Bhaghawat Gita,
Swami Sivananda Saraswati (Edizioni Mediterranee, 2005); there are other translations, such as the one by ed. Luni, (*'Bhagavadgītā. With commentary by Sri Sankaracarya'), or the one by Adelphi (from 1976).*

Lukoff, D.
"Making a Place in the DSM-IV for Spiritual Emergency", in *The Journal of Humanistic Psychology*, 1998

Maddaloni, C. (all in Italian):
Notes on Medical Pharmacology, Ecig ed., 1978
The Stars Within, Spirito Libero ed., 2010
Myths and Yoga, the Way Back, Youcanprint ed., 2010
Guide to the World of Dreams, Youcanprint ed., 2011
You Can Fly, Edizioni Ipsa, 2012

Dying Alive, a New Look at Panic Attacks, Youcanprint ed., 2015
The Church of Life, Mohicans ed., 2016
Crazy Things, Youcanprint ed., 2020
I Found Myself, The Divine Comedy as a Map for Awakening, Alpes ed., 2022
Astrology and Yoga, Om editions, 2024

Charles Brisset – Henri Ey – Paul Bernard, Masson ed., 1977
Handbook of Psychiatry

Franco Giberti, Romolo Rossi, ed. Vallardi, 1972
Manual of Psychiatry

Piero Sarteschi – Carlo Maggini ed. Monduzzi 1982
Manual of Psychiatry

Maslow A., (1971)
Towards a Psychology of Being, Ubaldini, 1971, Rome (translation of *Toward a Psychology of Being*, 1962)
The Farther Reaches of Human Nature, 1971
Motivation and Personality, 1954

Mazzarella, A.
Alla ricerca di Beatrice, (i.e., In Search of Beatrice), In/Out editions, 1991

Millon, Th.
Masters of the Mind, Wiley ed., 2004

Naranjo, C.
The Kundalini Process and the Hero's Journey, Revision ed., 1987

Luytens, M.
Krishnamurti: The Years of Awakening, Farrar, Straus and Giroux ed., 1975

Nelson, John E.
Healing the Split: Madness or Transcendence?, by J.P.Tarcher inc, '90,
The book proposes an evolutionary scheme of the conditions of consciousness i.e. SAC by proposing these differentiated diagnostic and therapeutic interventions. K. Wilber's preface claims that it is a truly valuable and unique book, and I agree.[1]

Neumann, E.
The Great Mother, Astrolabe ed., 1981

Ovid, Publius Naso
Le metamorfosi, (i.e., *The Metamorphoses*), Einaudi, 2000

Palacios, M.A.
Dante e l'Islâm, Parma, Nuove Pratiche Editrice, 1994

Paramahamsa Yogananda
Autobiography of a Yogi, Astrolabium, 2000
L'eterna ricerca dell'uomo, Astrolabio, 1980
Bhagavad Gita, Spiritual Interpretation, Vidyananda Editions, 1992

Pasotti, Andrea
Near Death Experiences, NDEs: The Proof of Survival, Paperback, 2019

Patañjali
Aphorisms of Yoga, Magnanelli, 1991

Pearls, F. S.
Gestalt Therapy: Excitement and Growth in the Human Personality, 1951 – Frederick S. Perls, Ralph F. Hefferline, Paul Goodman, Julian Press
Gestalt Therapy Verbatim, 1969 – Frederick S. Perls, Bantam Books

Pianigiani, O.
Online Etymological Dictionary

Ram Dass
Journey Of Awakening: A Meditator's Guidebook, Bantam Books, 1978

Rogers, C.
Client-Centered Therapy: Its Current Practice, Implications, and Theory, 1951, ed. Houghton Mifflin
Person-Centered Psychotherapy, 1968 – ed. Constable
On Becoming a Person, 1961

Pollan, M.
How to Change Your Mind, Penguin Press, 2018

Rafael
The Path of Non-Duality (Advaitavada), Ashram Vidya editions, 1997

Reich, W.
The Function of the Orgasm, 1927, SugarCo Editions; *Character Analysis*, 1933, SugarCo Editions

Reich, T.
Narcotics and Forbidden: The Way of the Master Plants, Amrita, 2021

Rilke, R. M.
Elegie duinesi, Einaudi, 1978

Samorini, G.
https://samorini.it/

Sannella, L.
Kundalini: Psychosis or Transcendence, 1976, Integral Publishing;
translated into Italian, was published by ed Hurrà associated with Hohm Press in 1987 under the title: *Kundalini, Psychosis or Transcendence*

Sarteschi, others
Treatise on Psychiatry

Segal, S.
Collision With the Infinite: A Life Beyond the Personal Self, 1966, ed. Blue Dove

Sukumari Bhattacharji
The Indian Theogony: Brahma, Visnu, Shiva, Penguin books, 1970

Swami Rama
Path of Fire and Light, Himalayan Publishers, Honesdale 1986

Sovatsky, S.
Energetic Transmutations in the Kundalini Process, ed. Kundalini Research Network, 1998

Tart, C.T.
Transpersonal Psychologies, vol. I, 1994, Chrysalis, Spigno Saturnia

Taylor, S.
"Beyond the Pre/Trans Fallacy: The Validity of Pre-Egoic Spiritual Experience", *The Journal of Transpersonal Psychology*, 2009

Edited by B. Scotton, A. Chinen, J. Baptist, from Basic Books, 1996[2]
Textbook of Transpersonal Psychiatry and Psychology

VBT, Vigyana Bhairava Tantra,
Motilal Banarsidass Publishers, Various editions, e.g. 1991
The Book of Secrets: 112 Meditations to Discover the Mystery Within Osho Media International, 1974

Vinardi, L.
"Healing and Self Healing", Arcoteso ed., 2000

Von Franz, M. L.
Projection and Recollection in Jungian Psychology: Reflections of the Soul, Open Court Publishing, 1980
Shadow and Evil in Fairy Tales, Shambhala publications, 1995
The Interpretation of Fairy Tales, Shambhala publications, 1996
The Interpretation of Fairy Tales, Shambhala publications, 2001

Watson, John B.,
"Psychology as Seen by a Behaviourist", 1913 article

Weitbrecht
Psychosis, Feltrinelli, 1962

Weil, P.
Man without Frontiers, 1996, Chrysalis, Spigno Saturnia

Wilber, K.
The Spectre of Consciousness, Chrysalis, Spigno Saturnia, 1993
The Holographic Paradigm and other Paradoxes, 1982 for the New Science Library;
Sex, Ecology, Spirituality (SES), 1995;
Kosmos Trilogy.
A Brief History of Everything, 1996
Integral Psychology, 1999
A Theory of Everything, 2000
Integral Spirituality, 2006
Transformations of Consciousness. Transpersonal Psychology and Human Development written with Jack Engler and Daniel P. Brown, published in English in 1986, and published in Italy by Astrolabio-Ubaldini Editore (1989) "The

Developmental Spectrum and Psychopathology: Part II, Treatment Modalities", published in the *Journal of Transpersonal Psychology* (1984)

Whitaker, R.

Mad in America: Bad Science, Bad Medicine, and the Enduring Mistreatment of the Mentally Ill, 2001, Perseus Publishing

Anatomy of an Epidemic: Magic Bullets, Psychiatric Drugs, and the Astonishing Rise of Mental Illness in America, 2010, Crown Publishing Group;

Translated into Italian, "Inchiesta su una epidemia. *Lo straordinario aumento delle disabilità psichiatriche nell'epoca del boom degli psicofarmaci*", Giovanni Fioriti Editore, 2016

Psychiatry Under the Influence: Institutional Corruption, Social Injury, and Prescriptions for Reform (with Lisa Cosgrove), 2015, Palgrave Macmillan

Wu Li

Pathways, informative quarterly of the Tai Chi Research Centre Italy, Summer 2002

Yogananda

Autobiography of a Yogi, ed. Astrolabe

Yukteswar Sri Swami

Sacred Science, Ubaldini, 1994

Zachary F. Lansdowne, Ph.D (1986 S. Weiser, USA)

The Chakras and Esoteric Healing, Samuel Weiser ed., 1986

Recent books and articles useful for further exploration of the subject of Kundalini *in psychiatry*

- Ambrose, P. 2014. [Review of the book *Advanced spiritual intimacy: The yoga of deep Tantric sensuality*, by S. Sovatsky]. *International Journal of Transpersonal Studies*, *33*(1), 172–173.
- Greenwell, B. 2002. *Energies of Transformation: A Guide to the Kundalini Process*. Motilal Banarsidass.
- Greyson, B. 1993a. "The Physio-Kundalini Syndrome and Mental Illness". *The Journal of Transpersonal Psychology*, *25*(1), 43–58.
- Greyson, B. 1993b. "Near-death Experiences and the Physio-Kundalini Syndrome". *Journal of Religion and Health*, *32*, 277–290.
- Maxwell, R. W., & Katyal, S. 2022. "Characteristics of Kundalini-Related Sensory, Motor, and Affective Experiences During Tantric Yoga Meditation". *Frontiers in Psychology*, *13*, 863091.
- Rele, V. G. 1984. *The Mysterious Kundalini*. Health Research Books.
- Sanches, L., & Daniels, M. 2008. "Kundalini and Transpersonal Development: Development of a Kundalini Awakening Scale and a Comparison Between Groups". *Transpersonal Psychology Review*, *12*(1), 73–83.
- Shannahoff-Khalsa, D. 2007. *Kundalini Yoga Meditation: Techniques Specific for Psychiatric Disorders, Couples Therapy, and Personal Growth*. W. W. Norton.
- South, M. 2001. *The mystic fire of Teresa of Avila: A comparative study of mysticism and the Kundalini phenomenon* [Doctoral dissertation, University of Ottawa, Canada].

- Sovatsky, S. 2009. "Kundalini and the Complete Maturation of the Ensouled Body". *The Journal of Transpersonal Psychology*, *41*(1), 1–21.
- Swain, D. L. 2019. *Re-visioning kundalini: Exploring experiences of kundalini from a Jungian and archetypal perspective* [Doctoral dissertation, Pacifica Graduate Institute].
- Thaler, M. 2024. "Pathology or Transcendence? Kundalini's Interpretation as Spiritual Emergency and Rebirth Process". In L. K. Pokorny & Mattes, A. (eds.), *Taking Seriously, Not Taking Sides* (pp. 263–285). Brill Schöningh.
- Willson, S. 2021. *Her breath in our holy bones: An intuitive inquiry into the lived experience of kundalini awakenings in Aotearoa, New Zealand from a critical health psychology perspective* [Doctoral dissertation, Massey University, New Zealand].

Web references

For classical and transpersonal psychiatry, in Italy and abroad

For those who wish to explore further, there are many useful online resources, including articles, journals, organisations and other sources of information. Here are some resources that may be of interest:

Batgap, by Rick Archer

Rick Archer is the founder and main host of Buddha at the Gas Pump (BATGAP), an online archive of more than 700 interviews to people who passed through spiritual awakening or transformation of consciousness. This site has become an important reference point for those seeking to understand various spiritual paths and the process of personal enlightenment, as it hosts recorded interviews from a wide range of spiritual teachers, masters and ordinary people whose life journey has led to greater spiritual awareness and realisation. The interviews are available on the official Buddha at the Gas Pump website, YouTube and other streaming platforms.

Conscious TV, by Iain and Renate McNay

Conscious TV is a UK-based online TV channel offering many one-hour interviews and conversations with experts, spiritual teachers, authors and people who have significant experience in the field of mindfulness, personal growth and spiritual development. The platform is dedicated to exploring topics ranging from spirituality to self-healing, meditation, transpersonal psychology and more.

Psychiatry online: www.psychiatryonline.it/, italian site offering study and sharing material on the field of psychiatry psychoanalysis psychotherapy.

The Transpersonal Associations[3]

- *The first association of transpersonal psychology* was founded in the United States in 1969, *the Association of Transpersonal Psychology (ATP)*, by personalities such as: Charlotte Buhler, Abraham Maslow, Allan Watts, Arthur Koestler, Viktor Frankl.

- *The Journal of Transpersonal Psychology* (JTP) was published, founded by Anthony J. Sutich, to which all the major American exponents of the transpersonal movement contributed.[4]
- *The ITA, the International Transpersonal Association,* would later emerge from the ATP.
- Several years later, in 1975, Robert Frager founded *the (Californian) Institute of Transpersonal Psychology in Palo Alto,* which has remained an advanced point in the fields of Transpersonal education, research and therapy for over thirty years. Publishes the "International Journal of Transpersonal Studies (IJTS)".
- *By this time, the Transpersonal orientation had begun to emerge across many branches of science and other areas of human endeavour.* Thus, the ITA conference programme included not only psychologists, psychiatrists and psychotherapists, but also physicists, biologists, doctors of anthropology, mythologists, philosophers, mathematicians, artists, spiritual teachers, educators, politicians, economists and many others.
- The ITA has held its conferences in many cities around the world.
- *All over the world* the transpersonal movement is quite active and well-known; in Brazil, for example, it has been present since the 1970s. It has developed in the academic sphere and has given birth to completely innovative methods and models.[5]
- *In Europe, Eurotas* (*European Transpersonal Association*) and ETPA (*European Transpersonal Psychology Association*) operate. They have a training school, which is somewhat expensive, and a periodical journal.[6] *Eurotas* holds regular annual international conferences, which are very well attended and stimulating.[7]

Notes

1 *Healing the Split: Integrating Spirit into Our Understanding of the Mentally Ill,* published in 1994. Over the years, this American author has written a beautiful, comprehensive, documented, clinically significant, and expert book in which he proposes a restructuring of the psychiatric medical modality in the management of psychiatric disorders. The book, of no less than 440 pages, is unique in my opinion for its complexity and depth; it thoroughly investigates psychosis, provides explanations in line with TP psychology, and should be translated and known also in Italy.

The text explores the connection between spirituality and mental health, and discusses the historical divide between science and spirituality, based on the traditional biomedical model of psychiatry, and how this division has negatively influenced the understanding and treatment of mental disorders.

The book explores various altered states of consciousness, such as those induced by meditation, spiritual practices, even the use of psychedelic substances, and their role in promoting healing and personal growth.

A range of therapeutic approaches are presented that integrate traditional techniques with spiritual practices, such as meditation, dreamwork and regression therapy.

Nelson explores how different cultures and spiritual traditions have historically understood and treated mental illness, recognizing the central role of spirituality in healing.

2 *Textbook of Transpersonal Psychiatry and Psychology*, published by Basic Books, 1996, with an introduction by Wilber. This is a very interesting contribution, an important aid to transpersonal psychiatry coming from a group of American scholars, who together published a collection of essays on transpersonal psychiatry. The '*Textbook*' collects contributions of numerous authors from various American regions, who jointly propose a different approach in TP psychiatry; it contains articles on theory and research, transcultural, clinical. It represents a milestone in the integration of spiritual and transcendental concepts into psychiatric and psychological practice. This book is a valuable resource for psychologists, psychiatrists and therapists interested in exploring and integrating transpersonal aspects into their clinical practice. It provides a robust theoretical framework, practical examples and a critical analysis of the challenges and opportunities offered by this innovative approach to understanding the human mind.

The book introduces transpersonal psychiatry and psychology, tracing their historical and conceptual roots. It explores the evolution of these disciplines from humanistic psychology and psychoanalysis. A range of therapeutic approaches are presented that integrate traditional techniques with spiritual practices, such as meditation, dream and regression therapy. Peak experiences, moments of joy and enlightenment that transcend the ordinary state of consciousness are explored. Altered states of consciousness induced by meditation, hypnosis, psychedelic substances and other spiritual practices are analysed. Near-death experiences and how consciousness evolves through different stages of development from ego to transcendence are examined. Guidelines are provided for the diagnosis and treatment of mental disorders from a transpersonal perspective. At the end of the *Textbook* there is an annotated bibliography of TP literature, compiled by Batista.

3 In 1967, a small working group comprising Abraham Maslow, Anthony Sutich, Stanislav Grof, James Fadiman, Miles Vich, and Sonya Margulies met in Menlo Park, California, with the intention of creating a new psychology that would honour the full spectrum of human experience, including various non-ordinary states of consciousness. During these discussions Maslow and Sutich followed Grof's suggestion and called the new discipline "transpersonal psychology". This term took the place of the original appellation 'transhumanistic' or 'directed beyond humanistic issues'.

4 Among them were *Ken Wilber, Stan Grof, Stanley Krippner, Lawrence Le Shan, Michael Murphy, Charles T. Tart, Frances E. Vaughan, and others.*

5 Since its inception in the late 1960s, *the Association for Transpersonal Psychology (ATP)* has held regular annual conferences in *Asilomar,* California. As interest in the movement grew and spread beyond the San Francisco Bay Area and outside the United States, *occasional international meetings on the transpersonal* were organised *in various parts of the world* (In Boston, Massachusetts; Melbourne, Australia; Bombay, India; Davos, Switzerland; Kyoto, Japan; Santa Rosa, California; Eugene, Oregon; Prague, Czechoslovakia; Killarney, Ireland; Santa Clara, California; Manaus, Brazil; and Palm Spring, California, USA). The first two took place in Bifrost, Iceland; the third in Inari, Finland; and the fourth in Belo Horizonte, Brazil.

By the time of the Brazilian meeting these conferences were so popular and well attended that it was decided to formalise them by creating an institution to organise them, *the International Transpersonal Association (ITA)*. The ITA was inaugurated by Stanislav Grof who became its founding president, joined by Michael Murphy and Richard Price; the latter two, in the early 1960s, started *the Esalen Institute in Big Sur,* California, the first centre for the development of human potential. Unlike the Association of Transpersonal Psychology, the ITA was explicitly international and interdisciplinary.

6 *Eurotas* includes names of researchers such as John Rowan, Laura Boggio Gilot, Vitor Rodrigues, Arturo De Luca, Ingo Benjamin Jahretz, Beata Bishop, Vladimir Maykov, Jure Biechonsky, Bernadette Blin, Judith Miller and Pierluigi Lattuada. Vitor Rodriguez is a psychologist from Lisbon who is a former president of Eurotas, has written numerous books and is active as a trainer. Personal website: https://vitorrodriguespsicologo.weebly.com/ . John Rowan (1925–2003) English psychologist and psychotherapist, one of the pioneers of humanistic and integrative psychology.

7 The last one organised in Italy by *Pierluigi Lattuada* in S. Vincenzo (Livorno) in the summer of 2023, saw contributions from all over the world, not only Europeans, and over 450 participants.

Index

Note: Page numbers in **bold** indicate tables and those in *italics* indicate figures. Endnotes are indicated by the page number followed by "n" and the note number e.g., 111n5 refers to note 5 on page 111.